Teen Health Series

Brain Disorders
SOURCEBOOK

Third Edition

Health Reference Series

Third Edition

Brain
Disorders
SOURCEBOOK

*Basic Consumer Health Information about Acquired
and Traumatic Brain Injuries, Brain Tumors, Cerebral
Palsy and Other Genetic and Congenital Brain Disorders,
Infections of the Brain, Epilepsy, and Degenerative
Neurological Disorders Such as Dementia,
Huntington Disease, and Amyotrophic
Lateral Sclerosis (ALS)*

*Along with Information on Brain Structure and
Function, Treatment and Rehabilitation Options, a
Glossary of Terms Related to Brain Disorders, and a
Directory of Resources for More Information*

Edited by
Joyce Brennfleck Shannon

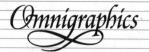

Omnigraphics

P.O. Box 31-1640, Detroit, MI 48231

Bibliographic Note
Because this page cannot legibly accommodate all the copyright notices, the Bibliographic
Note portion of the Preface constitutes an extension of the copyright notice.

Edited by Joyce Brennfleck Shannon

Health Reference Series

Karen Bellenir, *Managing Editor*
David A. Cooke, MD, FACP, *Medical Consultant*
Elizabeth Collins, *Research and Permissions Coordinator*
Cherry Edwards, *Permissions Assistant*
EdIndex, Services for Publishers, *Indexers*

* * *

Omnigraphics, Inc.
Matthew P. Barbour, *Senior Vice President*
Kevin M. Hayes, *Operations Manager*

* * *

Peter E. Ruffner, *Publisher*

Copyright © 2010 Omnigraphics, Inc.
ISBN 978-0-7808-1083-9

Library of Congress Cataloging-in-Publication Data

Brain disorders sourcebook : basic consumer health information about
acquired and traumatic brain injuries, brain tumors, cerebral palsy and
other genetic and congenital brain disorders, infections of the brain,
epilepsy, and degenerative neurological disorders such as dementia,
huntington disease, and amyotrophic lateral sclerosis (ALS) : along with
information on brain structure and function, treatment and rehabilitation
options, a glossary of terms related to brain disorders, and a directory
of resources for more information / edited by Joyce Brennfleck Shannon. --
3rd ed.
     p. cm. -- (Health reference series)
  Includes bibliographical references and index.
  ISBN 978-0-7808-1083-9 (hardcover : alk. paper) 1.
Brain--Diseases--Popular works. I. Shannon, Joyce Brennfleck.
  RC351.B735 2010
  616.8'3--dc22

                                                    2010017790

∞

Table of Contents

Visit www.healthreferenceseries.com to view *A Contents Guide to the Health Reference Series*, a listing of more than 15,000 topics and the volumes in which they are covered.

Part II: Diagnosing and Treating Brain Disorders

Part III: Genetic and Congenital Brain Disorders

Part IV: Brain Infections

Part V: Acquired and Traumatic Brain Injuries

Part VI: Brain Tumors

Part VII: Degenerative Brain Disorders

Part VIII: Seizures and Neurological Disorders of Sleep

Part IX: Additional Help and Information

Preface

About This Book

Millions of Americans and their families experience the daily challenges of living with physical, mental, or emotional difficulties that result from brain disorders caused by heredity, infection, injury, tumors, or degeneration. For example, an estimated four million people are currently living with the effects of stroke, which is the leading cause of serious, long-term disability in adults. Another 2.4 to 4.5 million individuals live with Alzheimer disease, and each year 1.4 million Americans suffer a traumatic brain injury. Although damage to the brain may result in permanent disability, with appropriate treatment and follow-up care, many affected individuals are able to participate fully in life's activities.

Brain Disorders Sourcebook, Third Edition provides readers with updated information about brain function, neurological emergencies such as a brain attack (stroke) or seizure, and symptoms of brain disorders. It describes the diagnosis, treatment, and rehabilitation therapies for genetic and congenital brain disorders, brain infections, brain tumors, seizures, traumatic brain injuries, and degenerative neurological disorders such as Alzheimer disease and other dementias, Parkinson disease, and amyotrophic lateral sclerosis (ALS). A glossary of related terms is also included along with a directory of additional resources about brain disorders.

How to Use This Book

This book is divided into parts and chapters. Parts focus on broad areas of interest. Chapters are devoted to single topics within a part.

Part I: Brain Basics describes the human brain and how the aging process and the environment may contribute to brain disorders. Symptoms of brain disorders and details about identifying neurological emergencies are discussed. Facts about coma, other states of impaired consciousness, and brain death are also included.

Part II: Diagnosing and Treating Brain Disorders reviews common neurological tests and describes current treatments, including the use of steroids, chemotherapy, radiation therapy, and brain surgery. Information about cognitive recovery, measurements of brain function, and guidelines for finding rehabilitation facilities is also presented.

Part III: Genetic and Congenital Brain Disorders offers information about adrenoleukodystrophy, Batten disease, and other neurological conditions that create severe disability and often shorten the lifespan. It also reviews congenital disorders that affect brain function throughout life, but which are not always progressively debilitating. These include cerebral palsy, cephalic disorders, and other birth defects.

Part IV: Brain Infections describes inflammatory diseases caused by bacteria, viruses, or parasites that affect the brain and related structures. These ailments, which can cause severe illness—and even death—in otherwise healthy individuals, include encephalitis, meningitis, and neurocysticercosis.

Part V: Acquired and Traumatic Brain Injuries offers guidelines for identifying traumatic head injuries and offering first aid. Facts about concussions are provided, and detailed information about traumatic brain injury (TBI) is given to help individuals and families affected by a TBI deal with difficulties such as cognition problems, fatigue, emotional disturbances, sleep disorders, and employment-related concerns. Separate chapters present information about acquired (non-traumatic) brain injuries, including brain aneurysm, cavernous angioma, hydrocephalus, and stroke.

Part VI: Brain Tumors describes the symptoms and treatments for primary, metastatic, pituitary, and childhood brain tumors as well as benign and tumor-associated brain cysts. It offers tips for managing treatment side effects, fatigue, cognitive changes, and work-related concerns.

Part VII: Degenerative Brain Disorders discusses neurological disorders that often lead to progressive deterioration of physical or mental functioning. These include Alzheimer disease and other dementias, amyotrophic lateral sclerosis (ALS), Creutzfeldt-Jakob disease, Huntington disease, multiple sclerosis (MS), Parkinson disease, and progressive supranuclear palsy (PSP).

Part VIII: Seizures and Neurological Disorders of Sleep describes epileptic and non-epileptic seizure disorders, myoclonus, restless legs syndrome, and narcolepsy. The chapters in this section review available treatments, including medication, surgery, vagus nerve stimulation, and the Ketogenic diet.

Part VI: Additional Help and Information provides a glossary of terms related to brain disorders and a directory of organizations and resources for additional information.

Bibliographic Note

This volume contains documents and excerpts from publications issued by the following U.S. government agencies: Agency for Toxic Substances and Disease Registry; Centers for Disease Control and Prevention (CDC); Genetics Home Reference; *Morbidity and Mortality Weekly Report* (MMWR); National Cancer Institute (NCI); National Center for Infectious Diseases; National Heart, Lung, and Blood Institute (NHLBI); National Institute of Environmental Health Sciences (NIEHS); National Institute of Mental Health (NIMH); National Institute of Neurological Disorders and Stroke (NINDS); National Institute on Aging (NIA); National Institute on Drug Abuse (NIDA); National Institutes of Health (NIH); U.S. Department of Labor; and the U.S. Department of Veterans Affairs (VA)

In addition, this volume contains copyrighted documents from the following organizations and individuals: A.D.A.M., Inc.; Alzheimer's Association; American Brain Tumor Association; Angioma Alliance; Brain Injury Resource Center; Children's National Medical Center; Epilepsy.com; Haygoush Kalinian, PhD; Lewy Body Dementia Association; Lifespan; National Association of State Head Injury Administrators; National Stroke Association; Nemours Foundation; Traumatic Brain Injury Model Systems National Data and Statistical Center; United Leukodystrophy Foundation; University of Washington Model

System Knowledge Translation Center; and Wolters Kluwer Health/ Lippincott Williams and Wilkins.

Acknowledgements

In addition to the listed organizations, agencies, and individuals who have contributed to this *Sourcebook*, special thanks go to managing editor Karen Bellenir, research and permissions coordinator Liz Collins, and document engineer Bruce Bellenir for their help and support.

About the Health Reference Series

The *Health Reference Series* is designed to provide basic medical information for patients, families, caregivers, and the general public. Each volume takes a particular topic and provides comprehensive coverage. This is especially important for people who may be dealing with a newly diagnosed disease or a chronic disorder in themselves or in a family member. People looking for preventive guidance, information about disease warning signs, medical statistics, and risk factors for health problems will also find answers to their questions in the *Health Reference Series*. The *Series*, however, is not intended to serve as a tool for diagnosing illness, in prescribing treatments, or as a substitute for the physician/patient relationship. All people concerned about medical symptoms or the possibility of disease are encouraged to seek professional care from an appropriate health care provider.

A Note about Spelling and Style

Health Reference Series editors use *Stedman's Medical Dictionary* as an authority for questions related to the spelling of medical terms and the *Chicago Manual of Style* for questions related to grammatical structures, punctuation, and other editorial concerns. Consistent adherence is not always possible, however, because the individual volumes within the *Series* include many documents from a wide variety of different producers and copyright holders, and the editor's primary goal is to present material from each source as accurately as is possible following the terms specified by each document's producer. This sometimes means that information in different chapters or sections may follow other guidelines and alternate spelling authorities. For example, occasionally a copyright holder may require that eponymous terms be shown in possessive forms (Crohn's disease *vs.* Crohn disease) or that British spelling norms be retained (leukaemia *vs.* leukemia).

Locating Information within the Health Reference Series

The *Health Reference Series* contains a wealth of information about a wide variety of medical topics. Ensuring easy access to all the fact sheets, research reports, in-depth discussions, and other material contained within the individual books of the *Series* remains one of our highest priorities. As the *Series* continues to grow in size and scope, however, locating the precise information needed by a reader may become more challenging.

A Contents Guide to the Health Reference Series was developed to direct readers to the specific volumes that address their concerns. It presents an extensive list of diseases, treatments, and other topics of general interest compiled from the Tables of Contents and major index headings. To access *A Contents Guide to the Health Reference Series*, visit www.healthreferenceseries.com.

Medical Consultant

Medical consultation services are provided to the *Health Reference Series* editors by David A. Cooke, MD, FACP. Dr. Cooke is a graduate of Brandeis University, and he received his MD degree from the University of Michigan. He completed residency training at the University of Wisconsin Hospital and Clinics. He is board-certified in Internal Medicine. Dr. Cooke currently works as part of the University of Michigan Health System and practices in Ann Arbor, MI. In his free time, he enjoys writing, science fiction, and spending time with his family.

Our Advisory Board

We would like to thank the following board members for providing guidance to the development of this *Series*:

- Dr. Lynda Baker, Associate Professor of Library and Information Science, Wayne State University, Detroit, MI

- Nancy Bulgarelli, William Beaumont Hospital Library, Royal Oak, MI

- Karen Imarisio, Bloomfield Township Public Library, Bloomfield Township, MI

- Karen Morgan, Mardigian Library, University of Michigan-Dearborn, Dearborn, MI

- Rosemary Orlando, St. Clair Shores Public Library, St. Clair Shores, MI

Health Reference Series Update Policy

The inaugural book in the *Health Reference Series* was the first edition of *Cancer Sourcebook* published in 1989. Since then, the *Series* has been enthusiastically received by librarians and in the medical community. In order to maintain the standard of providing high-quality health information for the layperson the editorial staff at Omnigraphics felt it was necessary to implement a policy of updating volumes when warranted.

Medical researchers have been making tremendous strides, and it is the purpose of the *Health Reference Series* to stay current with the most recent advances. Each decision to update a volume is made on an individual basis. Some of the considerations include how much new information is available and the feedback we receive from people who use the books. If there is a topic you would like to see added to the update list, or an area of medical concern you feel has not been adequately addressed, please write to:

Editor
Health Reference Series
Omnigraphics, Inc.
P.O. Box 31-1640
Detroit, MI 48231-1640
E-mail: editorial@omnigraphics.com

Part One

Brain Basics

Chapter 1

Inside the Human Brain

Basics of the Healthy Brain

The brain is a remarkable organ. Seemingly without effort, it allows us to carry out every element of our daily lives. It manages many body functions, such as breathing, blood circulation, and digestion, without our knowledge or direction. It also directs all the functions we carry out consciously. We can speak, hear, see, move, remember, feel emotions, and make decisions because of the complicated mix of chemical and electrical processes that take place in our brains.

The brain is made of nerve cells and several other cell types. Nerve cells also are called neurons. The neurons of all animals function in basically the same way, even though animals can be very different from each other. Neurons survive and function with the help and support of glial cells, the other main type of cell in the brain. Glial cells hold neurons in place, provide them with nutrients, rid the brain of damaged cells and other cellular debris, and provide insulation to neurons in the brain and spinal cord. In fact, the brain has many more glial cells than neurons—some scientists estimate even ten times as many.

Another essential feature of the brain is its enormous network of blood vessels. Even though the brain is only about 2% of the body's weight, it receives 20% of the body's blood supply. Billions of tiny blood

Text in this chapter is excerpted from "Alzheimer's Disease: Unraveling the Mystery," National Institute on Aging (NIA), October 27, 2009. Also included are excerpts from, "NIH Launches the Human Connectome Project to Unravel the Brain's Connections," National Institutes of Health (NIH), July 15, 2009.

vessels, or capillaries, carry oxygen, glucose (the brain's principal source of energy), nutrients, and hormones to brain cells so they can do their work. Capillaries also carry away waste products.

Parts of the Human Brain

The main players: Two cerebral hemispheres account for 85% of the brain's weight. The billions of neurons in the two hemispheres are connected by thick bundles of nerve cell fibers called the corpus callosum. Scientists now think that the two hemispheres differ not so much in what they do (the logical versus artistic notion), but in how they process information. The left hemisphere appears to focus on details (such as recognizing a particular face in a crowd). The right

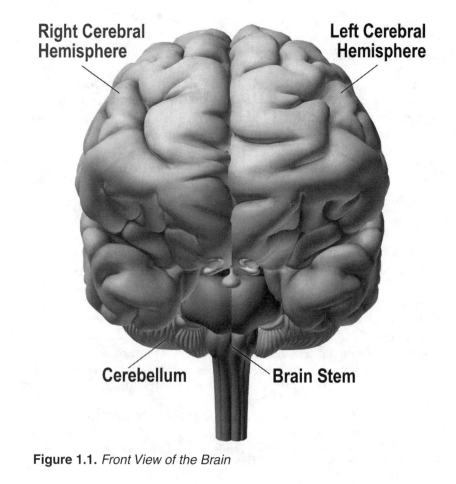

Figure 1.1. *Front View of the Brain*

hemisphere focuses on broad background (such as understanding the relative position of objects in a space). The cerebral hemispheres have an outer layer called the cerebral cortex. This is where the brain processes sensory information received from the outside world, controls voluntary movement, and regulates cognitive functions, such as thinking, learning, speaking, remembering, and making decisions. The hemispheres have four lobes, each of which has different roles:

- The frontal lobe, which is in the front of the brain, controls executive function activities like thinking, organizing, planning, and problem solving, as well as memory, attention, and movement.

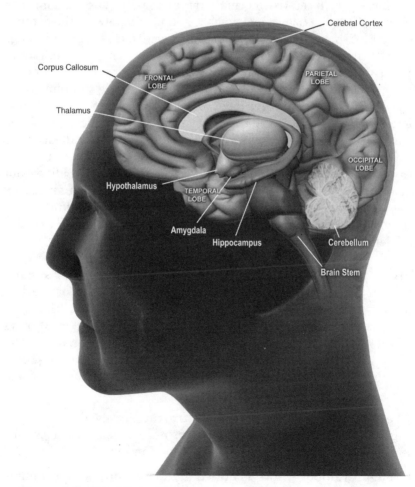

Figure 1.2. *Side View of the Brain*

- The parietal lobe, which sits behind the frontal lobe, deals with the perception and integration of stimuli from the senses.

- The occipital lobe, which is at the back of the brain, is concerned with vision.

- The temporal lobe, which runs along the side of the brain under the frontal and parietal lobes, deals with the senses of smell, taste, and sound, and the formation and storage of memories.

The cerebellum sits above the brain stem and beneath the occipital lobe. It takes up a little more than 10% of the brain. This part of the brain plays roles in balance and coordination. The cerebellum has two hemispheres, which receive information from the eyes, ears, and muscles and joints about the body's movements and position. Once the cerebellum processes that information, it sends instructions to the body through the rest of the brain and spinal cord. The cerebellum's work allows us to move smoothly, maintain our balance, and turn around without even thinking about it. It also is involved with motor learning and remembering how to do things like drive a car or write your name.

The brain stem sits at the base of the brain. It connects the spinal cord with the rest of the brain. Even though it is the smallest of the three main players, its functions are crucial to survival. The brain stem controls the functions that happen automatically to keep us alive—our heart rate, blood pressure, and breathing. It also relays information between the brain and the spinal cord, which then sends out messages to the muscles, skin, and other organs. Sleep and dreaming are also controlled by the brain stem.

Other crucial parts of the brain: Several other essential parts of the brain lie deep inside the cerebral hemispheres in a network of structures called the limbic system. The limbic system links the brain stem with the higher reasoning elements of the cerebral cortex. It plays a key role in developing and carrying out instinctive behaviors and emotions and also is important in perceiving smells and linking them with memory, emotion, and instinctive behaviors. The limbic system includes the following:

- The amygdala, an almond-shaped structure involved in processing and remembering strong emotions such as fear. It is located in the temporal lobe just in front of the hippocampus.

- The hippocampus, which is buried in the temporal lobe, is important for learning and short-term memory. This part of the brain is thought to be the site where short-term memories are converted into long-term memories for storage in other brain areas.

- The thalamus, located at the top of the brain stem, receives sensory and limbic information, processes it, and then sends it to the cerebral cortex.

- The hypothalamus, a structure under the thalamus, monitors activities such as body temperature and food intake. It issues instructions to correct any imbalances. The hypothalamus also controls the body's internal clock.

The brain in action: Sophisticated brain-imaging techniques allow scientists to monitor brain function in living people and to see how various parts of the brain are used for different kinds of tasks. This is opening up worlds of knowledge about brain function and how it changes with age or disease. One of these imaging techniques is called positron emission tomography, or PET scanning. Some PET scans measure blood flow and glucose metabolism throughout the brain. Scientists can use PET scans to see what happens in the brain when a person is engaged in a physical or mental activity, at rest, or even while sleeping or dreaming. Certain tracers can track the activity of brain chemicals, for example neurotransmitters such as dopamine and serotonin. Some of these neurotransmitters are changed with age, disease, and drug therapies.

Neurons and Their Jobs

The human brain is made up of billions of neurons. Each has a cell body, an axon, and many dendrites. The cell body contains a nucleus, which controls much of the cell's activities. The cell body also contains other structures, called organelles that perform specific tasks.

The axon, which is much narrower than the width of a human hair, extends out from the cell body. Axons transmit messages from neuron to neuron. Sometimes, signal transmissions—like those from head to toe—have to travel over very long distances. Axons are covered with an insulating layer called myelin (also called white matter because of its whitish color). Myelin, which is made by a particular kind of glial cell, increases the speed of nerve signal transmissions through the brain. Dendrites also branch out from the cell body. They receive messages from the axons of other neurons. Each neuron is connected to thousands of other nerve cells through its axon and dendrites.

Groups of neurons in the brain have special jobs. For example, some are involved with thinking, learning, and memory. Others are responsible for receiving information from the sensory organs (such as the eyes and ears) or the skin. Still others communicate with muscles, stimulating them into action. Several processes all have to work smoothly together for neurons, and the whole organism, to survive and stay healthy. These processes are communication, metabolism, and repair.

Communication: Imagine the many miles of fiber-optic cables that run under our streets. Day and night, millions of televised and telephonic messages flash at incredible speeds, letting people strike deals, give instructions, share a laugh, or learn some news. Miniaturize it, multiply it many-fold, make it much more complex, and you have the brain. Neurons are the great communicators, always in touch with their neighbors.

Neurons communicate with each other through their axons and dendrites. When a dendrite receives an incoming signal (electrical or chemical), an action potential, or nerve impulse, can be generated in the cell body. The action potential travels to the end of the axon, and once there, the passage of either electrical current or, more typically, the release of chemical messengers, called neurotransmitters, can be triggered. The neurotransmitters are released from the axon terminal and move across a tiny gap, or synapse, to specific receptor sites on the receiving, or post-synaptic, end of dendrites of nearby neurons. A typical neuron has thousands of synaptic connections, mostly on its many dendrites, with other neurons. Cell bodies also have receptor sites for neurotransmitters.

Once the post-synaptic receptors are activated, they open channels through the cell membrane into the receiving nerve cell's interior or start other processes that determine what the receiving nerve cell will do. Some neurotransmitters inhibit nerve cell function (that is, they make it less likely that the nerve cell will send an electrical signal down its axon). Other neurotransmitters stimulate nerve cells, priming the receiving cell to become active or send an electrical signal down the axon to more neurons in the pathway. A neuron receives signals from many other neurons simultaneously, and the sum of a neuron's neurotransmitter inputs at any one instant will determine whether it sends a signal down its axon to activate or inhibit the action of other neighboring neurons. During any one moment, millions of these signals are speeding through pathways in the brain, allowing the brain to receive and process information, make adjustments, and send out instructions to various parts of the body.

Metabolism: All cells break down chemicals and nutrients to generate energy and form building blocks that make new cellular molecules such as proteins. This process is called metabolism. To maintain metabolism, the brain needs plenty of blood constantly circulating through its billions of capillaries to supply neurons and other brain cells with oxygen and glucose. Without oxygen and glucose, neurons will quickly die.

Repair: Nerve cells are formed during fetal life and for a short time after birth. Unlike most cells, which have a fairly short lifespan, neurons in the brain live a long time. These cells can live for up to 100 years or longer. To stay healthy, living neurons must constantly maintain and repair themselves. In an adult, when neurons die because of disease or injury, they are not usually replaced. Research, however, shows that in a few brain regions, new neurons can be generated, even in the old brain.

NIH Launches the Human Connectome Project to Unravel the Brain's Connections

The National Institutes of Health (NIH) Blueprint for Neuroscience Research is launching a $30 million project that will use cutting-edge brain imaging technologies to map the circuitry of the healthy adult human brain. By systematically collecting brain imaging data from hundreds of subjects, the Human Connectome Project (HCP) will yield insight into how brain connections underlie brain function, and will open up new lines of inquiry for human neuroscience.

"The HCP is truly a grand and critical challenge: to map the wiring diagram of the entire, living human brain. Mapping the circuits and linking these circuits to the full spectrum of brain function in health and disease is an old challenge but one that can finally be addressed rigorously by combining powerful, emerging technologies," says Thomas Insel, MD, director of the National Institute of Mental Health (NIMH), which is part of the NIH Blueprint.

"Neuroscientists have only a piecemeal understanding of brain connectivity. If we knew more about the connections within the brain—and especially their susceptibility to change—we would know more about brain dysfunction in aging, mental health disorders, addiction, and neurological disease," says Story Landis, PhD, director of the National Institute of Neurological Disorders and Stroke (NINDS), also part of the NIH Blueprint. For example, there is evidence that the growth of abnormal brain connections during early life contributes to autism and schizophrenia. Changes in connectivity also appear to occur when neurons degenerate, either as a consequence of normal aging or of diseases such as Alzheimer disease.

In addition to brain imaging, the HCP will involve collection of deoxyribonucleic acid (DNA) samples, demographic information, and behavioral data from the subjects. Together, these data could hint at how brain connectivity is influenced by genetics and the environment, and in turn, how individual differences in brain connectivity relate to individual differences in behavior. Primarily, however, the data will serve as a baseline for future studies. These data will be freely available to the research community.

The complexity of the brain and a lack of adequate imaging technology have hampered past research on human brain connectivity. The brain is estimated to contain more than 100 billion neurons that form trillions of connections with each other. Neurons can connect across distant regions of the brain by extending long, slender projections called axons—but the trajectories that axons take within the human brain are almost entirely uncharted.

In the HCP, researchers will optimize and combine state-of-the-art brain imaging technologies to probe axonal pathways and other brain connections. In recent years, sophisticated versions of magnetic resonance imaging (MRI) have emerged that are capable of looking beyond the brain's gross anatomy to find functional connections. Functional MRI (fMRI), for example, uses changes in blood flow and oxygen consumption within the brain as markers for neuronal activity, and can highlight the brain circuits that become active during different behaviors.

"Human connectomics has been gaining momentum in the research community for a few years," says Michael Huerta, PhD, associate director of NIMH and the lead NIH contact for the HCP. "The data, the imaging tools, and the analytical tools produced through the HCP will play a major role in launching connectomics as a field."

Chapter 2

Brain Changes Related to Healthy Aging

In the past several decades, investigators have learned much about what happens in the brain when people have a neurodegenerative disease such as Parkinson disease, Alzheimer disease (AD), or other dementias. Their findings also have revealed much about what happens during healthy aging. Researchers are investigating a number of changes related to healthy aging in hopes of learning more about this process so they can fill gaps in our knowledge.

As a person gets older, changes occur in all parts of the body, including the brain:

- Certain parts of the brain shrink, especially the prefrontal cortex (an area at the front of the frontal lobe) and the hippocampus. Both areas are important to learning, memory, planning, and other complex mental activities.

- Changes in neurons and neurotransmitters affect communication between neurons. In certain brain regions, communication between neurons can be reduced because white matter (myelin-covered axons) is degraded or lost.

- Changes in the brain's blood vessels occur. Blood flow can be reduced because arteries narrow and less growth of new capillaries occurs.

Excerpted from "Alzheimer's Disease: Unraveling the Mystery," National Institute on Aging (NIA), updated November 25, 2008.

11

- In some people, structures called plaques and tangles develop outside of and inside neurons, respectively, although in much smaller amounts than in AD.

- Damage by free radicals increases (free radicals are a kind of molecule that reacts easily with other molecules).

- Inflammation increases (inflammation is the complex process that occurs when the body responds to an injury, disease, or abnormal situation).

What effects does aging have on mental function in healthy older people? Some people may notice a modest decline in their ability to learn new things and retrieve information, such as remembering names. They may perform worse on complex tasks of attention, learning, and memory than would a younger person. However, if given enough time to perform the task, the scores of healthy people in their 70s and 80s are often similar to those of young adults. In fact, as they age, adults often improve in other cognitive areas, such as vocabulary and other forms of verbal knowledge.

It also appears that additional brain regions can be activated in older adults during cognitive tasks, such as taking a memory test. Researchers do not fully understand why this happens, but one idea is that the brain engages mechanisms to compensate for difficulties that certain regions may be having. For example, the brain may recruit alternate brain networks in order to perform a task. These findings have led many scientists to believe that major declines in mental abilities are not inevitable as people age. Growing evidence of the adaptive (what scientists call plastic) capabilities of the older brain provide hope that people may be able to do things to sustain good brain function as they age. A variety of interacting factors, such as lifestyle, overall health, environment, and genetics also may play a role.

Another question that scientists are asking is why some people remain cognitively healthy as they get older while others develop cognitive impairment or dementia. The concept of cognitive reserve may provide some insights. Cognitive reserve refers to the brain's ability to operate effectively even when some function is disrupted. It also refers to the amount of damage that the brain can sustain before changes in cognition are evident. People vary in the cognitive reserve they have, and this variability may be because of differences in genetics, education, occupation, lifestyle, leisure activities, or other life experiences. These factors could provide a certain amount of tolerance and ability to adapt to change and damage that occurs during aging. At some point, depending on a person's cognitive reserve and unique mix of genetics, environment, and life experiences, the balance may tip in favor of a disease process that will ultimately lead to dementia. For another person, with a different reserve and a different mix of genetics, environment, and life experiences, the balance may result in no apparent decline in cognitive function with age.

Scientists are increasingly interested in the influence of all these factors on brain health, and studies are revealing some clues about actions people can take that may help preserve healthy brain aging. Fortunately, these actions also benefit a person's overall health:

- Controlling risk factors for chronic disease, such as heart disease and diabetes (for example, keeping blood cholesterol and blood pressure at healthy levels and maintaining a healthy weight)

- Enjoying regular exercise and physical activity

- Eating a healthy diet that includes plenty of vegetables and fruits

- Engaging in intellectually stimulating activities and maintaining close social ties with family, friends, and community

Advanced Cognitive Training for Independent and Vital Elderly *(ACTIVE) Study May Provide Clues to Help Older Adults Stay Mentally Sharp*

The phrase "use it or lose it" may make you think of your muscles, but scientists who study brain health in older people have found that it may apply to cognitive skills as well. In 2006, scientists funded by National Institute on Aging (NIA) and the National Institute of Nursing Research completed a study of cognitive training in older adults. This study, the *Advanced Cognitive Training for Independent and Vital Elderly* (ACTIVE) study, was the first randomized controlled trial to demonstrate long-lasting, positive effects of brief cognitive training in older adults.

The ACTIVE study included 2,802 healthy adults age 65 and older who were living independently. Participants were randomly assigned to four groups. Three groups took part in up to ten computer-based training sessions that targeted a specific cognitive ability—memory, reasoning, and speed of processing (in other words, how fast participants could respond to prompts on a computer screen). The fourth group (the control group) received no cognitive training. Of those who

13

completed the initial training, 60% also took part in 75-minute booster sessions 11 months later. These sessions were designed to maintain improvements gained from the initial training.

The investigators tested the participants at the beginning of the study, after the initial training and booster sessions, and once a year for five more years. They found that the improvements from the training roughly counteracted the degree of decline in cognitive performance that would be expected over a 7- to 14-year period among older people without dementia:

- Immediately after the initial training, 87% of the processing-speed group, 74% of the reasoning group, and 26% of the memory group showed improvement in the skills taught.

- After five years, people in each group performed better on tests in their respective areas of training than did people in the control group. The reasoning and processing-speed groups who received booster training had the greatest benefit.

The researchers also looked at the training's effects on participants' everyday lives. After five years, all three groups who received training reported less difficulty than the control group in tasks such as preparing meals, managing money, and doing housework. However, these results were statistically significant for only the group that had the reasoning training.

As they get older, many people worry about their mental skills getting rusty. The ACTIVE study offers hope that cognitive training may be useful because it showed that relatively brief and targeted cognitive exercises can produce lasting improvements in the skills taught. Next steps for researchers are to determine ways to generalize the training benefits beyond the specific skills taught in ACTIVE and to find out whether cognitive training programs could prevent, delay, or diminish the effects of Alzheimer disease and other dementias.

Chapter 3

How Toxins Affect the Brain

Chapter Contents

Section 3.1

Impact of Drug Abuse and Addiction on the Brain

Excerpted from "Understanding Drug Abuse and Addiction," *NIDA InfoFacts*, June 2008, National Institute on Drug Abuse (NIDA).

Addiction is a chronic, often relapsing brain disease that causes compulsive drug seeking and use despite harmful consequences to the individual who is addicted and to those around them. Drug addiction is a brain disease because the abuse of drugs leads to changes in the structure and function of the brain. Although it is true that for most people the initial decision to take drugs is voluntary, over time the changes in the brain caused by repeated drug abuse can affect a person's self control and ability to make sound decisions, and at the same time send intense impulses to take drugs.

It is because of these changes in the brain that it is so challenging for a person who is addicted to stop abusing drugs. Fortunately, there are treatments that help people to counteract addiction's powerful disruptive effects and regain control. Research shows that combining addiction treatment medications, if available, with behavioral therapy is the best way to ensure success for most patients. Treatment approaches that are tailored to each patient's drug abuse patterns and any co-occurring medical, psychiatric, and social problems can lead to sustained recovery and a life without drug abuse. Similar to other chronic, relapsing diseases, such as diabetes, asthma, or heart disease, drug addiction can be managed successfully. And, as with other chronic diseases, it is not uncommon for a person to relapse and begin abusing drugs again. Relapse, however, does not signal failure—rather, it indicates that treatment should be reinstated, adjusted, or that alternate treatment is needed to help the individual regain control and recover.

What happens to your brain when you take drugs?

Drugs are chemicals that tap into the brain's communication system and disrupt the way nerve cells normally send, receive, and process information. There are at least two ways that drugs are able to do this: (1) by imitating the brain's natural chemical messengers, and/or (2) by overstimulating the reward circuit of the brain.

Nearly all drugs, directly or indirectly, target the brain's reward system by flooding the circuit with dopamine. Dopamine is a neurotransmitter present in regions of the brain that control movement, emotion, motivation, and feelings of pleasure. The overstimulation of this system which normally responds to natural behaviors that are linked to survival (eating, spending time with loved ones, and so forth) produces euphoric effects in response to the drugs. This reaction sets in motion a pattern that teaches people to repeat the behavior of abusing drugs.

As a person continues to abuse drugs, the brain adapts to the overwhelming surges in dopamine by producing less dopamine or by reducing the number of dopamine receptors in the reward circuit. As a result, dopamine's impact on the reward circuit is lessened, reducing the abuser's ability to enjoy the drugs and the things that previously brought pleasure. This decrease compels those addicted to drugs to keep abusing drugs in order to attempt to bring their dopamine function back to normal. And, they may now require larger amounts of the drug than they first did to achieve the dopamine high—an effect known as tolerance.

Long-term abuse causes changes in other brain chemical systems and circuits as well. Glutamate is a neurotransmitter that influences the reward circuit and the ability to learn. When the optimal concentration of glutamate is altered by drug abuse, the brain attempts to compensate, which can impair cognitive function. Drugs of abuse facilitate unconscious (conditioned) learning, which leads the user to experience uncontrollable cravings when they see a place or person they associate with the drug experience, even when the drug itself is not available. Brain imaging studies of drug-addicted individuals show changes in areas of the brain that are critical to judgment, decision-making, learning and memory, and behavior control. Together, these changes can drive an abuser to seek out and take drugs compulsively despite adverse consequences—in other words, to become addicted to drugs.

Why do some people become addicted and others do not?

No single factor can predict whether or not a person will become addicted to drugs. Risk for addiction is influenced by a person's biology, social environment, and age or stage of development. The more risk factors an individual has, the greater the chance that taking drugs can lead to addiction.

- **Biology:** The genes that people are born with—in combination with environmental influences—account for about half of their addiction vulnerability. Additionally, gender, ethnicity, and the presence of other mental disorders may influence risk for drug abuse and addiction.

- **Environment:** A person's environment includes many different influences—from family and friends to socioeconomic status and quality of life in general. Factors such as peer pressure, physical and sexual abuse, stress, and parental involvement can greatly influence the course of drug abuse and addiction in a person's life.

- **Development:** Genetic and environmental factors interact with critical developmental stages in a person's life to affect addiction vulnerability, and adolescents experience a double challenge. Although taking drugs at any age can lead to addiction, the earlier that drug use begins, the more likely it is to progress to more serious abuse. And because adolescents' brains are still developing in the areas that govern decision-making, judgment, and self-control, they are especially prone to risk-taking behaviors, including trying drugs of abuse.

Prevention Is the Key

Drug addiction is a preventable disease. Results from National Institute on Drug Abuse (NIDA)-funded research have shown that prevention programs that involve families, schools, communities, and the media are effective in reducing drug abuse. Although many events and cultural factors affect drug abuse trends, when youths perceive drug abuse as harmful, they reduce their drug taking. It is necessary, therefore, to help youth and the general public to understand the risks of drug abuse, and for teachers, parents, and healthcare professionals to keep sending the message that drug addiction can be prevented if a person never abuses drugs.

Section 3.2

Mercury and Neurodevelopment

This section includes excerpts from "Mercury," Centers for Disease Control and Prevention (CDC), November 2009; and excerpts from "Mercury and Neurodevelopment," National Institute of Environmental Health Sciences (NIEHS), November 9, 2007.

Mercury

Mercury is an element and a metal that is found in air, water, and soil. It exists in three forms that have different properties, usage, and toxicity. The three forms are called elemental (or metallic) mercury, inorganic mercury compounds, and organic mercury compounds.

Elemental mercury is liquid at room temperature. It is used in some thermometers, dental amalgams, fluorescent light bulbs, some electrical switches, mining, and some industrial processes. It is released into the air when coal and other fossil fuels are burned.

Inorganic mercury compounds are formed when mercury combines with other elements, such as sulfur or oxygen, to form compounds or salts. Inorganic mercury compounds can occur naturally in the environment. Inorganic mercury compounds are used in some industrial processes and in the making of other chemicals. Outside the United States, inorganic mercury salts have been used in cosmetic skin creams.

Organic mercury compounds are formed when mercury combines with carbon. Microscopic organisms in water and soil can convert elemental and inorganic mercury into an organic mercury compound, methylmercury, which accumulates in the food chain. Thimerosal and phenylmercuric acetate are other types of organic mercury compounds made in small amounts for use as preservatives.

How People Are Exposed to Mercury

Elemental mercury: People may be exposed when they breathe air containing elemental mercury vapors. Vapors may be present in such workplaces as dental offices, smelting operations, and locations where mercury has been spilled or released. In the body, elemental mercury can be converted to inorganic mercury.

Inorganic mercury: People may be exposed if they work where inorganic mercury compounds are used.

Organic mercury: People may be exposed when they eat fish or shellfish contaminated with methylmercury. Methylmercury can pass through the placenta, exposing the developing fetus.

How Mercury Affects People's Health

Elemental mercury: The human health effects from exposure to low environmental levels of elemental mercury are unknown. Very high mercury vapor concentrations can quickly cause severe lung damage. At low vapor concentrations over a long time, neurological disturbances, memory problems, skin rash, and kidney abnormalities may occur.

Inorganic mercury: When eaten in large amounts, some inorganic mercury compounds can be very irritating and corrosive to the digestive system. If repeatedly eaten or applied to the skin over long periods of time, some inorganic mercury compounds can cause effects similar to what is seen with long-term mercury vapor exposure, including neurological disturbances, memory problems, skin rash, and kidney abnormalities.

Organic mercury: Large amounts of methylmercury eaten over weeks to months have caused damage to the nervous system. Infants born to women who were poisoned with methylmercury had developmental abnormalities and cerebral palsy.

Levels of Mercury in the U.S. Population

In the *Fourth National Report on Human Exposure to Environmental Chemicals (Fourth Report)*, Centers for Disease Control and Prevention (CDC) scientists measured total mercury in the blood of 8,373 participants aged one year and older who took part in the National Health and Nutrition Examination Survey (NHANES) during 2003–2004. Total blood mercury is mainly a measure of methyl mercury exposure. In the same 2003–2004 NHANES, CDC scientists measured mercury in the urine of 2,538 participants aged six years and older. Mercury in the urine is a measure of inorganic mercury exposure. By measuring mercury in blood and in urine, scientists can estimate the amount of mercury that has entered people's bodies.

- CDC scientists found measurable mercury in most of the participants. Both blood and urine mercury levels tend to increase with age.

- Defining safe levels of mercury in blood continues to be an active research area.

- Blood and urine mercury in the U.S. population were similar to levels seen in other developed countries.

Finding a measurable amount of mercury in blood or urine does not mean that levels of mercury cause an adverse health effect. Bio-monitoring studies on levels of mercury provide physicians and public health officials with reference values so that they can determine whether people have been exposed to higher levels of mercury than are found in the general population. Bio-monitoring data can also help scientists plan and conduct research about exposure and health effects.

Mercury and Neurodevelopment

Mercury is a naturally occurring metallic element that is extremely toxic to the brain, kidneys, and developing fetus. Numerous studies have shown that methylmercury is a developmental neurotoxin that readily passes through the placenta and damages the fetal nervous system. In the early 1990s, National Institute of Environmental Health Sciences (NIEHS)-funded researchers at the University of Rochester conducted a nine-year study on children in the Republic of the Seychelles to assess the developmental effects of low-dose exposure to methylmercury. The researchers tested 779 children at intervals of 6, 19, 29, and 66 months of age, whose mothers ate an average of 12 fish meals per week while pregnant. The test results revealed no ill effects from the high-fish diet.

However, results of studies funded jointly by the NIEHS and the European Commission's Climate Research Programme have shown some evidence of a link between mercury and developmental deficits. Cognitive tests performed on seven-year-old Faroe Islands children, whose mothers' diets of fish and whale blubber exposed them to high levels of methylmercury during her pregnancy, revealed significant impairments in language, attention, and memory. The researchers also noted similar cognitive deficits in these children when tested at 14 years of age.

The NIEHS is funding additional studies to determine whether nutritional factors associated with fish consumption might protect the fetal brain from the adverse effects of environmental toxicants. Researchers are also conducting studies on the possible interaction between methylmercury and polychlorinated biphenyls, toxic pollutants that were also present in the whale meat and blubber consumed by the Faroe Island subjects.

These studies have provided regulatory agencies with evidence of the developmental effects of mercury at environmentally relevant doses. This has resulted in the establishment of national fish consumption advisories for at-risk groups including women who are pregnant, those who might become pregnant, and nursing mothers.

Section 3.3

Dangers of Lead Exposure

"Spotlight on Lead," Centers for Disease Control and Prevention (CDC), November 2009.

Lead is a soft, dense, blue-gray metal. Lead occurs naturally in the earth's crust, where it combines with other elements such as oxygen and sulfur. It is used to make batteries and metal mixtures. Lead is also contained in some ammunitions, old pipes and their soldered connections, automotive radiators, pewter, pottery, folk medicines, leaded crystal glass, and as a contaminant in trace amounts in many products. Because of health concerns, lead is no longer added to gasoline and house paints. Lead solder for sealing tin food cans has been eliminated in the United States.

Exposure: People can be exposed to small amounts of lead by breathing air, drinking water, eating food, or swallowing dust or dirt that contains lead. For adults, the diet is the source of most general low-level environmental exposure to lead. Children can be exposed to more lead than adults. Children are commonly exposed to lead from hand-to-mouth activities involving contaminated dust and soils around older homes that contain lead-based paint or from eating paint chips that contain lead. Less common sources of lead exposure include folk medicines, cosmetics, ceramic and metal cookware, unusual clay-eating behaviors, and imported toys. Workers may be exposed in industries that involve lead, such as smelting and battery manufacturing. Workers can also secondarily expose household members by bringing lead home on their clothes.

Health effects: No safe blood lead level has been identified. For infants and young children, lead levels of ten micrograms or more in a deciliter of blood are levels of concern and can damage ability to learn. (A microgram is one millionth of a gram. A deciliter is about half a cup of liquid.) Of all people, young children face the most danger from exposure to lead because their growing bodies are more prone to harm and also children absorb lead more easily than do adults' bodies. Pregnant women and women of childbearing age should avoid exposure to lead because lead ingested by a mother can affect the unborn child. At much higher blood lead levels lead can damage people's kidneys, blood, and nervous system and progress to coma, convulsions, or death.

U.S. population levels of lead: In the *Fourth National Report on Human Exposure to Environmental Chemicals (Fourth Report)*, Centers for Disease Control and Prevention (CDC) scientists measured lead in the blood of 8,373 participants aged one year and older and in the urine of 2543 participants aged six years and older who took part in the National Health and Nutrition Examination Survey (NHANES) during 2003–2004. Prior survey periods of 1999–2000 and 2001–2002 are also included in the *Fourth Report*. By measuring lead in blood and urine, scientists can estimate the amount of lead that has entered people's bodies.

- During the period of 1999–2004, 1.4% of children aged 1–5 years had blood lead levels of concern—for example, ten micrograms per deciliter or higher. This finding is lower than the 4.4% seen in the period of 1988–1994.

- This finding shows that public health efforts to reduce the number of children with elevated blood lead levels in the general population continue to be successful. However, special populations of children at high risk for lead exposure (for example, children living in homes containing lead-based paint or lead-contaminated dust) have higher rates of elevated blood lead levels and lead remains a major public health concern.

Bio-monitoring: Studies on levels of lead provide physicians and public health officials with reference values so that they can determine whether people have been exposed to higher levels of lead than are found in the general population. Bio-monitoring data can also help scientists plan and conduct research on exposure and health effects.

Section 3.4

Manganese and Brain Damage

This section includes excerpts from "Public Health Statement: Manganese," Agency for Toxic Substances and Disease Registry, October 30, 2008; and excerpts from "Manganese and Brain Damage," National Institute of Environmental Health Sciences (NIEHS), November 9, 2007.

Public Health Statement on Manganese

The Environmental Protection Agency (EPA) identifies the most serious hazardous waste sites in the nation. These sites are then placed on the National Priorities List (NPL) and are targeted for long-term federal clean-up activities. Manganese has been found in at least 869 of the 1,699 current or former NPL sites. Although the total number of NPL sites evaluated for this substance is not known, the possibility exists that the number of sites at which manganese is found may increase in the future as more sites are evaluated. This information is important because these sites may be sources of exposure and exposure to this substance may harm you.

When a substance is released either from a large area, such as an industrial plant, or from a container, such as a drum or bottle, it enters the environment. Such a release does not always lead to exposure. You can be exposed to a substance only when you come in contact with it. You may be exposed by breathing, eating, or drinking the substance, or by skin contact.

If you are exposed to manganese, many factors will determine whether you will be harmed. These factors include the dose (how much), the duration (how long), and how you come in contact with it. You must also consider any other chemicals you are exposed to and your age, sex, diet, family traits, lifestyle, and state of health.

What is manganese?

Manganese is a naturally occurring substance found in many types of rocks and soil. Pure manganese is a silver-colored metal; however, it does not occur in the environment as a pure metal. Rather, it occurs combined with other substances such as oxygen, sulfur, and chlorine. Manganese is a trace element and is necessary for good health.

Manufacturing uses: Manganese is used principally in steel production to improve hardness, stiffness, and strength. It is used in carbon steel, stainless steel, high-temperature steel, and tool steel, along with cast iron and super-alloys.

Consumer products: Manganese occurs naturally in most foods and may be added to food or made available in nutritional supplements. Manganese is also used in a wide variety of other products, including: fireworks, dry-cell batteries, fertilizer, paints, a medical imaging agent, and cosmetics. It may also be used as an additive in gasoline to improve the octane rating of the gas. Small amounts of manganese are used in a pharmaceutical product called mangafodipir trisodium (MnDPDP) to improve lesion detection in magnetic resonance imaging of body organs.

How might I be exposed to manganese?

Food: The primary way you can be exposed to manganese is by eating food or manganese-containing nutritional supplements. Vegetarians who consume foods rich in manganese such as grains, beans and nuts, as well as heavy tea drinkers, may have a higher intake of manganese than the average person.

Workplace air: Certain occupations like welding or working in a factory where steel is made may increase your chances of being exposed to high levels of manganese.

Water and soil: Because manganese is a natural component of the environment, you are always exposed to low levels of it in water, air, soil, and food. Manganese is routinely contained in groundwater, drinking water, and soil at low levels. Drinking water containing manganese, or swimming or bathing in water containing manganese, may expose you to low levels of this chemical.

Air: Air also contains low levels of manganese, and breathing air may expose you to it. Releases of manganese into the air occur from industries using or manufacturing products containing manganese, mining activities, and automobile exhaust.

How can manganese affect my health?

The most common health problems in workers exposed to high levels of manganese involve the nervous system. These health effects include behavioral changes and other nervous system effects, which include movements that may become slow and clumsy. This combination of symptoms when sufficiently severe is referred to as manganism. Other less severe nervous system effects such as slowed hand movements have been observed in some workers exposed to lower concentrations in the work place.

The inhalation of a large quantity of dust or fumes containing manganese may cause irritation of the lungs which could lead to pneumonia. Also, loss of sex drive and sperm damage has been observed in men exposed to high levels of manganese in workplace air.

The manganese concentrations that cause effects such as slowed hand movements in some workers are approximately twenty thousand times higher than the concentrations normally found in the environment. Manganism has been found in some workers exposed to manganese concentrations about a million times higher than normal air concentrations of manganese.

Affects on children: Studies in children have suggested that extremely high levels of manganese exposure may produce undesirable effects on brain development, including changes in behavior and decreases in the ability to learn and remember. In some cases, these same manganese exposure levels have been suspected of causing severe symptoms of manganism disease (including difficulty with speech and walking).

How can families reduce the risk of exposure to manganese?

High levels of airborne manganese are observed in certain occupational settings such as steel factories or welding areas. You should take precautions to prevent inhalation of manganese by wearing an appropriate mask to limit the amount of manganese you breathe. Avoid wearing manganese dust-contaminated work clothing in your home or car. Avoid inhalation of welding fumes at home.

Children are not likely to be exposed to harmful amounts of manganese in the diet. However, higher-than-usual amounts of manganese may be absorbed if their diet is low in iron. It is important to provide your child with a well-balanced diet.

While tap and bottled water generally contain safe levels of manganese, well water may sometimes be contaminated with sufficiently high levels of manganese to create a potential health hazard. If drinking water is obtained from a well water source, it may be wise to have the water checked for manganese to ensure the level is below the current guideline level established by the Environmental Protection Agency (EPA).

Is there a medical test to determine whether I have been exposed to manganese?

Several tests are available to measure manganese in blood, urine, hair, or feces. Because manganese is normally present in our body, some is always found in tissues or fluids. Normal ranges of manganese levels are about 4–15 µg/L in blood, 1–8 µg/L in urine, and 0.4–0.85 µg/L in serum (the fluid portion of the blood). Because excess manganese is usually removed from the body within a few days, past exposures are difficult to measure with common laboratory tests.

Manganese and Brain Damage

The National Institute of Environmental Health Sciences (NIEHS) has supported a number of studies to better understand the potential health effects associated with exposure to manganese. These studies show that long-term occupational exposure to manganese results in irreversible damage to areas of the brain that control body movements. These findings have resulted in federal standards that limit the amount of manganese in drinking water, and new approaches for the prevention and treatment of neurological damage caused by manganese exposure. Study results show the following:

- In 1999, the NIEHS funded a study on the health consequences of occupational exposure to manganese. The results showed that miners and steel workers exposed to high levels of manganese in occupational settings developed problems with balance, movement, and fine motor coordination characteristic of Parkinson disease (PD), and were at much greater risk of developing PD itself.

- Effects of manganese exposure on 10-year-old children in Bangladesh, where groundwater levels of the toxic metal are relatively high showed that children who received the highest doses of manganese in their drinking water had significantly lower scores on tests of intellectual function.

- Results from a recent study revealed that people who inhaled manganese from automobile emissions, and had high levels of the compound in their blood, showed signs of neurological problems that were similar to those reported in occupationally exposed individuals.

- Research designed to identify the underlying causes of manganese's effects on brain function shows that manganese exposure produces the same pattern of brain cell death as that seen in PD patients. The loss of these cells results in reduction of a critical neurotransmitter called dopamine, the chemical messenger responsible for coordinated muscle movement. These insights into the impact of manganese exposure on critical brain functions will eventually pave the way for new strategies designed to protect these dopamine-producing neurons from manganese-induced damage.

Chapter 4

Signs and Symptoms of Brain Disorders

Chapter Contents

Section 4.1

Symptom Overview

"Symptoms of Brain Disorder," © 2005 Haygoush Kalinian, PhD. For additional information about neurological disorders and neuropsychological evaluation, along with information about contacting Dr. Kalinian, visit www.neuropsychconsultant.com. Reviewed in January, 2010 by David A. Cooke, MD, FACP, Diplomate, American Board of Internal Medicine.

Note: A number of different medical conditions can impact mental performance. The cause may be straightforward in some cases, but in others it may be quite difficult to identify. Consulting with a neuropsychologist may help yield an accurate diagnosis. (David A. Cooke, MD, FACP, 2010.)

Symptoms of Brain Disorder

If you are experiencing any of these symptoms, consult with a neuropsychologist.

Attention and Concentration Difficulties

- Highly distractible
- Lose my train of thought easily
- Become easily confused and disoriented
- Blackout spells (fainting)
- My mind goes blank
- Aura (strange feelings)
- Don't feel very alert or aware of things
- Other concentration or awareness problems

Memory

- Forgetting where I leave things (keys, gloves, and so forth)

- Forgetting names
- Forgetting what I should be doing
- Forgetting where I am or where I am going
- Forgetting events that happened quite recently (for example, my last meal)
- Need someone to give me a hint so I can remember things
- Relying more and more on notes to remember how to do things
- Forgetting how to do things, but I can remember facts
- Forgetting faces of people I know (when they are not present)
- Frequently forgetting appointments
- Other memory problems

Difficulty Solving Everyday Problems

- Difficulty figuring out how to do new things
- Difficulty planning ahead
- Difficulty figuring out problems that most other people can do
- Difficulty thinking as quickly as needed
- Difficulty doing things in the right order (sequence problems)
- Difficulty verbally describing the steps involved in doing something
- Difficulty changing a plan or activity in a reasonable amount of time
- Difficulty completing an activity in a reasonable amount of time
- Difficulty doing more than one this at a time
- Difficulty switching from one activity to another activity
- Easily frustrated
- Other problem solving difficulties

Speech, Language, and Math Skills

- Difficulty finding the right word to say
- Difficulty understanding what others are saying

- Unable to speak
- Difficulty staying with one idea
- Difficulty writing letters or words (not due to motor problems)
- Slurred speech
- Odd or unusual speech sound
- Difficulty with math (for example, checkbook balancing, making change)
- Difficulty understanding what I read
- Difficulty speaking
- Other speech, language, or math problems

Nonverbal Skills

- Difficulty telling right from left
- Difficulty doing things I should automatically be able to do (such as brushing teeth)
- Problems drawing or copying
- Difficulty dressing (not due to physical difficulty)
- Problems finding my way around places I've been to before
- Difficulty recognizing objects or people
- Parts of my body do not seem as if they belong to me
- Unaware of time (such as, time of day, season, year)
- Slow reaction to time
- Other nonverbal problems

Motor and Coordination Symptoms

- Fine motor control problems (for example, using a pencil or key)
- Weakness on one side of my body
- Difficulty holding onto things
- Tremor or shakiness
- Muscle tick or strange movements

- My writing is very small
- My writing is very large
- Walking more slowly than other people
- Feeling stiff
- Balance problems
- Difficulty starting to move
- Jerky muscles
- Muscles tire quickly
- Often bumping into things
- Other motor or coordination problems

Sensory Symptoms

- Loss of feeling or numbness
- Tingling or strange skin sensations
- Difficulty telling hot from cold
- Problems seeing on one side
- Blurred vision
- Blank spots in vision
- Brief periods of blindness
- "Seeing stars" or flashes of light
- Double vision
- Difficulty looking quickly from one object to another object
- Need to squint or move closer to see clearly
- Losing hearing
- Ringing in my ears or hearing strange sounds
- Difficulty tasting food
- Difficulty smelling
- Smelling strange odors
- Other sensory problems

Physical Symptoms

- Headaches
- Dizziness
- Nausea or vomiting
- Urinary incontinence
- Loss of bowel control
- Excessive tiredness
- Sensitivity to bright lights
- Sensitivity to loud noises
- Other physical problems

Mood/Emotion Symptoms

- Sadness or depression
- Anxiety or nervousness
- Stress
- Sleeping problems (such as falling asleep, staying asleep)
- Become angry more easily
- Euphoria (feeling on top of the world)
- Much more emotional (for example, crying more easily)
- Feel as if I just don't care anymore

Behavior Symptoms

- Doing things automatically (without awareness)
- Less inhibited (to do things I would not do before)
- Difficulty being spontaneous
- Change in eating habits
- Change in interest in sex
- Loss of energy
- Increase of energy
- Experiencing nightmares on a daily/weekly basis

- Loss of sexual desire
- Increase in weight
- Loss of weight
- Lack of interest in pleasurable activities
- Increase in irritability
- Increase in aggression
- Other recent changes in behavior or personality

Section 4.2

Headache

Excerpted from "Headache: Hope through Research,"
National Institute of Neurological Disorders and Stroke (NINDS),
NIH Publication No. 09–158, updated December 21, 2009.

Anyone can experience a headache. Nearly two out of three children will have a headache by age 15. More than nine in ten adults will experience a headache sometime in their life. Headache is our most common form of pain and a major reason cited for days missed at work or school as well as visits to the doctor. Without proper treatment, headaches can be severe and interfere with daily activities. Certain types of headache run in families. Episodes of headache may ease or even disappear for a time and recur later in life. It's possible to have more than one type of headache at the same time.

Primary headaches occur independently and are not caused by another medical condition. It's uncertain what sets the process of a primary headache in motion. Migraine, cluster, and tension-type headache are the more familiar types of primary headache.

Secondary headaches are symptoms of another health disorder that causes pain-sensitive nerve endings to be pressed on or pulled or pushed out of place. They may result from underlying conditions including fever, infection, medication overuse, stress or emotional conflict, high blood pressure, psychiatric disorders, head injury or trauma, stroke, tumors, and nerve disorders (particularly trigeminal neuralgia, a chronic pain condition that typically affects a major nerve on one side of the jaw or cheek).

When to See a Doctor

Not all headaches require a physician's attention. But headaches can signal a more serious disorder that requires prompt medical care. Immediately call or see a physician if you or someone you're with experience any of these symptoms:

- Sudden, severe headache that may be accompanied by a stiff neck

- Severe headache accompanied by fever, nausea, or vomiting that is not related to another illness

- First or worst headache, often accompanied by confusion, weakness, double vision, or loss of consciousness

- Headache that worsens over days or weeks or has changed in pattern or behavior

- Recurring headache in children

- Headache following a head injury

- Headache and a loss of sensation or weakness in any part of the body, which could be a sign of a stroke

- Headache associated with convulsions

- Headache associated with shortness of breath

- Two or more headaches a week

- Persistent headache in someone who has been previously headache-free, particularly in someone over age 50

- New headaches in someone with a history of cancer or human immunodeficiency virus/acquired immunodeficiency syndrome (HIV/AIDS)

Primary Headache Disorders

Primary headache disorders are divided into four main groups: migraine, tension-type headache, trigeminal autonomic cephalgias (a group of short-lasting but severe headaches), and a miscellaneous group.

Migraine headaches: One form of vascular headaches characterized by throbbing and pulsating pain caused by the activation of nerve fibers that reside within the wall of brain blood vessels traveling within the meninges. Migraines involve recurrent attacks of moderate to severe pain that is throbbing or pulsing and often strikes one side of the head. Untreated attacks last from 4–72 hours. Other common symptoms are increased sensitivity to light, noise, and odors; and nausea and vomiting. Many people feel exhausted or weak following a migraine but are usually symptom-free between attacks.

Tension-type headache: Previously called muscle contraction headache, tension-type headache is the most common type of headache. The pain is usually mild to moderate and feels as if constant pressure is being applied to the front of the face or to the head or neck. It also may feel as if a belt is being tightened around the head. Most often the pain is felt on both sides of the head.

Trigeminal autonomic cephalgias: Some primary headaches are characterized by severe pain in or around the eye on one side of the face and autonomic (or involuntary) features on the same side, such as red and teary eye, drooping eyelid, and runny nose. These disorders, called trigeminal autonomic cephalgias (cephalgia meaning head pain), differ in attack duration and frequency, and have episodic and chronic forms.

Cluster headache: The most severe form of primary headache—involves sudden, extremely painful headaches that occur in clusters, usually at the same time of the day and night for several weeks. They strike one side of the head, often behind or around one eye, and may be preceded by a migraine-like aura and nausea.

Paroxysmal hemicrania is a rare form of primary headache that usually begins in adulthood. Pain and related symptoms may be similar to those felt in cluster headaches, but with shorter duration. Attacks typically occur 5–40 times per day, with each attack lasting 2–45 minutes. Severe throbbing, claw-like, or piercing pain is felt on one side of the face-in, around, or behind the eye and occasionally reaching to the back of the neck.

Short-lasting, **u**nilateral, **n**euralgiform headache attack with **c**onjunctival injection and **t**earing (**SUNCT**): A very rare type of headache with bursts of moderate to severe burning, piercing, or throbbing pain that is usually felt in the forehead, eye, or temple on one side of the head.

Miscellaneous primary headaches that are not caused by other disorders include: Chronic daily headache, primary stabbing headache, primary exertional headache, and hypnic headache.

Secondary Headache Disorders

Secondary headache disorders are caused by an underlying illness or condition that affects the brain. Secondary headaches are usually diagnosed based on other symptoms that occur concurrently and the characteristics of the headaches. Some of the more serious causes of secondary headache include the following:

Brain tumor: A tumor that is growing in the brain can press against nerve tissue and pain-sensitive blood vessel walls, disrupting communication between the brain and the nerves or restricting the supply of blood to the brain.

Disorders of blood vessels in the brain, including stroke: Several disorders associated with blood vessel formation and activity can cause headache. Most notable among these conditions is stroke. Headache itself can cause stroke or accompany a series of blood vessel disorders that can cause a stroke.

- Hemorrhagic stroke: Occurs when an artery in the brain bursts, spilling blood into the surrounding tissue. A hemorrhagic stroke is usually associated with disturbed brain function and an extremely painful headache that develops suddenly and may worsen with physical activity, coughing, or straining.

- Ischemic stroke: Occurs when an artery supplying the brain with blood becomes blocked, suddenly decreasing or stopping blood flow and causing brain cells to die. Headache that accompanies ischemic stroke can be caused by several problems with the brain's vascular system. Headache is prominent in individuals with clots in the brain's veins. Head pain occurs on the side of the brain in which the clot blocks blood flow and is often felt in the eyes or on the side of the head.

Exposure to a substance or its withdrawal: Headaches may result from toxic states such as drinking alcohol, following carbon monoxide poisoning, or from exposure to toxic chemicals and metals, cleaning products or solvents, and pesticides. In the most severe cases, rising toxin levels can cause a pulsing, throbbing headache that, if left untreated, can lead to systemic poisoning, organ failure, and permanent neurological damage. The withdrawal from certain medicines or caffeine after frequent or excessive use can also cause headaches.

Head injury: Headaches are often a symptom of a concussion or other head injury. The headache may develop either immediately or months after a blow to the head, with pain felt at the injury site or throughout the head. Emotional disturbances may worsen headache pain. In most cases, the cause of post-traumatic headache is unknown. Subdural hematoma may occur after head trauma but also occurs spontaneously in elderly persons or in individuals taking anticoagulant medications.

Increased intracranial pressure: A growing tumor, infection, or hydrocephalus (an extensive build up of cerebrospinal fluid in the brain) can raise pressure in the brain and compress nerves and blood vessels, causing headaches. Headache attributed to idiopathic intracranial hypertension, previously known as pseudotumor cerebri (meaning false brain tumor), is associated with severe headache.

Inflammation from meningitis, encephalitis, and other infections: Inflammation from infections can harm or destroy nerve cells and cause dull to severe headache pain, brain damage, or stroke, among other conditions. Inflammation of the brain and spinal cord (meningitis and encephalitis) requires urgent medical attention Headaches may also occur with a fever or a flu-like infection. A headache may accompany a bacterial infection of the upper respiratory tract that spreads to and inflames the lining of the sinus cavities.

Seizures: Migraine-like headache pain may occur during or after a seizure. Moderate to severe headache pain may last for several hours and worsen with sudden movements of the head or when sneezing, coughing, or bending.

Spinal fluid leak: About one-fourth of people who undergo a lumbar puncture (which involves a small sampling of the spinal fluid being removed for testing) develop a headache due to a leak of cerebrospinal fluid following the procedure.

Structural abnormalities of the head, neck and spine: Headache pain and loss of function may be triggered by structural abnormalities in the head or spine, restricted blood flow through the neck, irritation to nerves anywhere along the path from the spinal cord to the brain, or stressful or awkward positions of the head and neck.

Trigeminal neuralgia: The trigeminal nerve conducts sensations to the brain from the upper, middle, and lower portions of the face, as well as inside the mouth. The presumed cause of trigeminal neuralgia is a blood vessel pressing on the nerve as it exits the brain stem, but other causes have been described. Symptoms include headache and intense shock-like or stabbing pain that comes on suddenly and is typically felt on one side of the jaw or cheek. Muscle spasms may occur on the affected side of the face.

Section 4.3

Memory Loss (Amnesia)

Definition: Memory loss (amnesia) is unusual forgetfulness.

Considerations: The cause determines whether amnesia comes on slowly or suddenly, and whether it is temporary or permanent. Normal aging may lead to trouble learning new material or requiring a longer time to remember learned material. However, it does not lead to dramatic memory loss unless diseases are involved.

Causes

- Aging
- Alcoholism
- Alzheimer disease
- Brain damage due to disease or injury
- Brain growths (caused by tumors or infection)
- Brain infections such as Lyme disease or syphilis

- Depression or emotional trauma
- Drugs such as barbiturates or benzodiazepines
- Electroconvulsive therapy (especially if it is long-term)
- Encephalitis of any type (herpes, West Nile, Eastern Equine)
- General anesthetics such as halothane, isoflurane, and fentanyl
- Head trauma or injury
- Hysteria, often accompanied by confusion
- Illness that results in the loss of nerve cells (neurodegenerative illness)
- Nutritional problems (vitamin deficiencies such as low vitamin B12)
- Seizures
- Stroke or transient ischemic attack (TIA)
- Transient global amnesia
- Temporal lobe brain surgery

Home Care

The family should provide support. Reality orientation is recommended—supply familiar music, objects, or photos, to help the person stay oriented. Some people may need support to help them relearn.

Any medication schedules should be written down so the person does not have to rely on memory.

Extended care facilities, such as nursing homes, should be considered for people whose basic needs cannot be met in any other way, or whose safety or nutrition is in jeopardy.

When to Contact a Medical Professional

Call your health care provider if you have any unexplained memory loss.

What to Expect at Your Office Visit

The doctor will perform a thorough examination and take a medical history. This may require asking questions of family members and friends.

Medical history questions may include:

Type

- Can the person remember recent events? (Is there impaired short-term memory?)

- Can the person remember events from further in the past? (Is there impaired long-term memory?)

- Is there a loss of memory about events that occurred before a specific experience (anterograde amnesia)?

- Is there a loss of memory about events that occurred soon after a specific experience (retrograde amnesia)?

- Is there only a minimal loss of memory?

- Does the person make up stories to cover gaps in memory (confabulation)?

- Is the person suffering from low moods that impair concentration?

Time Pattern

- Has the memory loss been getting worse over years?

- Has the memory loss been developing over weeks or months?

- Is the memory loss present all the time or are there distinct episodes of amnesia?

- If there are amnesia episodes, how long do they last?

Aggravating or Triggering Factors

- Has there been a head injury in the recent past?

- Has the person experienced an event that was emotionally traumatic?

- Has there been a surgery or procedure requiring general anesthesia?

- Does the person use alcohol? How much?

- Does the person use illegal or illicit drugs? How much? What type?

Other Symptoms

- What other symptoms does the person have?

- Is the person confused or disoriented?
- Can they independently eat, dress, and perform similar self-care activities?
- Have they had seizures?

The physical examination will include a detailed test of thinking and memory (mental status test), and an exams of the nervous system. Recent, intermediate, and long-term memory will be tested.

Diagnostic tests that may be performed include the following:

- Blood tests for specific diseases that are suspected (such as low vitamin B12 or thyroid disease)
- Cerebral angiography
- Cognitive tests (psychometric tests)
- Computed tomography (CT) scan or magnetic resonance imaging (MRI) of the head
- Electroencephalogram (EEG)
- Lumbar puncture

Reference

Knopman DS. *Regional cerebral dysfunction: higher mental functions.* In: Goldman L, Ausiello D, eds. Cecil Medicine. 23rd ed. Philadelphia, Pa: Saunders Elsevier; 2007: chap 424.

Chapter 5

Neurological Emergencies

Chapter Contents

Section 5.1

Brain Attack: Know the Signs, Act in Time

Excerpted from "Know Stroke. Know the Signs. Act in Time."
National Institute of Neurological Disorders and Stroke (NINDS),
NIH Publication No. 08–4872, updated December 18, 2009.

Know Stroke

Stroke is the third leading cause of death in the United States and a leading cause of serious, long-term disability in adults. About 600,000 new strokes are reported in the U.S. each year. The good news is that treatments are available that can greatly reduce the damage caused by a stroke. However, you need to recognize the symptoms of a stroke and get to a hospital quickly. Getting treatment within 60 minutes can prevent disability.

A stroke, sometimes called a brain attack, occurs when blood flow to the brain is interrupted. When a stroke occurs, brain cells in the immediate area begin to die because they stop getting the oxygen and nutrients they need to function.

Although stroke is a disease of the brain, it can affect the entire body. The effects of a stroke range from mild to severe and can include paralysis, problems with thinking, problems with speaking, and emotional problems. Patients may also experience pain or numbness after a stroke.

Know the Signs

Because stroke injures the brain, you may not realize that you are having a stroke. To a bystander, someone having a stroke may just look unaware or confused. Stroke victims have the best chance if someone around them recognizes the symptoms and acts quickly.

The symptoms of stroke are distinct because they happen quickly:

- Sudden numbness or weakness of the face, arm, or leg (especially on one side of the body)

- Sudden confusion, trouble speaking or understanding speech

- Sudden trouble seeing in one or both eyes
- Sudden trouble walking, dizziness, loss of balance or coordination
- Sudden severe headache with no known cause

If you believe someone is having a stroke—if he or she suddenly loses the ability to speak, or move an arm or leg on one side, or experiences facial paralysis on one side—call 911 immediately.

Act in Time

Stroke is a medical emergency. Every minute counts when someone is having a stroke. The longer blood flow is cut off to the brain, the greater the damage. Immediate treatment can save people's lives and enhance their chances for successful recovery.

Ischemic strokes, the most common type of strokes, can be treated with a drug called t-PA, that dissolves blood clots obstructing blood flow to the brain. The window of opportunity to start treating stroke patients is three hours, but to be evaluated and receive treatment, patients need to get to the hospital within 60 minutes.

A five-year study by the National Institute of Neurological Disorders and Stroke (NINDS) found that some stroke patients who received t-PA within three hours of the start of stroke symptoms were at least 30% more likely to recover with little or no disability after three months.

The best treatment for stroke is prevention. There are several risk factors that increase your chances of having a stroke including high blood pressure, heart disease, smoking, diabetes, and high cholesterol. If you smoke—quit. If you have high blood pressure, heart disease, diabetes, or high cholesterol, getting them under control—and keeping them under control—will greatly reduce your chances of having a stroke.

Section 5.2

Brain Herniation

"Brain Herniation,"
© 2009 A.D.A.M., Inc. Reprinted with permission.

Alternative names: Herniation syndrome; transtentorial herniation; uncal herniation; subfalcine herniation; tonsillar herniation, herniation–brain

Definition: A brain herniation is when brain tissue, cerebrospinal fluid, and blood vessels are moved or pressed away from their usual position in the head.

Causes

A brain herniation occurs when something inside the skull produces pressure that moves brain tissues. This is most often the result of brain swelling from a head injury. Brain herniations are the most common side effect of tumors in the brain, including metastatic brain tumor and primary brain tumor. A brain herniation can also be caused by abscess, hemorrhage, hydrocephalus, or strokes that cause brain swelling. A brain herniation can occur between areas inside the skull, such as those separated by a rigid membrane called the tentorium; through a natural opening at the base of the skull called the foramen magnum; or through openings created during brain surgery.

Symptoms

- Cardiac arrest (no pulse)
- Coma
- Irregular breathing
- Irregular pulse
- Loss of all brainstem reflexes (blinking, gagging, pupils reacting to light)

- Progressive loss of consciousness
- Respiratory arrest (no breathing)

Exams and Tests

A neurological exam shows changes in alertness (consciousness). Depending on the severity of the herniation, there will be problems with one or more brain-related reflexes and cranial nerve functions. Patients with a brain herniation have irregular heart rhythms and difficulty breathing consistently.

Treatment

Brain herniation is a medical emergency. The goal of treatment is to save the patient's life. To help reverse or prevent a brain herniation, the medical team will treat increased swelling and pressure in the brain. Treatment may involve the following:

- Placing a drain placed into the brain to help remove fluid
- Corticosteroids such as dexamethasone, especially if there is a brain tumor
- Medications that remove fluid from the body such as mannitol or other diuretics, which reduce pressure inside the skull
- Placing a tube in the airway (endotracheal intubation) and increasing the breathing rate to reduce the levels of carbon dioxide (CO_2) in the blood
- Removing the blood if bleeding is causing herniation

Outlook (Prognosis)

The outlook varies and depends on where in the brain the herniation occurred. Death is possible. A brain herniation itself often causes massive stroke. There can be damage to parts of the brain that control breathing and blood flow. This can rapidly lead to death or brain death. Possible complications include brain death or permanent and significant neurologic problems.

When to contact a medical professional: Call your local emergency number (such as 911) or take the patient to a hospital emergency room if decreased alertness or other symptoms suddenly develop, especially if there has been a head injury or if the person has a brain tumor or blood-vessel malformation.

Prevention: Prompt treatment of increased intracranial pressure and related disorders may reduce the risk of brain herniation.

Reference

Nkwuo N, Schamban N, Borenstein M. Selected Oncologic Emergencies. In: Marx, JA, ed. *Rosen's Emergency Medicine: Concepts and Clinical Practice.* 6th ed. Philadelphia, Pa: Mosby Elsevier; 2006: chap 121.

Section 5.3

Cerebral Hypoxia

"Cerebral Hypoxia,"
© 2009 A.D.A.M., Inc. Reprinted with permission.

Alternative name: Hypoxic encephalopathy

Definition: Cerebral hypoxia technically means a lack of oxygen supply to the outer part of the brain, an area called the cerebral hemisphere. However, the term is more typically used to refer to a lack of oxygen supply to the entire brain.

Causes

There are many causes of cerebral hypoxia. These include, but are not limited to the following:

- Asphyxiation caused by smoke inhalation
- Carbon monoxide poisoning
- Cardiac arrest (when the heart stops pumping)
- Choking
- Complications of general anesthesia

- Compression of the windpipe (trachea)
- Diseases that cause a loss of movement (paralysis) of the breathing muscles
- Drowning
- Drug overdose
- High altitudes
- Injuries before, during, or soon after, birth
- Strangulation
- Stroke
- Very low blood pressure

Brain cells are extremely sensitive to oxygen deprivation. Some brain cells actually start dying less than five minutes after their oxygen supply disappears. As a result, brain hypoxia can rapidly cause death or severe brain damage.

Symptoms

Symptoms of mild cerebral hypoxia include change in attention (inattentiveness), poor judgment, and uncoordinated movement.

Symptoms of severe cerebral hypoxia include complete unawareness and unresponsiveness (coma), no breathing, and no response to light. If only blood pressure and heart function remain, then the brain may actually be completely dead.

Exams and Tests

Cerebral hypoxia can usually be diagnosed based on the person's medical history and a physical exam. Tests are done to determine the cause of the hypoxia, and may include the following:

- Blood work, including arterial blood gases and blood sugar level
- Echocardiogram
- Electrocardiogram (ECG), a measurement of the heart's electrical activity
- Electroencephalogram (EEG), a test of brain waves that can identify seizures and show how well brain cells work

- Evoked potentials, a test that determines whether certain sensations such as vision and touch reach the brain

- Magnetic resonance imaging (MRI)

Treatment

Cerebral hypoxia is an emergency condition that requires immediate treatment. The sooner the oxygen supply is restored to the brain, the lower the risk of severe brain damage and death.

Treatment depends on the underlying cause of the hypoxia. Basic life support is most important. Treatment involves:

- breathing assistance (mechanical ventilation);

- controlling the heart rate;

- fluids, blood products, or medications to control blood pressure; and

- medications including phenytoin, phenobarbital, valproic acid, and general anesthetics to calm seizures.

Sometimes cooling the person with cold blankets is used, because cooling slows down the activity of the brain cells and decreases their need for oxygen. However, the benefit of such treatment has not been firmly established.

Outlook (Prognosis)

The outlook depends on the extent of the brain injury, which is determined by how long the brain lacked oxygen. If the brain lacked oxygen for only a very brief period of time, a coma may be reversible and the person may have some return of function. However, this depends on the extent of injury. Some patients recover many functions, but have abnormal movements such as twitching or jerking. Seizures may sometimes occur, and may be continuous (status epilepticus).

Most people who make a full recovery were only briefly unconscious. The longer the person is unconscious, the higher the risk for death or brain death, and the lower the chances for a meaningful recovery.

Possible Complications

Complications of cerebral hypoxia include prolonged vegetative state—basic life functions such as breathing, blood pressure, sleep-wake cycle, and eye opening may be preserved, but the person is not alert and does not respond to their surroundings. Such patients usually die within a year, although some may survive longer.

Length of survival depends partly on how much care is taken to prevent other problems. Major complications may include bed sores, clots in the veins (deep vein thrombosis), improper nutrition, and lung infections (pneumonia).

When to contact a medical professional: Cerebral hypoxia is a medical emergency. Call 911 immediately if someone is losing consciousness or has other symptoms of cerebral hypoxia.

Prevention: Prevention depends on the specific cause of hypoxia. Unfortunately, hypoxia is usually unexpected. This makes the condition somewhat difficult to prevent. Cardiopulmonary resuscitation (CPR) can be lifesaving, especially when it is started right away.

Section 5.4

Subarachnoid Hemorrhage

"Subarachnoid Hemorrhage,"
© 2009 A.D.A.M., Inc. Reprinted with permission.

Definition: Subarachnoid hemorrhage (SAH) is bleeding in the area between the brain and the thin tissues that cover the brain. This area is called the subarachnoid space.

Causes

Subarachnoid hemorrhage can be caused by:

- bleeding from an arteriovenous malformation (AVM),
- bleeding disorder,
- bleeding from a cerebral aneurysm,
- head injury,

- unknown cause (idiopathic), and

- use of blood thinners.

Injury-related subarachnoid hemorrhage is often seen in the elderly who have fallen and hit their head. Among the young, the most common injury leading to subarachnoid hemorrhage is motor vehicle crashes.

Subarachnoid hemorrhage due to rupture of a cerebral aneurysm occurs in approximately 10–15 out of 10,000 people. Subarachnoid hemorrhage due to rupture of a cerebral aneurysm is most common in persons age 20 to 60. It is slightly more common in women than men.

Risks include:

- aneurysms in other blood vessels,

- fibromuscular dysplasia (FMD) and other connective tissue disorders associated with aneurysm or weakened blood vessels,

- high blood pressure,

- history of polycystic kidney disease, and

- smoking.

A strong family history of aneurysms may also increase your risk.

Symptoms

The main symptom is a severe headache that starts suddenly and is often worse near the back of the head. Patients often describe it as the worst headache ever and unlike any other type of headache pain. The headache may start after a popping or snapping feeling in the head.

Other symptoms are:

- sudden or decreased consciousness and alertness;

- difficulty or loss of movement or feeling;

- mood and personality changes, including confusion and irritability;

- muscle aches (especially neck pain and shoulder pain);

- nausea and vomiting;

- photophobia (light bothers or hurts the eyes);

- seizure;

- stiff neck; and

- vision problems, including double vision, blind spots, or temporary vision loss in one eye.

Additional symptoms that may be associated with this disease are:

- eyelid drooping;

- eyes, pupils different size;

- sudden stiffening of back and neck, with arching of the back (Opisthotonos; not very common); and

- seizures.

Exams and Tests

A physical exam may show a stiff neck due to irritation by blood of the meninges, the tissues that cover the brain. Except those in a deep coma, persons with a subarachnoid hemorrhage may resist neck movement.

A neurological exam may show signs of decreased nerve and brain function (focal neurologic deficit).

An eye exam will be performed. Decreased eye movements can be a sign of damage to the cranial nerves. In milder cases, no problems may be seen on an eye exam.

If your doctor thinks you may have a subarachnoid hemorrhage, a head computed tomography (CT) scan (without dye contrast) should be immediately done. In some cases, the scan may be normal, especially if there has only been a small bleed. If the CT scan is normal, a lumbar puncture (spinal tap) must be performed. Patients with SAH will have blood in their spinal fluid.

CT scan angiography (using contrast dye) may be done to look for evidence of an aneurism.

Cerebral angiography of blood vessels of the brain is better than CT angiography to show small aneurysms or other vascular problems. This test can pinpoint the exact location of the bleed and can tell if there are blood vessel spasms.

Transcranial Doppler ultrasound is used to look at blood flow in the arteries of the brain that run inside the skull. The ultrasound beam is directed through the skull. It can also detect blood vessel spasms and may be used to guide treatment.

Magnetic resonance imaging (MRI) and magnetic resonance angiography (MRA) are occasionally used to diagnose a subarachnoid hemorrhage or find other associated conditions.

Treatment

The goals of treatment are to save your life, repair the cause of bleeding, relieve symptoms, and prevent complications such as permanent brain damage (stroke).

If the hemorrhage is due to an injury, surgery is done only to remove large collections of blood or to relieve pressure on the brain. If the hemorrhage is due to the rupture of an aneurysm, surgery is needed to repair the aneurysm. If the patient is critically ill, surgery may have to wait until the person is more stable. Surgery may involve a craniotomy (cutting a hole in the skull) and aneurysm clipping, which closes the aneurysm, or endovascular coiling, a procedure in which coils are placed within the aneurysm to reduce the risk of further bleeding. If no aneurysm is found, the person should be closely watched by a health care team and may need repeated imaging tests.

Treatment for coma or decreased alertness status may be needed. This may include special positioning, life support, and methods to protect the airway. A draining tube may be placed into the brain to relieve pressure.

If the person is conscious, strict bed rest may be advised. The person will be told to avoid activities that can increase pressure inside the head. Such activities include bending over, straining, and suddenly changing position. The doctor may prescribe stool softeners or laxatives to prevent straining during bowel movements. Blood pressure will be strictly controlled. This requires medicines given through an intervenous (IV) line. The medicine often requires frequent adjustments. A medicine called calcium channel blocker is used to prevent blood vessel spams. Pain killers and anti-anxiety medications may be used to relieve headache and reduce intracranial pressure. Phenytoin or other medications may be used to prevent or treat seizures.

Outlook (Prognosis)

How well a patient with subarachnoid hemorrhage does depends on a number of different factors, including the location and extent of the bleeding, as well as any complications. Older age and more severe symptoms from the beginning are associated with a poorer prognosis. Complete recovery can occur after treatment, but death may occur in some cases even with aggressive treatment.

Possible complications: Repeated bleeding is the most serious complication. If a cerebral aneurysm bleeds for a second time, the outlook is significantly worsened. Changes in consciousness and alertness due to a subarachnoid hemorrhage may become worse and lead to coma or death. Other complications include stroke, seizures, medication side effects, and complications of surgery.

When to contact a medical professional: Go to the emergency room or call the local emergency number (such as 911) if you have symptoms of a subarachnoid hemorrhage.

Prevention: Identification and successful treatment of an aneurysm would prevent subarachnoid hemorrhage.

Reference

Zivin J. Hemorrhagic cerebrovascular disease. In: Goldman L, Ausiello D, eds. *Cecil Medicine. 23rd ed.* Philadelphia, Pa: Saunders Elsevier; 2007:chap 432.

Section 5.5

First Aid for Seizures

Centers for Disease Control and Prevention (CDC), March 20, 2009.

First aid for seizures involves responding in ways that can keep the person safe until the seizure stops by itself. Here are a few things you can do to help someone who is having a generalized tonic-clonic (grand mal) seizure:

- Keep calm and reassure other people who may be nearby.

- Prevent injury by clearing the area around the person of anything hard or sharp.

- Ease the person to the floor and put something soft and flat, like a folded jacket, under his head.

- Remove eyeglasses and loosen ties or anything around the neck that may make breathing difficult.

- Time the seizure with your watch. If the seizure continues for longer than five minutes without signs of slowing down or if a person has trouble breathing afterwards, appears to be injured, in pain, or recovery is unusual in some way, call 911.

- Do not hold the person down or try to stop his movements.

- Contrary to popular belief, it is not true that a person having a seizure can swallow his tongue. Do not put anything in the person's mouth. Efforts to hold the tongue down can injure the teeth or jaw.

- Turn the person gently onto one side. This will help keep the airway clear.

- Don't attempt artificial respiration except in the unlikely event that a person does not start breathing again after the seizure has stopped.

- Stay with the person until the seizure ends naturally and he is fully awake.

- Do not offer the person water or food until fully alert.

- Be friendly and reassuring as consciousness returns.

- Offer to call a taxi, friend, or relative to help the person get home if he seems confused or unable to get home without help.

Here are a few things you can do to help someone who is having a seizure that appears as blank staring, loss of awareness, and/or involuntary blinking, chewing, or other facial movements.

- Stay calm and speak reassuringly.

- Guide him away from dangers.

- Block access to hazards, but don't restrain the person.

- If he is agitated, stay a distance away, but close enough to protect him until full awareness has returned.

Consider a seizure an emergency and call 911 if any of the following occurs:

- The seizure lasts longer than five minutes without signs of slowing down or if a person has trouble breathing afterwards, appears to be in pain, or recovery is unusual in some way.

- The person has another seizure soon after the first one.

- The person cannot be awakened after the seizure activity has stopped.
- The person became injured during the seizure.
- The person becomes aggressive.
- The seizure occurs in water.
- The person has a health condition like diabetes or heart disease or is pregnant.

Section 5.6

Delirium (Acute Onset Cognitive Changes)

"Delirium," © 2009 A.D.A.M., Inc. Reprinted with permission.

Alternative names: Acute confusional state, acute brain syndrome

Definition: Delirium is sudden severe confusion and rapid changes in brain function that occur with physical or mental illness.

Causes

Delirium is most often caused by physical or mental illness and is usually temporary and reversible. Many disorders cause delirium, including conditions that deprive the brain of oxygen or other substances. Causes include drug abuse; infections such as urinary tract infections or pneumonia (in people who already have brain damage from stroke or dementia); poisons; and, fluid/electrolyte or acid/base disturbances. Patients with more severe brain injuries are more likely to get delirium from another illness.

Symptoms

Delirium involves a quick change between mental states (for example, from lethargy to agitation and back to lethargy).

Symptoms include the following:

- Changes in alertness (usually more alert in the morning, less alert at night)

- Changes in feeling (sensation) and perception

- Changes in level of consciousness or awareness

- Changes in movement (for example, may be inactive or slow moving)

- Changes in sleep patterns, drowsiness

- Confusion (disorientation) about time or place

- Decrease in short-term memory and recall (for example, being unable to remember events since delirium began [anterograde amnesia], or unable to remember past events [retrograde amnesia])

- Disrupted or wandering attention (for example, inability to think or behave with purpose, or problems concentrating)

- Disorganized thinking (speech that doesn't make sense [incoherent], or inability to stop speech patterns or behaviors)

- Emotional or personality changes (anger, anxiety, apathy, depression, euphoria, irritability)

- Movements triggered by changes in the nervous system (psychomotor restlessness)

Exams and Tests

The following tests may have abnormal results:

- An exam of the nervous system (neurologic examination)

- Psychologic studies

- Tests of feeling (sensation), thinking (cognitive function), and motor function

The following tests may also be done:

- Ammonia levels

- B12 level

- Blood chemistry (chem-20)

- Blood gas analysis

- Chest x-ray

- Cerebrospinal fluid (CSF) analysis

- Creatine phosphokinase (CPK) level

- Drug, alcohol levels (toxicology screen)

- Electroencephalogram (EEG)

- Glucose test

- Head computed tomography (CT) scan

- Head magnetic resonance imaging (MRI) scan

- Liver function tests

- Mental status test

- Serum calcium

- Serum electrolytes

- Serum magnesium

- Thyroid function tests

- Thyroid stimulating hormone level

- Urinalysis

Treatment

The goal of treatment is to control or reverse the cause of the symptoms. Treatment depends on the condition causing delirium. Diagnosis and care should take place in a pleasant, comfortable, nonthreatening, physically safe environment. The person may need to stay in the hospital for a short time.

Stopping or changing medications that worsen confusion, or that are not necessary, may improve mental function. Medications that may worsen confusion include:

- alcohol and illegal drugs,

- analgesics,

- anticholinergics,

- central nervous system depressants,

- cimetidine, and

- lidocaine.

Disorders that contribute to confusion should be treated. These may include:

- heart failure,

- decreased oxygen (hypoxia),

- high carbon dioxide levels (hypercapnia),

- thyroid disorders,

- anemia,

- nutritional disorders,

- infections,

- kidney failure,

- liver failure, and

- psychiatric conditions (such as depression).

Treating medical and mental disorders often greatly improves mental function. Medications may be needed to control aggressive or agitated behaviors. These are usually started at very low doses and adjusted as needed.

Medications include:

- dopamine blockers (haloperidol, olanzapine, risperidone, clozapine),

- mood stabilizers (fluoxetine, imipramine, citalopram),

- sedating medications (clonazepam or diazepam),

- serotonin-affecting drugs (trazodone, buspirone), and

- thiamine.

Some people with delirium may benefit from hearing aids, glasses, or cataract surgery. Other treatments that may be helpful are behavior modification to control unacceptable or dangerous behaviors, or reality orientation to reduce disorientation.

Outlook (Prognosis)

Acute conditions that cause delirium may occur with chronic disorders that cause dementia. Acute brain syndromes may be reversible by treating the cause. Delirium often lasts only about one week, although it may take several weeks for mental function to return to normal levels. Full recovery is common.

Possible complications include:

- loss of ability to function or care for self,

- loss of ability to interact,

- progression to stupor or coma, and

- side effects of medications used to treat the disorder.

When to contact a medical professional: Call your health care provider if there is a rapid change in mental status.

Prevention: Treating the conditions that cause delirium can reduce its risk.

Chapter 6

Impaired Consciousness

Chapter Contents

Section 6.1

Coma

"What Is Coma?" October 2008, reprinted with permission from www. kidshealth.org. Copyright © 2008 The Nemours Foundation. This information was provided by KidsHealth, one of the largest resources online for medically reviewed health information written for parents, kids, and teens. For more articles like this one, visit www.KidsHealth.org or www. TeensHealth.org.

What is a coma?

What do you think about when you hear the word coma (say: ko-muh)? Does it make you think of someone in a deep sleep, or the way you feel after eating too much Thanksgiving turkey? Does the word remind you of a television (TV) soap opera, where it seems that at least one character is always in a coma?

A coma can be difficult to understand, especially because people sometimes jokingly use the words coma and comatose (say: ko-muh-tose, which means in a coma or coma-like state) to describe people who aren't paying attention or who are drowsy or sleeping. But a coma is a serious condition that has nothing to do with sleep.

What happens when someone is in a coma?

Someone who is in a coma is unconscious and will not respond to voices, other sounds, or any sort of activity going on nearby. The person is still alive, but the brain is functioning at its lowest stage of alertness. You can't shake and wake up someone who is in a coma like you can someone who has just fallen asleep.

What can cause a coma?

Comas can be caused by different things, including:

- a severe injury to the head that hurts the brain,
- seizures,
- infections involving the brain,

- brain damage caused by a lack of oxygen for too long,

- an overdose (taking too much) of medicine or other drugs,

- a stroke.

When one of these things happens, it can mess up how the brain's cells work. This can hurt the parts of the brain that make someone conscious, and if those parts stop working, the person will stay unconscious.

How do people take care of someone in a coma?

Someone in a coma usually needs to be cared for in the intensive care unit (ICU) of the hospital. There, the person can get extra care and attention from doctors, nurses, and other hospital staff. They make sure the person gets fluids, nutrients, and any medicines needed to keep the body as healthy as possible. These are sometimes given through a tiny plastic tube inserted in a vein or through a feeding tube that brings fluids and nutrients directly to the stomach.

Some comatose people are unable to breathe on their own and need the help of a ventilator (say: ven-tih-lay-ter), a machine that pumps air into the lungs through a tube placed in the windpipe. The hospital staff also tries to prevent bedsores in someone who is comatose. Bedsores are open sores on the body that come from lying in one place for too long without moving at all.

It can be very upsetting and frustrating for a person's family to see someone they love in a coma, and they may feel scared and helpless. But they can help take care of the person. Taking time to visit the hospital and read to, talk to, and even play music for the patient are important because it's possible that the person may be able to hear what's going on, even if he or she can't respond.

What happens after a coma?

Usually, a coma does not last more than a few weeks. Sometimes, however, a person stays in a coma for a long time—even years—and will be able to do very little except breathe on his or her own.

Most people do come out of comas, however. Some of them are able to return to the normal lives they had before they got sick. On TV, someone in a coma usually wakes up right away, looks around, and is able to think and talk normally. But in real life, this rarely happens. When coming out of a coma, a person will often be confused and can only slowly respond to what's going on. It will take time for the person to start feeling better.

Whether someone fully returns to normal after being in a coma depends on what caused the coma and how badly the brain may have been hurt. Sometimes people who come out of comas are just as they were before—they can remember what happened to them before the coma and can do everything they used to do. Other people may need therapy to relearn basic things like tying their shoes, eating with a fork or spoon, or learning to walk all over again. They may also have problems with speaking or remembering things.

Over time and with the help of therapists, however, many people who have been in a coma can make a lot of progress. They may not be exactly like they were before the coma, but they can do a lot of things and enjoy life with their family and friends.

Section 6.2

Facts about the Vegetative and Minimally Conscious States

Sherer M, Vaccaro M, Whyte J, Giacino JT, and the Consciousness Consortium. *Facts about the Vegetative and Minimally Conscious States after Severe Brain Injury 2007*. Houston: The Consciousness Consortium. Reprinted with permission.

Severe brain injury causes a change in consciousness. Consciousness refers to awareness of the self and the environment. Brain injury can cause a wide range of disturbances of consciousness. Some injuries are mild and may cause relatively minor changes in consciousness such as brief confusion or disorientation.

The most severe injuries cause profound disturbance of consciousness. Twenty to 40% of persons with injuries this severe do not survive. Some persons who survive have a period of time of complete unconsciousness with no awareness of themselves or the world around them. The diagnosis given these people depends on whether their eyes are always closed or whether they have periods when their eyes are open. The state of complete unconsciousness with no eye opening is called coma. The state of complete unconsciousness with some eye opening and periods of wakefulness and sleep is called the vegetative state. As people recover from severe brain injury, they usually pass through various phases of recovery. Recovery can stop at any one of these phases.

Characteristics of Coma

1. No eye-opening.

2. Unable to follow instructions.

3. No speech or other forms of communication.

4. No purposeful movement.

Characteristics of the Vegetative State

1. Return of a sleep-wake cycle with periods of eye opening and eye closing.

2. May moan or make other sounds especially when tight muscles are stretched.

3. May cry or smile or make other facial expressions without apparent cause.

4. May briefly move eyes toward persons or objects.

5. May react to a loud sound with a startle.

6. Unable to follow instructions.

7. No speech or other forms of communication.

8. No purposeful movement.

Persons in coma or vegetative state require extensive care that may include:

1. Feeding using a feeding tube.

2. Turning in bed to prevent pressure sores.

3. Special bedding to help prevent pressure sores.

4. Assistance with bowel and bladder relief using catheter and/or diapers.

5. Management of breathing such as suctioning of secretions; this may include care for a tracheostomy tube.

6. Management of muscle tone (excessive tightness of muscles).

7. Special equipment that may include a wheelchair or special bedding to help with proper posture and decrease muscle tightness.

8. Management of infections such as pneumonia or urinary tract infections.

9. Management of other medical issues such as fever, seizures, and so forth.

What happens after coma and vegetative state?

When people start to regain consciousness, they may:

- follow simple instructions from others such as, "Open your eyes," "Squeeze my hand," "Say your name," and so forth;

- communicate by speaking words or by indicating yes or no by head nods or gestures; and/or

- use a common object in a normal way such as brushing hair with a brush, using a straw to drink, or holding a phone to the ear.

Persons with brain injury transition through the period of unconsciousness and subsequent stages of recovery at a slower or faster rate, largely depending on the severity of injury. Those with less severe injuries may transition through these stages more rapidly and some of the stages described here may be poorly recognized or not occur at all. Those with very severe injuries may stall at one or another stage and not be able to make the transition to a higher level of recovery.

For persons with more prolonged periods of unconsciousness, emergence from unconsciousness is a gradual process. Coma rarely lasts more than four weeks. Some patients move from coma to the vegetative state but others may move from coma to a period of partial consciousness. It would be very rare for a person to move directly from coma, or vegetative state, to a state of full consciousness.

Persons who have shorter periods of unconsciousness likely had less severe brain injuries initially. Consequently, they are likely to go on to make better recoveries than persons who had longer periods of unconsciousness.

Traumatic brain injury refers to damage to the brain caused by external force such as a car crash or a fall. About 50% of persons who are in a vegetative state one month after traumatic brain injury eventually recover consciousness. They are likely to have a slow course of recovery and usually have some ongoing cognitive and physical impairments and disabilities. People in a vegetative state due to stroke, loss of oxygen to the brain (anoxia), or some types of severe medical illness, may not recover as well as those with traumatic brain injury. Those few persons who remain in a prolonged vegetative state may survive for an extended period of time but they often experience medical complications such as pneumonia, respiratory failure, infections, and so forth which may reduce life expectancy.

People who have a slow recovery of consciousness continue to have a reduced level of self-awareness or awareness of the world around them. They have inconsistent and limited ability to respond and communicate. This condition of limited awareness is called the minimally conscious state.

Characteristics of the Minimally Conscious State

1. Sometimes follows simple instructions.

2. May communicate yes or no by talking or gesturing.

3. May speak some understandable words or phrases.

4. May respond to people, things, or other events by: crying, smiling, or laughing; making sounds or gesturing; reaching for objects; trying to hold or use an object; or, keeping the eyes focused on people or things for a sustained period of time whether they are moving or staying still.

People in a minimally conscious state do these things inconsistently. For example, one time the person might be able to follow a simple instruction and another time they might not be able to follow any instructions at all. This makes it difficult to distinguish the vegetative state from the minimally conscious state. While in a minimally conscious state, people need extensive care similar to that needed by people in a vegetative state.

Emergence from the Minimally Conscious State

Once a person can communicate, follow instructions, or use an object such as a comb or pencil consistently, they are no longer in a minimally conscious state. Some people remain minimally conscious indefinitely, but many improve. The longer a person remains in a minimally conscious state, the more permanent impairments he or she is likely to have. This is because vegetative and minimally conscious states are caused by severe damage to multiple brain areas. Following emergence from the minimally conscious state, people almost always experience confusion. Sometimes people move directly from coma to this confusional state.

Table 6.1. Comparison of Coma, Vegetative State, and Minimally Conscious State

	Coma	Vegetative State	Minimally Conscious State
Eye opening	No	Yes	Yes
Sleep/wake cycles	No	Yes	Yes
Visual tracking	No	No	Often
Object recognition	No	No	Inconsistent
Command following	No	No	Inconsistent
Communication	No	No	Inconsistent
Contingent emotion	No	No	Inconsistent

Characteristics of the Confusional State

1. Disorientation (inability to keep track of the correct date and place).

2. Severe impairment in attention, memory and other mental abilities.

3. Fluctuation in level of responsiveness.

4. Restlessness.

5. Nighttime sleep disturbance.

6. Excessive drowsiness and sleeping during the day.

7. Delusions or hallucinations.

As with the vegetative and minimally conscious states, the rate and extent of recovery from the confused state vary from person to person. However, almost all people who reach the confused state go on to make further progress. The main factors that determine the eventual degree of recovery are the initial severity of the brain injury and some types of additional medical problems. The shorter the time the person is in the confused state, the better the eventual recovery will be. Mild medical complications such as sleep disturbance or urinary tract infection may prolong the confused state but do not necessarily influence the final outcome.

Once the confusional state resolves, people are usually much better able to pay attention, orient themselves to place and time, and retain memories for day to day experiences. Nevertheless, they are very likely to have some significant cognitive problems such as impaired memory or slowed thinking. These cognitive problems are likely to continue to improve as time passes. Some people make limited progress, while others make a good deal of progress.

Patterns of Recovery after Very Severe Brain Injury

Some individuals rapidly emerge from coma and briefly remain in the minimally conscious state before recovering a higher level of consciousness with mild impairments. Others may have a longer period in the minimally conscious state after emerging from the vegetative state and then usually have a greater degree of long-term impairment. Occasionally, persons remain in the vegetative or minimally conscious state for an extended period of time and, in rare cases, these conditions may be permanent.

What treatments are used with people in the vegetative or minimally conscious state?

Currently, there is no treatment that has been proven to speed up or improve recovery from the vegetative or minimally conscious state. However, there is general agreement that the primary focus of medical care is to prevent or treat any factors that might hinder recovery (such as hydrocephalus, a build up of fluid on the brain, or use of sedating drugs for other conditions), and to preserve bodily health (such as treating infections or stiffness of joints). Medical facilities and clinicians vary in the extent to which they try various treatments such as medications or sensory stimulation to promote recovery of consciousness. Because the amount of recovery from disorders of consciousness varies so greatly, it is difficult to judge the value of these and other treatments outside of research studies. You can inquire about your physician or program's philosophy about using these types of treatments.

Transitions to Different Levels of Care

At various points in the process of recovery, persons in the minimally conscious or vegetative state may receive care in a wide range of settings. Initially, the person with severely impaired consciousness is most likely to be treated in an acute care hospital where the focus is primarily on saving his or her life and stabilizing him or her medically. Once that is achieved, the next focus is on recovery of function to whatever level is possible. Sometimes this happens in an acute rehabilitation hospital, which provides a high intensity program of rehabilitation services, including physical therapy, occupational therapy, speech and language therapy, recreational therapy, neuropsychological services, and medical services.

Some patients do not transition from the acute care hospital to an acute rehabilitation program. These people may go directly to a skilled nursing facility, a sub-acute rehabilitation program, a nursing home, or even home with family. Persons discharged from an acute rehabilitation program usually go to one of these places as well. Skilled nursing facilities, sub-acute rehabilitation programs, and nursing homes vary widely in the quantity and quality of medical management, nursing care, and rehabilitation therapy services they provide.

Many factors influence decisions about where a person with severe impairment of consciousness or other severe impairments may go after discharge from the acute care hospital or discharge from the acute rehabilitation program. Some of these factors are the person's medical condition, health insurance coverage and other benefits, the person's ability to tolerate rehabilitation therapies, the doctor's philosophy about where people should go to continue to recover after severe injuries, the family's ability to care for the person at home, the family's wishes, and practical matters such as that the distance the family has to travel to visit the person at the facility.

The names used to describe levels of care and the settings in which they are provided, vary across the country. It is helpful to work with a social worker or case manager in the facility where your loved one is currently receiving services to plan whatever transitions are necessary. Do not be afraid to ask questions to make sure that you obtain the information you need to help you make the best possible decision.

Things to Look for when Considering a Setting to Care for Your Loved One

At various points in the process of recovery, persons in the minimally conscious or vegetative state may receive care in a wide range of settings. These include in-patient rehabilitation facilities, skilled nursing facilities, and long-term acute care facilities. The following are some considerations for selecting a place for care:

1. Your family member's current treatment team has had good experiences with the program when they have referred others there.

2. The staff at the facility makes you feel comfortable, is accessible to talk with about your concerns, and answers your questions.

3. The program and medical staff have experience working with the same kinds of problems that your family member has.

4. The facility is informed about the specifics of the care your loved one needs and is able to meet these care needs. You can have a role in ensuring that a detailed nursing plan of care is developed.

5. The program includes case management to assist in planning for the next level of service, whether it is transition to a rehabilitation program, a facility for long-term care, or home.

6. The program provides education and training for future caregivers.

7. The program uses specific procedures to measure progress.

If support services can be arranged, some persons in the minimally conscious or vegetative state can be cared for at home.

Thoughts from Families Who Have Been There

Family members who have a loved one in a minimally conscious or vegetative state have identified a number of important issues:

1. **Communicating with healthcare providers:** Be sure to ask questions, share your observations, and express your opinions.

2. **Managing medical equipment and supplies:** It is important to be knowledgeable about your loved one's equipment and supplies, and know how to communicate with the companies who provide these items.

3. **Providing care:** Family members often provide some of the care for their loved ones. The amount of care you provide will depend on your role in providing care (this can range from providing most of the care yourself to simply directing the care provided by others); the people such as sitters, attendants,

nurses, and family members who are available to help you with providing care; the setting (this could be your home or a skilled nursing facility); and the guidance you receive from health care providers. It is desirable to obtain as much training as possible to provide whatever elements of care you chose to provide and are able to manage. These might include bathing, grooming, bowel and bladder management, mobility, range of motion, and other medical issues that your loved one may have.

4. **Learning about financial resources:** You may initially feel overwhelmed when you start to learn about various financial resources that may be appropriate for your loved one. However, with patience, persistence, and some help from others, you will be able to figure out which programs apply and find your way through the application processes. Programs you will want to learn about include: healthcare programs such as Medicare and Medicaid; income replacement or financial assistance programs such as SSDI (Social Security Disability Insurance), SSI (Supplemental Security Income), or possibly disability insurance policies that you loved one may have had through work; and services to help with community living such as state agencies that assist people in these areas. It might not be possible to find someone who knows everything about how to access these various services and programs. The key is to keep asking questions and following up to make sure that you and your loved one get all the benefits that are available. People who may be helpful to you are social workers, therapists, case managers, the local social security office, your state brain injury association chapter, family members or friends who are disabled or who have family who are disabled, or the human resources (personnel) department at your loved one's employer.

5. **Guardianship:** Since your loved one is not able to fully make decisions for himself or herself, it may be helpful for you, or someone else, to be appointed guardian. This may make it easier to handle medical decision making or management of your loved one's financial matters. If you think that your loved one may need to have a guardian appointed, you will need to contact an attorney to get assistance. Guardianship can be reversed when it is no longer needed.

How to Interact with Your Loved One Who Is Unconsciousness or at a Low Level of Responsiveness

The most natural way of interacting is to talk to your loved one, even though he or she may not respond or understand. Simple things like telling him or her about recent events in your life, what is going on in your family or neighborhood, or the latest news might make you feel a sense of connection. Talking with your loved one about what you are doing as you provide care can increase your comfort with the process of care giving. For example, telling your loved one that you are going to move his or her arms and legs to help prevent joint tightness might make you feel more comfortable with this task. Only do this range-of-motion type activity if you have been instructed to do so by the doctor, nurse, or therapist.

Physical touch is another way of having a sense of connection. Some family members have said that the act of giving a massage or applying lotion to the hands or face helps them to feel close to their loved one. It is also important to avoid the risk of overstimulation as this may result in rapid breathing, tightening of the muscles, grinding of the teeth, restlessness, and fatigue.

Taking Care of Yourself and Other Family Members

Family members of a person in a vegetative or minimally conscious state often feel a sense of loss or grief for the relationship they had prior to the injury. There can be a number of ways to cope with these feelings. A person in a minimally conscious or vegetative state may make very slow progress or go for periods of time with no apparent progress. Sometimes keeping a journal of the changes you have observed may be comforting. This may give you a chance to look back and see ways in which he or she is more able to respond than he or she was at an earlier point in time.

Having a loved one who is in a vegetative or minimally conscious state can be physically and emotionally draining. Managing this alone can be too much to ask of one person. It is important to rely on support from others, looking to existing supports and developing new ones. You might find help from supports you have relied on in the past, such as family, friends, and religious groups.

Other resources to consider include support groups, support agencies, and the Internet. A good way to learn more about these possible supports is to make a contact with the Brain Injury Association of America's National Brain Injury Information Center (www.biausa.org,

800-444-6443) and obtain contact information for the closest state brain injury association (BIAA) chapter. Health care providers such as doctors, therapists, social workers, and others can be good sources of information about supports available to you.

Even the most committed caregiver needs to have some private time. If your loved one is at home, this can range from having a friend or family member give you a two-hour break to go do something for yourself, to having full-time caregivers for a week, or having your loved one spend a brief time in a nursing care facility or hospital. If your loved one is still in the hospital or living in a nursing care facility, having a rotating visitation schedule can give you some breaks while giving other friends and family a chance to spend time with him or her.

When your loved one was first injured you were likely to be in crisis mode, focusing on the problems, and putting the rest of life on hold. As time goes by, you will need to shift from crisis management mode, and begin to take care of the concerns of everyday life such as paying bills, maintaining relationships with other family members, and taking care of your own physical and mental health. While it is natural to focus on your injured loved one, other members of your family will have needs too. For some people, formal counseling with a therapist or member of the clergy can be an important part of making adjustments to life changes that have occurred as a result of your loved one's injury.

While caring for a person in a vegetative or minimally conscious state is an enormous challenge, use of appropriate resources, as described, can be a big help. Each person will respond differently to this challenge, but almost everyone can cope and move forward. Many family members have a deep sense of personal satisfaction in making life as comfortable and pleasant as possible for a loved one who has sustained a severe injury.

Chapter 7

Brain Death

The History of Brain Death

For thousands of years, the term death meant the permanent stopping of the heart and breathing. However, when Bjorn Ibsen from Denmark invented the artificial respirator in the 1950s, breathing and heartbeat could be continued when people were in a deep coma. This invention and the rise of better medicine and medical care forced doctors to rethink the old definition of death. In 1959, French doctors Mollaret and Goulon first described what is now called brain death. In 1968, the rules for deciding brain death were first put in place with guidelines called the Harvard criteria. These were developed by anesthesiologist and early bioethicist Henry K. Beecher. Following Christian Barnard's first transplant of a human heart in 1967, Beecher wrote that organ donation from those who were "hopelessly unconscious" would be beneficial.

How do physicians declare a patient brain dead?

In a study reported in the January 2008 issue of *Neurology®*, Greer and co-authors studied this question by looking at the top 50 U.S. neurology and neurosurgery programs. They compared the official

"Are We Equal in Death? Avoiding diagnostic error in brain death: 10 Ways to Improve Communication with Your Doctor," Steven Laureys, MD, PhD, and Joseph J. Fins, MD, FACP, *Neurology*, Jan. 2008, 70(4), e14–e15. © 2008 Lippincott Williams and Wilkins, Inc. Reprinted with permission.

medical guidelines from these top hospitals against guidelines used by the American Academy of Neurology (AAN) published in 1995 (see Table 7.1).

Table 7.1. "Gold standard" guidelines for the diagnosis of brain death as published by the American Academy of Neurology (1995)

- Demonstration of coma

- Evidence for the cause of coma

- Absence of confounding factors, including hypothermia, drugs, electrolyte, and endocrine disturbances

- Absence of brainstem reflexes

- Absent motor responses

- Apnea

- A repeat evaluation in six hours is advised, but the time period is considered arbitrary

- Confirmatory lab tests are only required when specific components of the clinical testing cannot be reliably evaluated

What did the authors find?

The good news is that doctors in most of these programs closely followed the AAN guidelines in the examination of brain death. All hospitals correctly defined brain death as irreversible coma with absent brainstem reflexes (such as reactions of the pupils to light and other automatic reflexes). However, many centers' policies did not follow AAN guidelines on rules for testing. Programs were not the same in the attention they paid to low body temperature (hypothermia), sedative or paralytic medicines, or the presence of severe metabolic disorders that might confuse the diagnosis of brain death.

Although careful and standardized testing of the absence of breathing—called apnea testing—is needed for the diagnosis of brain death, the centers were a bit different in how they did apnea testing. Programs were also different in the number of required examinations and the required time between them, the use of extra tests, and in deciding who makes the diagnosis. The best person to make the diagnosis should be a trained and experienced neurologist, but the medical staffing at many U.S. hospitals might make this difficult.

Why is this study important?

This study is important because it provides facts about current practices that can help improve the 13-year-old guidelines from the AAN; in addition, the authors mention areas where there are too many differences between current practices and the AAN guidelines. We need to make practices more similar so that doctors can keep the trust of patients and their families. Also, a definite assessment of death is needed for organ donation so that organs are taken at the right time.

All of these things together are needed for the successful continuation—and growth—of organ donor programs. Finally, studies like this one also give families better information about potential outcomes from coma. By better understanding the future—both good and bad—of patients in coma, families can make informed choices about continuing or stopping life-sustaining therapy. By improving the diagnosis of brain death, doctors can provide strong proof in cases when further treatment would not be helpful or ethical.

Where do we go from here?

Doctors should make every effort to make the correct diagnosis for patients in coma. A patient who is brain dead or who will always be in a vegetative state should be correctly diagnosed. Also, doctors should not make a mistake when saying that a patient will always be in a vegetative state. A patient who is vegetative is in a state of wakeful unresponsiveness in which the eyes are open but there is no awareness of self or others. Such patients have reflex movements, including random eye movements, but are unconscious (Laureys S. Eyes open, brain shut: the vegetative state. *Scientific American* 2007;4:32–37).

Here, doctors need to make all efforts to make sure there is no consciousness left and also exclude the diagnosis of a minimally conscious state (MCS). MCS patients show limited and changing signs of awareness as evidenced by occasional but inconsistent purposeful movements such as following a command or speaking. These responses are not simple reflexes. However, MCS patients cannot reliably communicate (spoken or non-spoken) their thoughts and feelings. We also need to improve our understanding of how the different types of injury (from trauma, or from lack of oxygen to the brain) influence how the brain moves from coma through the vegetative state and onto MCS.

Another diagnosis that should not be missed is that of the locked-in syndrome (LIS). Here patients awaken from their coma, fully conscious, but are unable to move or speak; they can communicate only by blinking or moving their eyes. Jean Dominique Bauby (whose story

The Diving Bell and the Butterfly has been in U.S. theaters) probably was the world's best-known locked-in patient. His book and movie are about the importance of doctors not missing this diagnosis and how a meaningful life can be missed through misdiagnosis.

All physicians have an ethical obligation to make correct diagnoses in brain death. We thank Greer and co-authors for pointing the way toward the improvement of these clinical assessments through careful study.

Part Two

Diagnosing and Treating Brain Disorders

Chapter 8

Neurological Tests and Procedures

Chapter Contents

Section 8.1

Mental Status Tests

"Mental Status Tests," © 2009 A.D.A.M., Inc.
Reprinted with permission.

Definition: Mental status tests are used to determine whether a disease or condition is affecting a person's thinking abilities, and whether a person's mental condition is improving or getting worse.

How the Test Is Performed

The following tests may be performed:

Appearance: The health care provider will check the person's physical appearance, including: age, dress, general level of comfort, gender, grooming, and height and weight.

Orientation: The health care provider will ask questions that may include: the person's name, age, and job; the place where the person lives, type of building, city, and state; and the time, date, and season.

Attention span: The provider will test the person's ability to finish a thought, either through conversation, or by asking the person to follow a series of directions.

Recent memory: The provider will ask questions related to recent people, places, and events in the person's life or in the world.

Remote memory: The provider will ask about the person's childhood, school, or historical events that occurred earlier in life.

Word comprehension: The provider will point to everyday items in the room and ask the person to name them.

Judgment: To test the person's judgment and ability to solve a problem or situation, the provider might ask questions such as:

- "If you found a driver's license on the ground, what would you do?"

- "If a police officer approached you from behind in a car with lights flashing, what would you do?"

How to Prepare for the Test

No preparation is necessary for these tests. All responses should be natural, spontaneous, and honest. Preparation, especially by a highly intelligent person, could change the results of the test by making it seem that mental function has not declined when it actually has.

How the test will feel: There is no physical discomfort.

Normal Results

- Orientation to person, place, and time
- Normal attention span
- Normal judgment
- Normal recent memory
- Normal remote memory
- Normal word comprehension, reading, and writing

What Abnormal Results Mean

Each test can identify different possible problems.

Orientation: Typically, orientation to time is first to be lost, followed by orientation to place, then to person. There are many possible causes for disorientation:

- Alcohol intoxication

- Drugs such as atropine, chloroquine, cimetidine, central nervous system depressants in large doses, cycloserine, indomethacin, lidocaine, oral digitalis medicines, or withdrawal from narcotics and barbiturates

- Environmental causes such as heat stroke, heavy metal poisoning, hypothermia, or methanol poisoning

- Fluid and electrolyte imbalance

- Head trauma or concussion

- Low blood sugar

- Low oxygen in the blood (hypoxemia)

- Nutritional deficiencies, especially lack of niacin, thiamine, vitamin B12, or vitamin C

- Organic brain syndrome

Attention span: People who are unable to complete a thought, or are easily distracted, may have an abnormal attention span. This may have a number of causes, including attention deficit disorder (ADD), confusion, histrionic personality disorder, manic depressive illness, and schizophrenia.

Recent and remote memory: A medical disorder may cause loss of recent memory but keep remote memory intact. Remote memory is lost when damage to the upper part of the brain occurs in diseases such as Alzheimer disease.

Word comprehension, reading, and writing: These tests screen for language disorder (aphasia). Some causes of aphasia include head trauma, senile dementia (Alzheimer type), stroke, and transient ischemic attack.

Judgment: The ability to decide the right course of action is important to survival in many situations. The following are some causes of impaired judgment: emotional dysfunction, mental retardation, organic brain syndrome, and schizophrenia.

Risks

There are no risks with these tests.

Considerations

Some tests that screen for language problems using reading or writing do not account for people who may never have been able to read or write. If you know that the person being tested has never been able to read or write, tell the health care provider in advance.

If your child is having any of these tests performed, it is important to help him or her understand the reasons for the tests.

Section 8.2

Common Screening and Diagnostic Tests for Neurological Disorders

Excerpted from "Neurological Diagnostic Tests and Procedures,"
National Institute of Neurological Disorders and Stroke (NINDS),
updated December 18, 2009.

Diagnostic tests and procedures are vital tools that help physicians confirm or rule out the presence of a neurological disorder or other medical condition. Researchers and physicians use a variety of diagnostic imaging techniques and chemical and metabolic analyses to detect, manage, and treat neurological disease. Some procedures are performed in specialized settings, conducted to determine the presence of a particular disorder or abnormality. Many tests that were previously conducted in a hospital are now performed in a physician's office or at an outpatient testing facility, with little if any risk to the patient. Depending on the type of procedure, results are either immediate or may take several hours to process.

What are some of the more common screening tests?

Laboratory screening tests of blood, urine, or other substances are used to help diagnose disease, better understand the disease process, and monitor levels of therapeutic drugs. Certain tests, ordered by the physician as part of a regular check-up, provide general information, while others are used to identify specific health concerns. For example, blood and blood product tests can detect brain and/or spinal cord infection, bone marrow disease, hemorrhage, blood vessel damage, toxins that affect the nervous system, and the presence of antibodies that signal the presence of an autoimmune disease. Blood tests are also used to monitor levels of therapeutic drugs used to treat epilepsy and other neurological disorders. Genetic testing of deoxyribonucleic acid (DNA) extracted from white cells in the blood can help diagnose Huntington disease and other congenital diseases. Analysis of the fluid that surrounds the brain and spinal cord can detect meningitis, acute and chronic inflammation, rare infections, and some cases of multiple

89

sclerosis. Chemical and metabolic testing of the blood can indicate protein disorders, some forms of muscular dystrophy and other muscle disorders, and diabetes. Urinalysis can reveal abnormal substances in the urine or the presence or absence of certain proteins that cause diseases including the mucopolysaccharidoses.

Genetic testing or counseling can help parents who have a family history of a neurological disease determine if they are carrying one of the known genes that cause the disorder or find out if their child is affected. Genetic testing can identify many neurological disorders. Genetic tests include amniocentesis, chorionic villus sampling (CVS), and uterine ultrasound.

What is a neurological examination?

A neurological examination assesses motor and sensory skills, the functioning of one or more cranial nerves, hearing and speech, vision, coordination and balance, mental status, and changes in mood or behavior, among other abilities. Items including a tuning fork, flashlight, reflex hammer, ophthalmoscope, and needles are used to help diagnose brain tumors, infections such as encephalitis and meningitis, and diseases such as Parkinson disease, Huntington disease, amyotrophic lateral sclerosis (ALS), and epilepsy. Some tests require the services of a specialist to perform and analyze results. X-rays of the patient's chest and skull are often taken as part of a neurological work-up. Fluoroscopy is a type of x-ray that uses a continuous or pulsed beam of low-dose radiation to produce continuous images of a body part in motion. Fluoroscopy can be used to evaluate the flow of blood through arteries.

What are some diagnostic tests used to diagnose neurological disorders?

Based on the result of a neurological exam, physical exam, patient history, x-rays of the patient's chest and skull, and any previous screening or testing, physicians may order one or more of the following diagnostic tests to determine the specific nature of a suspected neurological disorder or injury. These diagnostics generally involve either nuclear medicine imaging, in which very small amounts of radioactive materials are used to study organ function and structure, or diagnostic imaging, which uses magnets and electrical charges to study human anatomy.

The following list of available procedures—in alphabetical rather than sequential order—includes some of the more common tests used to help diagnose a neurological condition.

Angiography is a test used to detect blockages of the arteries or veins. A cerebral angiogram can detect the degree of narrowing or obstruction of an artery or blood vessel in the brain, head, or neck. It is used to diagnose stroke and to determine the location and size of a brain tumor, aneurysm, or vascular malformation. (See section 8.3 for more information about angiography.)

Biopsy involves the removal and examination of a small piece of tissue from the body. Muscle or nerve biopsies are used to diagnose neuromuscular disorders and may also reveal if a person is a carrier of a defective gene that could be passed on to children. A brain biopsy, used to determine tumor type, requires surgery to remove a small piece of the brain or tumor. Performed in a hospital, this operation is riskier than a muscle biopsy and involves a longer recovery period.

Brain scans are imaging techniques used to diagnose tumors, blood vessel malformations, or hemorrhage in the brain. These scans are used to study organ function or injury or disease to tissue or muscle. Types of brain scans include computed tomography, magnetic resonance imaging, and positron emission tomography.

Cerebrospinal fluid analysis involves the removal of a small amount of the fluid that protects the brain and spinal cord. The fluid is tested to detect any bleeding or brain hemorrhage, diagnose infection to the brain and/or spinal cord, identify some cases of multiple sclerosis and other neurological conditions, and measure intracranial pressure. (See section 8.5 for more information)

Computed tomography (CT) scan is a noninvasive, painless process used to produce rapid, clear two-dimensional images of organs, bones, and tissues. Neurological CT scans are used to view the brain and spine. They can detect bone and vascular irregularities, certain brain tumors and cysts, herniated discs, epilepsy, encephalitis, spinal stenosis (narrowing of the spinal canal), a blood clot or intracranial bleeding in patients with stroke, brain damage from head injury, and other disorders. (See section 8.3 for detailed CT information.)

Electroencephalography (EEG) monitors brain activity through the skull. EEG is used to help diagnose certain seizure disorders, brain tumors, brain damage from head injuries, inflammation of the brain and/or spinal cord, alcoholism, certain psychiatric disorders, and metabolic and degenerative disorders that affect the brain. EEGs are also used to evaluate sleep disorders, monitor brain activity when a patient has been fully anesthetized or loses consciousness, and confirm brain death. In order to learn more about brain wave activity, electrodes may be inserted through a surgical opening in the skull and into the brain to reduce signal interference from the skull.

This painless, risk-free test can be performed in a doctor's office or at a hospital or testing facility. Prior to taking an EEG, the person must avoid caffeine intake and prescription drugs that affect the nervous system. A series of cup-like electrodes are attached to the patient's scalp, either with a special conducting paste or with extremely fine needles. The electrodes (also called leads) are small devices that are attached to wires and carry the electrical energy of the brain to a machine for reading. A very low electrical current is sent through the electrodes and the baseline brain energy is recorded. Patients are then exposed to a variety of external stimuli—including bright or flashing light, noise or certain drugs—or are asked to open and close the eyes, or to change breathing patterns. The electrodes transmit the resulting changes in brain wave patterns. Since movement and nervousness can change brain wave patterns, patients usually recline in a chair or on a bed during the test, which takes up to an hour. Testing for certain disorders requires performing an EEG during sleep, which takes at least three hours.

Electromyography (EMG) is used to diagnose nerve and muscle dysfunction and spinal cord disease. It records the electrical activity from the brain and/or spinal cord to a peripheral nerve root (found in the arms and legs) that controls muscles during contraction and at rest.

During an EMG, very fine wire electrodes are inserted into a muscle to assess changes in electrical voltage that occur during movement and when the muscle is at rest. The electrodes are attached through a series of wires to a recording instrument. Testing usually takes place at a testing facility and lasts about an hour but may take longer, depending on the number of muscles and nerves to be tested. Most patients find this test to be somewhat uncomfortable.

An EMG is usually done in conjunction with a nerve conduction velocity (NCV) test, which measures electrical energy by assessing the nerve's ability to send a signal. This two-part test is conducted most often in a hospital. A technician tapes two sets of flat electrodes on the skin over the muscles. The first set of electrodes is used to send small pulses of electricity (similar to the sensation of static electricity) to stimulate the nerve that directs a particular muscle. The second set of electrodes transmits the responding electrical signal to a recording machine. The physician then reviews the response to verify any nerve damage or muscle disease. Patients who are preparing to take an EMG or NCV test may be asked to avoid caffeine and not smoke for 2 to 3 hours prior to the test, as well as to avoid aspirin and non-steroidal anti-inflammatory drugs for 24 hours before the EMG. There is no discomfort or risk associated with this test.

Electronystagmography (ENG) describes a group of tests used to diagnose involuntary eye movement, dizziness, and balance disorders, and to evaluate some brain functions. The test is performed at an imaging center. Small electrodes are taped around the eyes to record eye movements. If infrared photography is used in place of electrodes, the patient wears special goggles that help record the information. Both versions of the test are painless and risk-free.

Evoked potentials (also called evoked response) measure the electrical signals to the brain generated by hearing, touch, or sight. These tests are used to assess sensory nerve problems and confirm neurological conditions including multiple sclerosis, brain tumor, acoustic neuroma (small tumors of the inner ear), and spinal cord injury. Evoked potentials are also used to test sight and hearing (especially in infants and young children), monitor brain activity among coma patients, and confirm brain death.

Testing may take place in a doctor's office or hospital setting. It is painless and risk-free. Two sets of needle electrodes are used to test for nerve damage. One set of electrodes, which will be used to measure the electrophysiological response to stimuli, is attached to the patient's scalp using conducting paste. The second set of electrodes is attached to the part of the body to be tested. The physician then records the amount of time it takes for the impulse generated by stimuli to reach the brain. Under normal circumstances, the process of signal transmission is instantaneous.

- Auditory evoked potentials (also called brain stem auditory evoked response) are used to assess high-frequency hearing loss, diagnose any damage to the acoustic nerve and auditory pathways in the brainstem, and detect acoustic neuromas.

- Visual evoked potentials detect loss of vision from optic nerve damage (in particular, damage caused by multiple sclerosis).

- Somatosensory evoked potentials measure response from stimuli to the peripheral nerves and can detect nerve or spinal cord damage or nerve degeneration from multiple sclerosis and other degenerating diseases.

Magnetic resonance imaging (MRI) uses computer-generated radio waves and a powerful magnetic field to produce detailed images of body structures including tissues, organs, bones, and nerves. Neurological uses include the diagnosis of brain and spinal cord tumors, eye disease, inflammation, infection, and vascular irregularities that may lead to stroke. MRI can also detect and monitor degenerative disorders such as multiple sclerosis and can document brain injury from trauma. Functional MRI (fMRI) uses the blood's magnetic properties to produce real-time images of blood flow to particular areas of the brain. An fMRI can pinpoint areas of the brain that become active and note how long they stay active. It can also tell if brain activity within a region occurs simultaneously or sequentially. This imaging process is used to assess brain damage from head injury or degenerative disorders such as Alzheimer disease and to identify and monitor other neurological disorders, including multiple sclerosis, stroke, and brain tumors. (See section 8.3 for additional MRI information.)

Positron emission tomography (PET) scans provide two- and three-dimensional pictures of brain activity by measuring radioactive isotopes that are injected into the bloodstream. PET scans of the brain are used to detect or highlight tumors and diseased tissue, measure cellular and/or tissue metabolism, show blood flow, evaluate patients who have seizure disorders that do not respond to medical therapy and patients with certain memory disorders, and determine brain changes following injury or drug abuse, among other uses. PET may be ordered as a follow-up to a CT or MRI scan to give the physician a greater understanding of specific areas of the brain that may be involved with certain problems.

A polysomnogram measures brain and body activity during sleep. It is performed over one or more nights at a sleep center. Electrodes are pasted or taped to the patient's scalp, eyelids, and/or chin. Throughout the night and during the various wake/sleep cycles, the electrodes record brain waves, eye movement, breathing, leg and skeletal muscle activity, blood pressure, and heart rate. The patient may be videotaped to note any movement during sleep. Results are then used to identify any characteristic patterns of sleep disorders, including restless legs syndrome, periodic limb movement disorder, insomnia, and breathing disorders such as obstructive sleep apnea. Polysomnograms are noninvasive, painless, and risk-free.

Single photon emission computed tomography (SPECT) is a nuclear imaging test involving blood flow to tissue used to evaluate certain brain functions. The test may be ordered as a follow-up to an MRI to diagnose tumors, infections, degenerative spinal disease, and stress fractures.

Thermography uses infrared sensing devices to measure small temperature changes between the two sides of the body or within a specific organ. Also known as digital infrared thermal imaging, thermography may be used to detect vascular disease of the head and neck, soft tissue injury, various neuromusculoskeletal disorders, and the presence or absence of nerve root compression.

Ultrasound imaging, also called ultrasound scanning or sonography, uses high-frequency sound waves to obtain images inside the body. *Neurosonography* (ultrasound of the brain and spinal column) analyzes blood flow in the brain and can diagnose stroke, brain tumors, hydrocephalus (build-up of cerebrospinal fluid in the brain), and vascular problems. It can also identify or rule out inflammatory processes causing pain. It is more effective than an x-ray in displaying soft tissue masses and can show tears in ligaments, muscles, tendons, and other soft tissue masses in the back. Transcranial Doppler ultrasound is used to view arteries and blood vessels in the neck and determine blood flow and risk of stroke.

Section 8.3

Neurological Imaging

"Diagnostic Testing–Imaging: Parts I, II, and III," by Jack Hoch, © 2009 Angioma Alliance (www.angiomalliance.org). Reprinted with permission.

Note: This section describes common imaging technologies used for neurological tests and procedures, and specifically addresses the use of these technologies in the cavernous malformation diagnosis process.

Diagnostic Imaging Primer Part I

Medical diagnostic imaging is a complex field requiring highly trained and specialized medical professionals to administer these procedures and interpret the results. As technology and understanding of disease pathology evolves, combinations of diagnostic images are being used in an integrated and layered approach. In some cases, imaging technology, which has been around for a decade or more, is being altered and used in new ways. This can make the testing process easier and less invasive or lead to new approaches in the diagnosis of a disease.

This section describes the two most common imaging technologies and their use in the cavernous malformation diagnosis process.

Computed tomography (CT/CAT scan): For many years, the first line of diagnosis was the computed tomography (CT), or CAT scan (the "A" in CAT stands for axial, meaning looking at one's head from the top down). CT is a technology that has been in use for roughly 30 years, and has improved with time.

Initially slow and prone to patient movement artifacts, getting a sharp and detailed image was problematic. Regardless, it was worth the time and trouble because the process was non-invasive and gave doctors a good look at the soft tissue structures of the brain. CT is still widely used today, especially in emergency rooms where trauma doctors need to get a first look at a patient's problem. It helps that CT is less expensive than magnetic resonance imaging (MRI), and it's also adept at imaging fresh blood.

Drawbacks to the use of CT technology include the use of x-rays to create the resultant image, and the image detail is less than other technologies. Like MRI, CT may include the use of a contrast agent (dye) to enhance certain aspects of the image. Patients who don't like needles won't appreciate this portion of the test, but at least it's only a single injection.

Magnetic resonance imaging (MRI): MRI is the gold standard in diagnostic imaging. Invented in the late 1980s, MRI has revolutionized the diagnosis of certain diseases, including cavernous malformation (CCM). While the images generated by this technology appear similar to those produced by CT, the process by which these images are rendered is completely different.

There are two physical types of MRI—open and closed. Closed MRI requires the patient to enter a very narrow tube, and lie flat and still during the procedure which can take 30 minutes or more. For those who are claustrophobic, it can be extremely challenging.

Open MRI is not comprised of a closed tube, so there are really no problems for claustrophobic patients. There is, however, a trade-off; in most cases, open MRI is less precise than the closed counterpart. If a patient can handle the claustrophobic aspects of a closed MRI, then a closed MRI is the optimal procedure to undergo.

An MRI develops a very strong magnetic field resulting from the generation of radio waves focused at a certain part of the body. As of now, there are no known health problems from the occasional exposure to high strength magnetic fields. However, because of the generated magnetic field, no metal objects are allowed in the actual MRI room. Due to the high strength magnetic field, certain patients cannot undergo an MRI if they have an implanted pacemaker, or metal plates or screws surgically inserted somewhere in the body.

Although there are no preparation requirements (such as fasting or other restrictions) that must be met before the procedure, there is a requirement that the patient remain absolutely still during the imaging portion of the exam. Movement will result in blurred, useless images. Additionally, MRI is a noisy process and requires the use of hearing protection.

Like CT, MRI generates an image slice by slice. These slices are normally a few millimeters thick, so that the rendered image is detailed and clear. Likewise, the slicing orientation is controlled by the technician: axial (top of head looking down), coronal (back of head looking forward), and sagittal (side of head, looking toward other side of head). MRI scans can be run with a multitude of settings, depending upon the expected results and location of the mass or entity to be studied.

The garden variety MRI is the spin-echo MRI. Spin-echo refers to the type of MRI pulse that is used during the procedure. There are different weightings and spin-echo sequences that radiologists will use depending upon the individual case. In general, there are two weightings of spin-echo images which are most widely used: (1) T1– Longitudinal relaxation time: Hemorrhages, especially newer ones, appear brighter than surrounding brain tissue; and (2) T2–Transverse relaxation time: Hemorrhages appear darker than surrounding brain tissue.

Both T1 and T2 times are adjustable by the radiologist, so that the best contrast relative to background brain tissue can be depicted. Again, the settings will be optimized for the expected location of study in the brain, as well as the type of finding expected. In those cases where a brain scan is ordered without pre-existing knowledge of lesion, general template T1 and T2 settings are used to have the best chance of picking up abnormalities.

Gradient-echo and susceptibility weighted imaging (SWI) differ from spin-echo and allow detection of very small (punctuate or pin-sized) abnormalities. This is especially critical for potential cavernous malformation patients, as even small lesions can have big neurological consequences. For one's first diagnostic scan, when the root cause of clinical symptoms is yet unknown, performing a gradient-echo MRI or SWI MRI is highly recommended. When in doubt, be sure to ask that gradient-echo or SWI be specified by the MRI prescription issued by the referring doctor.

There are additional MRI sequences, such as turbo (fast) spin-echo and functional MRI (fMRI), among others. Turbo spin-echo is simply a quicker way of accomplishing a regular spin echo scan, yielding certain advantages (and disadvantages). Functional MRI is very useful in certain pre-surgical situations. These and other diagnostic tests, such as angiography, are highlighted later in this section.

Limitations of imaging and upcoming new technology: It has been established that people who suffer from claustrophobia, possess metallic implants, or who cannot remain still for an extended period of time may have difficulty undergoing a successful MRI examination. What about children? Young ones can also experience serious medical difficulties requiring diagnostic examination. Trying to keep kids from squirming during a 30 or 45 minute MRI procedure is practically impossible.

General anesthesia has been the fallback, but this is tough on the kids, not to mention their parents. If you've ever seen a preschooler regaining consciousness from an anesthesia-based procedure, it's an eye opener. There are side-effects, such as headache, and other dangers. For a non-invasive procedure, anesthesia seems like overkill, but until recently it was the only realistic alternative. Fortunately, new technology is on the horizon that hopefully will relegate general anesthesia to the trash bin for follow-up pediatric MRI. New technologies will reduce the negative effects of motion, resulting in high definition scans even with a squirmy kid. This means that many young children will no longer require sedation to undergo follow-up MRI. Also, the overall process is quicker, possibly cutting the exam duration by 40%–50%. So far, these new technologies use turbo spin-echo sequences, and they may not be the best choice for an initial scan, but they could be appropriate for follow-up and expectant management of cerebral cavernous malformation (CCM).

Diagnostic Imaging Primer Part II: Angiography

An angiogram (also known as an arteriogram) is a diagnostic test used to gauge the integrity of blood vessels within the body. It is an indispensable element in determining the root cause of a problem, either by positive identification or by ruling out certain possibilities. An angiogram will only see areas where there is blood flow above a specific threshold rate. As such, it cannot image cavernous malformations directly, but it may help to do so by process of elimination. When used in conjunction with an MRI, an angiogram provides an invaluable look at blood vessel irregularities previously viewable only through surgery or at autopsy. The combination of the two generally results in a diagnosis of high confidence.

Of course, nothing in life is ever easy, and that is the case with angiography. Technological advances have yielded additional angiography choices that can complicate the decision-making process, potentially adding stress or anxiety to an already confusing situation. Even so, it's nice to have alternatives, especially non-invasive ones, which weren't available 20 years ago.

Following are some details on the three different types of angiography commonly used in today's medical facilities: computed tomography angiography (CTA), magnet resonance angiography (MRA), and conventional angiography.

Computed tomography angiography (CTA): CTA is the least accurate and least expensive angiography alternative. In essence, its strengths and weaknesses are similar to the CT versus MRI comparison discussed previously. Basically, its availability is more widespread than MRA; it costs less, and there are fewer restrictions in that CTA can be used on patients with metal in their bodies (pacemakers, screws, rods, plates, and so forth). Unfortunately, like its CT cousin, the precision is not as high as with MRI, and it requires an iodine-based contrast injection, which can be detrimental to some at-risk patients.

Magnetic resonance angiography (MRA): MRA is rapidly becoming the diagnostic test of choice for blood vessel imaging. It can detect blood vessels that are bulging (aneurism) or narrowing (stenosis). Likewise, it can pick up high blood flow lesions such as arteriovenous malformations (AVM). CTA can do this as well, but not with the degree of precision found in MRA. The degree of precision is what gives MRA a big advantage over CTA in terms of early detection.

MRA also offers important advantages over conventional angiography. Unlike the latter, MRA is non-invasive and is much quicker. While the risks with an invasive procedure are relatively small, those risks are still present. MRA completely removes this concern.

Regardless, some of the more intransigent medical facilities consider MRA (and CTA) somewhat experimental and prefer to use conventional angiography.

Conventional angiography: Long the gold standard for blood vessel diagnostics, conventional angiography has been around a very long time. One can think of it as an x-ray of one's blood vessels. The procedure is more involved than that for MRA or CTA in that it requires an incision, normally in the femoral artery near the groin area (local anesthesia). Once this incision is made, a catheter is inserted into the artery and snaked into the blood vessel of concern. To image blood vessels in the brain, this requires the catheter to be guided through the torso and neck and into the head. Once the catheter is in place, contrast material is injected and images are taken of the affected area.

The advantage to conventional angiography is that the images are taken with close proximity perspective. Of all of the imaging methods, it is the most precise. This precision, however, comes at a higher relative risk of complications such as infection, hemorrhage from the catheter damaging a blood vessel, or even stroke. Also, there is a recovery time associated with the operation of at least four hours, which requires keeping one's leg immobilized for that period of time.

What's the Best Procedure?

No doubt, the cop-out answer is "it depends." In reality, most general cases can probably be handled by MRA as long as the hospital staff is well trained on the latest technology and diagnostic procedures. If one doctor recommends a conventional angiogram, ask why not an MRA? Good engineering practice always stipulates that one chooses the simplest and safest of two procedures if the expected results are the same. Ask the physician to explain to you why conventional angiography should be used in lieu of MRA.

Be aware that when discussing the darker side of medicine and inherent conflicts of interest, conventional angiography procedures receive a higher insurance reimbursement rate than do MRAs. All other factors being equal, some unscrupulous doctors may choose conventional angiography over MRA to grab that higher reimbursement rate. Also, don't lambaste emergency medical room staff if they order a CTA. In many cases, a CTA is a great first look at an emerging problem where time is of the essence.

The real kicker is that after having read all of this, if one's angiography is negative (normal), that only rules out high flow lesions such as arteriovenous malformation (AVM). If a lesion imaged by MRI is suspected as the underlying cause of symptoms, then the absence of anything unusual on an angiogram heightens the possibility that the lesion may be an angiographically occult vascular malformation (AOVM), such as a cavernous malformation, which by nature is low flow.

Diagnostic Imaging Primer Part III: Functional MRI and Other Techniques

Functional MRI (fMRI)

Functional MRI is a recently developed, and still advancing, procedure allowing the non-invasive measurement of blood flow in the brain. Images can be taken rapid-fire, allowing an almost movie-like synthesis of image frames so that doctors can identify currently active brain regions. This imaging and identification is usually done in conjunction with a patient task-oriented test. By assigning a task (playing a game, moving an arm or leg) to a patient and then immediately taking pictures of the brain, changes in blood flow rate and distribution can be measured. In this way, exact regions of the brain can be mapped as to function.

The key assumption here is that the flow of oxygenated blood, which fMRI indirectly measures, is directly related to the task demands and area of the brain requiring this enhanced flow. Except for the tasks, the fMRI procedure itself is very similar to a regular MRI, especially considering that one's head must remain immobilized during the imaging process.

Functional MRI is useful as a mapping tool prior to surgery. The surgeon can use the following fMRI procedures to differentiate between important tissue (for example, speech center, motor area) and tissue which is not as eloquent. This can make all of the difference in surgical success rate for those operations requiring a very low margin of error.

Types of fMRI

Functional MRI comes in different flavors, and the flavor of the day is dependent upon the particular aspect of the patient's case the attending physician wishes to study. Ideally, the following fMRI techniques involve measuring cerebral blood flow while performing a before and after mental state test of a patient. Hopefully, all other variables during this test are kept constant. The four main fMRI types in use today are: bold, perfusion, diffusion-weighted, and MRI spectroscopy.

Bold-fMRI: Depicts oxygenated blood in the brain as bright areas on the film. The assumption is that blood content high in oxygen is being delivered to those areas of the brain in use or needing it most at that given time. By giving a patient a singular and simple task (holding an object), the doctor can see the areas of the brain that are activated during the task. Images are rapidly taken before and during the task so that they may be contrasted with each other. Bold-fMRI is optimal for studying functions that can be quickly turned on and off like language, vision, movement, hearing, and memory.

Perfusion-fMRI: Like bold-fMRI, perfusion-fMRI attempts to measure blood flow in the brain. It differs in that it does not measure blood oxygenation.

There are two types of perfusion-fMRI: intravenous bolus tracking and arterial spin-labeling. The former uses an injection of a tracer substance such as gadolinium to depict relative blood flow. Gadolinium is the same contrast agent used during many standard MRI procedures. The tracer, or bolus, is then mapped as it courses through the cerebral bloodstream in the area of the brain being studied. More than one bolus can be administered in a session. Unfortunately, this is somewhat invasive (gadolinium injection) and is also limited by the ability of one's kidneys to process and eliminate the tracer substance without damage due to toxicity.

Arterial spin-labeling, on the other hand, is non-invasive and can be repeated as many times as necessary, plus, it can measure absolute blood flow. Absolute blood flow allows a series of images focusing on the same area to be taken during a specific fMRI session.

The biggest drawback is that this method is very slow, and individual images (slices) can only be generated every few minutes. This contrasts with bold-fMRI, which is rapid-fire. The longer the time between slices, the greater the chance of the patient's mental state changing in a non-controlled fashion, thereby introducing unwanted variables into the procedure.

Diffusion-weighted imaging: This procedure measures the relative mobility of water molecules in the brain. The natural, random motion of water molecules (for those of us who remember their days in physics class—Brownian motion) can be factored out such that abnormal movement of these molecules can be measured. For instance, during a de-myelinizing disease process such as multiple sclerosis, water molecules would more readily diffuse across the boundary of the myelin sheath since it is no longer intact. Most lesions and strokes cause disruption of the brain's white matter such that diffusion-weighted imaging can hone in on these areas.

MRI spectroscopy (MRIS): While basic MRI shows relative differences between areas of the brain, MRI spectroscopy allows for detailed chemical information about specific composition of individual brain areas. For instance, MRIS can tell the difference between a tumor, and dead tissue. Use and refinement of this technique continues to evolve and will most likely play a greater role in future diagnostic procedures.

Other Diagnostic Tools

There are a host of other image-oriented tools that doctors employ to diagnose suspected problems in the brain. Positron emission tomography (PET) and single photon emission computed tomography (SPECT) have been around for awhile. Their greatest attribute, relative to cavernous malformation (CCM) patients, is diagnosing/localizing epilepsy centers in the brain. Both of these procedures image the brain similar to fMRI, but PET and SPECT involve slower image acquisition times, are more costly, and include ionizing radiation as a byproduct of their use. Given these limitations, fMRI is almost always preferable.

Magnetoencephalogram (MEG) and electroencephalogram (EEG) measure the electrical activity of the brain. EEG requires long preparation time, especially in the placement of electrodes on the patient. MEG, while quicker, requires more expensive equipment.

Ultrasound uses inaudible (to the human ear) sound waves to image a particular area. Most are familiar with its use during mid-term pregnancy to predetermine the gender of the fetus and ensure normal gestation. Currently, ultrasound doesn't have much practical application in the diagnostic process of potential CCM patients.

Summary and the Future

MRI and fMRI will continue to be the imaging procedures of choice for the foreseeable future. While other imaging procedures exist, most are so specialized that they are either very costly or are not applicable to CCM patients. Others require significant invasiveness, such as a craniotomy, in order to be useful.

Probably the biggest near-term impact in the MRI world will be an increase in magnetic field strength. Currently, the standard field strength is 1.5 Tesla (T). Newer machines will easily double that and may possibly reach seven or eight T once it is determined that these higher field strengths are safe for humans. Quicker MRI procedures and much higher image resolutions will be the result.

Further in the future, more molecular-oriented imaging systems will be developed. If one follows the money in the medical research world, studies involving sub-cellular molecular structures and processes are getting their share of the funding. One day we may have readily available patient diagnostics that can show doctors changes on the molecular level. To put it another way, the imaging difference is similar to a satellite photographing the earth and viewing detail at city level versus using a different satellite to peer into a window and read the contents of a post-it note on someone's desk.

Technology is blazing the way for new and exciting developments in diagnostic imaging. The rapid pace of development is good news for those patients harboring brain lesions. Diagnosis is usually quicker and more accurate than in years past. The days of mistaking CCM for other diseases such as multiple sclerosis are fading fast. Even so, deployment of new imaging systems must pass stringent safety tests that can delay their clinical use. Just as important, medical professionals must be trained to use the new systems and properly interpret their output.

Section 8.4

Carotid Ultrasound

Excerpted from "Carotid Ultrasound,"
National Heart, Lung, and Blood Institute (NHLBI), May 2009.

Carotid ultrasound is a painless and harmless test that uses high-frequency sound waves to create pictures of the insides of the two large arteries in your neck. These arteries, called carotid arteries, supply your brain with oxygen-rich blood. You have one carotid artery on each side of your neck. Carotid ultrasound shows whether a substance called plaque (plak) has narrowed your carotid arteries. Plaque is made up of fat, cholesterol, calcium, and other substances found in the blood. Plaque builds up on the insides of your arteries as you age. This condition is called carotid artery disease.

You have two common carotid arteries—one on each side of your neck—that divide into internal and external carotid arteries. Too much plaque in a carotid artery can cause a stroke. The plaque can slow down or block the flow of blood through the artery, allowing a blood clot to form. A piece of the blood clot can break off and get stuck in the artery, blocking blood flow to the brain. This is what causes a stroke.

A standard carotid ultrasound shows the structure of your carotid arteries. Your carotid ultrasound test may include a Doppler ultrasound. Doppler ultrasound is a special test that shows the movement of blood through your blood vessels. Your doctor often will need results from both types of ultrasound to fully assess whether there's a problem with blood flow through your carotid arteries.

Your doctor may recommend a carotid ultrasound if you had a stroke or mini-stroke recently; or if you have an abnormal sound in your carotid artery called a carotid bruit. Your doctor can hear a carotid bruit with the help of a stethoscope put on your neck over the carotid artery. A bruit may suggest a partial blockage in your carotid artery that could lead to a stroke.

Your doctor also may recommend a carotid ultrasound if he or she suspects you may have blood clots that can slow blood flow in your carotid artery, or a split between the layers of your carotid artery wall that weakens the wall or reduces blood flow to your brain

Also, a carotid ultrasound also may be done to see whether carotid artery surgery, also called carotid endarterectomy, has restored normal blood flow through your carotid artery, or after surgery to check the position of the stent put in your carotid artery. (The stent, a small mesh tube, helps prevent the artery from becoming narrowed or blocked again.)

Sometimes carotid ultrasound is used as a preventive screening test in people who have medical conditions that increase their risk of stroke, including high blood pressure and diabetes.

What to expect: Carotid ultrasound is a painless test, and typically there is little to do in advance. Your doctor will tell you how to prepare for your carotid ultrasound. Carotid ultrasound usually is done in a doctor's office or hospital. The test is painless and often doesn't take more than 30 minutes.

The ultrasound machine includes a computer, a video screen, and a transducer. A transducer is a hand-held device that sends and receives ultrasound waves into and from the body. You will lie on your back on an exam table for the test. Your technician or doctor will put a gel on your neck where your carotid arteries are located. This gel helps the ultrasound waves reach the arteries better. Your technician or doctor will put the transducer against different spots on your neck and move it back and forth. The transducer gives off ultrasound waves and detects their echoes after they bounce off the artery walls and blood cells. Ultrasound waves can't be heard by the human ear. A computer uses the echoes to create and record pictures of the insides of the arteries (usually in black and white) and your blood flowing through them (usually in color; this is the Doppler ultrasound). A video screen displays these live images for your doctor to review.

Results: Often, your doctor will be able to tell you the results of the carotid ultrasound when it occurs or soon afterward. A carotid ultrasound can show whether plaque buildup has narrowed one or both of your carotid arteries and reduced blood flow to your brain. If plaque has narrowed your carotid arteries, you may be at risk of having a stroke. That risk depends on how much of your artery is blocked and how much blood flow is restricted. To reduce your risk for stroke, your doctor may recommend medical or surgical treatments to reduce or remove the plaque buildup in your carotid arteries.

Section 8.5

Lumbar Puncture (Spinal Tap)

"Lumbar Puncture," September 2008, reprinted with permission from www. kidshealth.org. Copyright © 2008 The Nemours Foundation. This information was provided by KidsHealth, one of the largest resources online for medically reviewed health information written for parents, kids, and teens. For more articles like this one, visit www.KidsHealth.org or www. TeensHealth.org.

Editor's note: This information was written for parents; however, the procedure is the same for children and adults.

What It Is

A lumbar puncture (also called a spinal tap) is a common medical test that involves taking a small sample of cerebrospinal fluid (CSF) for examination. CSF is a clear, colorless liquid that delivers nutrients and cushions the brain and spinal cord, or central nervous system. In a lumbar puncture, a needle is carefully inserted into the lower spine to collect the CSF sample.

Why It's Done

Medical personnel perform lumbar punctures and test the cerebrospinal fluid to detect or rule out suspected diseases or conditions. CSF testing looks for signs of possible infection by analyzing the white blood cell count, glucose levels, protein, and bacteria or abnormal cells that can help identify specific diseases in the central nervous system.

Most lumbar punctures are done to test for meningitis, but they also can determine if there is bleeding in the brain, detect certain conditions affecting the nervous system such as Guillain Barré syndrome and multiple sclerosis, and administer chemotherapy medications.

Preparation

After the procedure is explained to you, you'll be asked to sign an informed consent form—this states that you understand the procedure and its risks and give your permission for it to be performed. The doctor doing the lumbar puncture will know your child's medical history but might ask additional questions, such as whether your child is allergic to any medicines. You might be able to stay in the room with your child during the procedure, or you can step outside to a waiting area.

The Procedure

A lumbar puncture takes about 30 minutes. The doctor carefully inserts a thin needle between the bones of the lower spine (below the spinal cord) to withdraw the fluid sample. The patient will be positioned with the back curved out so the spaces between the vertebrae are as wide as possible. This allows the doctor to easily find the spaces between the lower lumbar bones (where the needle will be inserted). Older children may be asked to either sit on an exam table while leaning over with their head on a pillow or lie on their side. Infants and younger children are usually positioned on their sides with their knees under their chin.

A small puncture through the skin on the lower back is made and liquid anesthetic medicine is injected into the tissues beneath the skin to prevent pain. In many cases, before the injected anesthesia medication is given, a numbing cream is applied to the skin to minimize discomfort.

The spinal needle is thin and the length varies according to the size of the patient. It has a hollow core, and inside the hollow core is a "stylet," another type of thin needle that acts kind of like a plug. When the spinal needle is inserted into the lower lumbar area, the stylet is carefully removed, which allows the cerebrospinal fluid to drip out into the collection tubes.

After the CSF sample is collected (this usually takes about five minutes), the needle is withdrawn and a small bandage is placed on the site. Collected samples are sent to a lab for analysis and testing.

What to Expect

While some notice a brief pinch and some discomfort, most people don't consider a lumbar puncture to be painful. Depending on the doctor's recommendations, your child might have to lie on his or her back for a few hours after the procedure. Your child might feel tired and have a mild backache the day after the procedure.

Getting the Results

Some results from a lumbar puncture are available within 30 to 60 minutes. However, to look for specific bacteria growing in the sample, a bacterial culture is sent to the lab and these results are usually available in 48 hours. If it's determined there might be an infection, the doctor will start antibiotic treatment while waiting for the results of the culture.

Risks

A lumbar puncture is considered a safe procedure with minimal risks. Most of the time, there are no complications. In some instances, a patient may get a headache (it's recommended that patients lie down for a few hours after the test and drink plenty of fluids to help prevent headaches). And in rare cases, infection or bleeding can occur.

Helping Your Child

You can help prepare your child for a lumbar puncture by explaining that while the test might be uncomfortable, it shouldn't be painful and won't take long. Also explain the importance of lying still during the test, and let your child know that a nurse might hold him or her in place. After the procedure, make sure your child rests and follow any other instructions the doctor gives you.

If You Have Questions

It's important to understand any procedure your child undergoes. If you have questions or concerns about the lumbar puncture procedure, be sure to speak with your doctor.

Section 8.6

Intracranial Pressure Monitoring

"Intracranial Pressure Monitoring,"
© 2009 A.D.A.M., Inc. Reprinted with permission.

Intracranial pressure monitoring uses a device, placed inside the head, which senses the pressure inside the skull and sends its measurements to a recording device.

How the Test Is Performed

There are three ways to monitor pressure in the skull (intracranial pressure):

- A thin, flexible tube threaded into one of the two cavities, called lateral ventricles, of the brain (intraventricular catheter)

- A screw or bolt placed just through the skull in the space between the arachnoid membrane and cerebral cortex (subarachnoid screw or bolt)

- A sensor placed into the epidural space beneath the skull (epidural sensor)

The intraventricular catheter is thought to be the most accurate method, but if immediate access is needed, a subarachnoid bolt is typically used. If no qualified brain surgeon (neurosurgeon) is available to place a bolt, then an epidural sensor will probably be used.

To insert an intraventricular catheter, a burr hole is drilled through the skull and the catheter is inserted through the brain matter into the lateral ventricle, which normally contains liquid (cerebrospinal fluid [CSF]) that protects the brain and spinal cord. Not only can the intracranial pressure (ICP) be monitored, but it can be lowered by draining cerebral spinal fluid out through the catheter. This catheter may be difficult to get in place when there is increased intracranial pressure, since the ventricles change shape under increased pressure and are often quite small because the brain expands around them from injury and swelling.

A subarachnoid screw or bolt is a hollow screw that is inserted through a hole drilled in the skull and through a hole cut in the outermost membrane protecting the brain and spinal cord (dura mater).

The epidural sensor is placed through a burr hole drilled in the skull, just over the epidural covering. Since no hole is made in the epidural lining, this procedure is less invasive than other methods, but it cannot remove excess CSF.

Lidocaine or another local anesthetic will be injected at the site where the incision will be made. You will most likely get a sedative to help you relax. First the area is shaved and cleansed with antiseptic. After the area is dry, an incision is made and the skin is pulled back until the skull is visible. A drill is then used to cut through the bone to expose the epidural tissue.

If an epidural sensor is used, it is then inserted between the skull and epidural tissue. If a bolt is used, an incision is made to expose the subarachnoid space and the bolt is screwed into the bone. This allows the sensor to record from the subdural/subarachnoid space.

If an intraventricular catheter is used, it is threaded through the brain matter into one of the lateral ventricles. This type of catheter is effective and accurate at sensing intracranial pressure measurements.

How to prepare for the test: If you need this procedure done, you will be in the hospital and most likely in an intensive care unit. If you are conscious, your health care provider will explain the procedure and the risks, and (as with any surgery) you will have to sign a consent form.

How the test will feel: If the procedure is done while you are under general anesthesia, you will feel nothing until you wake from the anesthesia. At that time you will feel the normal side effects of anesthesia, plus the discomfort of the incision made in your skull.

If the procedure is performed under local anesthesia, you will feel a prick on your scalp like a bee sting as the local anesthetic is injected. You may feel a tugging sensation as the skin is cut and pulled back to expose the bone. You will hear a drill sound as it cuts through the skull. The amount of time this takes will depend on the type of drill that is used. You will also feel a tugging sensation as the surgeon sutures the skin back together after the procedure.

Your health care provider may prescribe mild pain medications for relief. You will not receive strong pain medications, so that your doctor can check for signs of brain function. Neurologic problems are common with increased intracranial pressure.

Why the Test Is Performed

This test or procedure is done to measure the intracranial pressure and to learn if you are at risk for injury from increased intracranial pressure. It also provides a sterile access for draining excess CSF.

Normal results: Normally, the ICP ranges from 1–15 millimeters of mercury (mm Hg). Note: Normal value ranges may vary slightly among different laboratories. Talk to your doctor about the meaning of your specific test results.

What abnormal results mean: Intracranial pressure monitoring is usually done in cases of severe head injury. It also may be done after surgery to remove a tumor or repair damage to a blood vessel (vascular lesion) if the surgical team is concerned about brain swelling.

Elevated intracranial pressure can be treated by draining CSF through the catheter. It also may be treated by changing ventilator settings (for people who are in critical condition and on a respirator) or by giving certain medications through a vein (intravenous).

Intracranial pressure monitoring is crucial to identify the problem and treat it right away. Raised intracranial pressure means that both nervous system (neural) and blood vessel (vascular) tissues are being compressed. If left untreated, it can result in permanent neurologic damage. In some cases, it can be fatal.

Risks: Bleeding; brain herniation or injury from the increased pressure despite the monitor; damage to the brain tissue with continued neurologic effects; inability to find the ventricle and accurately place catheter; infection; and risks of general anesthesia.

Reference

Fletcher JJ, Nathan BR. Cerebrospinal fluid and intracranial pressure. In: Goetz, CG, ed. *Textbook of Clinical Neurology*. 3rd ed. Philadelphia, Pa: Saunders Elsevier; 2007: chap 26.

Chapter 9

Steroids for Brain Disorders

Steroids are naturally occurring hormones. In brain tumor treatment, steroids are used to reduce the swelling, or edema, sometimes caused by the tumor or its treatment. The steroids given to brain tumor patients are corticosteroids—hormones produced by small glands, called adrenal glands, near the kidneys. They are not the same as the anabolic steroids used by athletes to build muscle.

Dexamethasone (Decadron) and prednisone are corticosteroid drugs. These steroids can temporarily relieve brain tumor symptoms, improve neurological symptoms, promote a feeling of well-being, and increase your appetite. Because steroids are hormones, their long-term use requires close monitoring. In this chapter, we'll share why steroids are given, how to manage the effects of steroids, and a few guidelines for their safe use.

About edema: Edema is the accumulation of fluids in the tissue around a tumor—it is a common occurrence in people who have a brain tumor. Edema happens when the blood brain barrier, an invisible protection around the brain, is disrupted by the tumor. Small blood vessels around the tumor can then leak fluids which collect in the surrounding tissue. Edema can also occur following surgery, radiation, or other treatment for a brain tumor.

"Steroids," © 2004 American Brain Tumor Association (www.abta.org). Reprinted with permission. Reviewed in January 2010 by Dr. David A. Cooke, MD, FACP, Diplomate, American Board of Internal Medicine.

When are steroids given?

Steroids may be prescribed before, during, or after surgery. They may be started at the time of diagnosis if edema is seen on a magnetic resonance imaging (MRI) scan, or if swelling is causing pressure on the brain. Steroids may be used to control edema caused by surgery. In this situation, they may be started just prior to surgery or during the procedure. If swelling occurs following surgery, as it sometimes does, steroids can be given at that time. If you were on steroids prior to surgery, your dose might be adjusted after surgery if increased swelling causes an increase in your symptoms.

Steroids are also used to treat edema caused by radiation therapy. Steroids may be started prior to radiation, or at the time of treatment. The steroids are continued until the brain appears to have healed from the acute effects of the therapy.

For people with a recurrent tumor, or those with a metastatic brain tumor (which spread to the brain from a cancer elsewhere in the body), steroids can help improve quality of life by reducing symptoms. When used in this way, steroids may increase a person's alertness, ability to be mobile, or perhaps increase their ability to communicate and interact with others.

Do steroids treat tumor cells?

Steroids are not intended to be a cytotoxic or cell-killing therapy. Their purpose is to reduce swelling, not cure the tumor. However, some researchers do believe steroids have some toxic effect on tumor cells. If true, this effect is probably not great enough to kill significant numbers of tumor cells or to make steroids an effective stand-alone therapy.

One particular tumor that is very sensitive to steroids is primary central nervous system lymphoma (PCNSL). If this type of tumor is suspected, steroids should not be used until after the diagnosis is made. There are other diseases that respond to steroids, and a pathology reading may be more difficult if the lymphoma was pre-treated with steroids. PCNSL can markedly decrease in size on scans taken immediately following the use of these drugs. Rather than controlling edema, steroids destroy lymphoma tumor cells, but they are not a long-term cure for this tumor.

How are steroids taken?

Although steroids can be started through an intravenous (IV) line or by injection into a muscle (IM), most people with a brain tumor take their steroids by mouth—also called orally. The pills come in doses that range from 0.25 milligram (mg) to 6.0 mg tablets, taken between two and four times a day. Your doctor will determine the starting dose of steroid based on your MRI scan and your symptoms. It will take 24–48 hours before you begin to see the effects of the medication, but the change is often remarkable. The dose may need to be adjusted—either increased or decreased slightly—depending on how your body reacts to them. To protect your stomach, take your steroids with food or milk. Your doctor may also prescribe an antacid to be taken daily.

If your doctor prescribes the long-term use of steroids, don't be disappointed if your steroid dose needs to be increased over time. The goal, of course, will be to find the lowest, most effective dose of medication that keeps your neurological symptoms at a minimum. With time, however, that most effective dose may need to be adjusted. The need to increase your medication does not automatically mean your tumor is growing, and it does not mean you've made errors in taking your medication.

You and your family can be of great help in this process by keeping your doctor aware of the way your body reacts to the steroids. If at any point the side effects become difficult to manage, please share your concerns with your nurse or doctor.

When your doctor feels you no longer require steroids, you will be given instructions for slowly stopping the drug. Do not abruptly stop taking your steroids. The tapering process slowly decreases your steroid dose. Your body needs this period of time to again begin producing its own steroids, and to avoid an emergency medical crisis. Lowering steroid levels too quickly can also cause a rebound increase in swelling.

Side Effects

Steroids can have several positive side effects. They can markedly decrease symptoms, give one an overall sense of well-being, temporarily increase thought and functioning abilities, and increase your appetite.

Steroids can also cause a wide range of effects that must be carefully monitored by your doctor. The most common side-effects are: weight gain; thinning of the skin; gastrointestinal upset; muscle weakness in your thighs, shoulders, and neck; susceptibility to infections; masking or hiding a fever; mood swings; insomnia; pneumonia; and increased blood sugar levels (especially if you have diabetes). Steroids can interact with some seizure medications, either increasing or lowering their levels in your blood, which can alter their effectiveness. Other, more serious side-effects can occur, although they are less common.

The benefits of steroid use almost always outweigh their potential side effects. If you have any questions about balancing risks and benefits, please talk with your doctor.

Managing Common Side Effects

Weight gain and increased blood sugar: After a few months of steroid use, you may begin to notice a significant weight gain. This is not the fatty weight of overeating—it is your body processing and storing food in a different way. You may notice your face looks puffy or moon-like, and you've developed a small hump on your back, just below the neck, called a buffalo hump. You may notice stretch marks across your abdomen as it increases in size, while your upper arms and legs seem to become thinner. These changes are due to your body storing more fat on the trunk of your body and less in your extremities. While this is an unavoidable effect of steroids, there are several things you can do to help manage this change in your body.

First, steroid weight gain gradually increases. If you gain more than five pounds in one week, please call your doctor. A sudden, large weight increase can signal medical problems that should be reported to your health care team.

Second, ask your doctor for a referral to a licensed registered dietician experienced in treating people on steroids. This may be a dietician who regularly works with cancer patients, or a dietician experienced in treating people with pituitary disorders. Either can be of help in outlining a healthy eating plan that will provide the nutrients important to your healing, yet limit those which your body has difficulty with right now. Since nutritional needs vary from person to person, a professional is your best resource for this help.

Third, it's important that your body maintain its ability to flush waste out of your system. Keep your kidneys and bowels in good shape—don't stop drinking water. It's a natural reaction to try to avoid adding liquids to your body right now, but that will only compound the problem.

Steroids may affect your blood sugar level, especially if you are diabetic. If your sugar levels increase, you may be referred to both an endocrinologist and a dietician. In some cases medication may need to be started or your existing medication may need to be adjusted.

Gastrointestinal problems: Steroids can cause an upset stomach. Be sure to take your medication with food, milk, or an antacid that your doctor prescribes for you. Call your doctor if you have stomach pains, run a temperature, are constipated, or notice any blood in your bowel movement. Avoid the use of non-steroidal anti-inflammatory drugs (NSAIDs such as Advil, Motrin, and Aleve) and aspirin unless directed by your doctor. While you are on steroids, it is especially important that you have regular bowel movements. If you become constipated, or experience diarrhea, call your health care team.

Insomnia: Sleep disturbances are a possible side effect of changing hormone levels. If you have difficulty sleeping, ask your doctor if your dosage can be adjusted so you take more medication in the morning and less after dinner. (Don't make this change on your own.) Healthful sleeping habits, such as avoiding bright light, caffeine, and sugar as bedtime approaches, and a regular nighttime routine may be of help.

Depression/mood changes: While taking steroids, you might experience depression, mood swings, irritability, or agitation. These symptoms are due to the steroid's effect on the natural hormone balance in your body, and can be treated. Let your doctor know how you are feeling. Medications may relieve some of these symptoms and can be particularly helpful if you remain on steroids for a long period of time. It is also helpful to discuss these effects with your family so they know what to expect and can be supportive.

Muscle weakness: Steroids sometimes cause weakness in the muscles of the legs, arms, neck, and chest. Leg weakness may be most noticeable when you get up from a sitting position and try to use the large muscles in your thighs. If leg weakness is a problem, ask for assistance when using the bathroom or getting up from a chair. Walk with another person who can get help should you stumble, or try an assistive device, such as a cane or walker. If the chest muscles are affected, you may experience difficulty breathing or pain when taking deep breaths—especially if you have a history of asthma, emphysema, or smoking. Please be sure your doctor is aware of your past medical history. Ask your doctor about exercises that may help strengthen your muscles, or for a referral for physical therapy.

Infections: Steroids have a tricky way of masking, or hiding, the beginning of an infection in your body. Be alert to anything that just doesn't seem right. An increase in temperature may be the first, or only, sign something is amiss. Because of that, some people on steroids take their temperature at the same time every day, regardless of how they feel. This is an easy way to keep a baseline check on your good health. Additionally, look at your tongue each time you brush your teeth—people on steroids are especially prone to yeast infections, or thrush, in their mouth. If you notice a thick white coating on your tongue, make your nurse or doctor aware.

Some people are prone to developing a certain type of pneumonia after they have been on steroids for awhile. Your doctor may start you on an antibiotic to prevent this from happening. Bactrim is a drug commonly used for this purpose, but please let your doctor know if you are allergic to sulfa-based drugs.

While you are on steroids, follow the health precautions used by people at higher risk for infection. Wash all fresh fruits and vegetables carefully. Wear gloves when using a kitchen knife. Cook meat and poultry until well done. Use gardening gloves when working outside. Avoid crowds and, in general, avoid sick people.

Call your doctor if:

- You are running a temperature—even if you feel well otherwise.

- You see any blood in your bowel movements.

- You have stomach pain.

- You gain more than five pounds in one week.

- You develop a rash.

- You are drinking and urinating a lot.

- You are falling.

- You have chest pains or difficulty breathing which may signal a medical emergency—call for emergency help.

The Next Steps

We hope that the information in this chapter helps you understand how these drugs work, and provides the knowledge you need to be more comfortable caring for yourself or your family member while they are on steroids. As stated, the goal of steroid treatment will be to use the minimal amount of medication necessary, and to wean you from the medication as soon as practical.

Regardless of where you are in your treatment, your task is becoming well again. Make appointments for your follow-up doctor visits or scans and mark them on your calendar. Find a support group if you'd like to meet others with brain tumors. See friends. Learn about your tumor. The information in this chapter is meant to help you communicate better with the people who are caring for you. The purpose is not to provide answers; rather, to encourage you to ask questions.

Chapter 10

Chemotherapy and the Brain

Chapter Contents

Section 10.1

Chemotherapy for Brain Tumors

"Chemotherapy," © 2008 American Brain Tumor
Association (www.abta.org). Reprinted with permission.

What is chemotherapy?

Chemotherapy is the use of drugs to treat cancer. Chemotherapy drugs are typically used to treat malignant or higher grade tumors, but may also be used to treat low grade and benign brain tumors.

Why is chemotherapy used?

Most cells in the body are capable of duplicating into two new cells when the body needs them. Those two cells double into four, the four into eight, and so on. This reproductive process is controlled by a set of internal switches which tell the body when new cells are needed, and signal the body to slow down this process when cells are not needed. If the body continues making unneeded cells, or if the new cells are abnormal and reproduction continues, the excess cells form a mass called a tumor.

The goals of chemotherapy are to stop tumor growth by making the cells unable to duplicate themselves, or to artificially start the normal process of cell death called apoptosis. In normal body organs, apoptosis controls the number of cells in our body at any given time. In cancer, the tumor cells may be resistant to the signals of apoptosis. Or the tumor cells may begin reproducing more rapidly than the number of cells dying, leading to overall tumor growth.

Chemotherapy drugs are used to stop this reproductive process or to alter the behavior of tumor cells. There are two broad categories of chemotherapy drugs: cytotoxic drugs, which are intended to lead to cell death, or cytostatic drugs, also called targeted or biologic drugs, which prevent cell reproduction.

How does chemotherapy work?

In order for a cell to split itself into two normal cells, the parent cell must complete several tasks in a very specific order. This list of tasks is called the cell cycle. It includes jobs such as making the proteins and enzymes needed to fuel the cell's reproductive process, duplicating the deoxyribonucleic acid (DNA) within the cell, and then separating that DNA into sets—one set for each new cell. Chemotherapy drugs can stop cells from starting or completing the cell cycle. Chemotherapy drugs that stop cells from starting the process of division are often called targeted or biologic agents. These treatments work differently than classic chemotherapy which affects the cell during the process of cell division.

Some chemotherapy drugs act during specific parts of the cell cycle; thus, those drugs are called cell-cycle specific drugs. Other drugs are effective at any time during the cell-cycle; those are called non cell-cycle specific drugs. Sometimes chemotherapy treatment plans use a combination of cell-cycle specific and non-cell cycle specific drugs in an attempt to treat a larger number of tumor cells.

When might chemotherapy not be recommended?

There are reasons why chemotherapy might not be suggested as a treatment for your tumor.

Not all brain tumors are sensitive to, or respond to chemotherapy: If it is known that your type of tumor does not respond to chemotherapy, or it becomes resistant to the drug that is being used, other treatments can be recommended. Your tumor may be able to be removed with surgery alone, or may be sensitive to radiation therapy. Some tumors respond to treatment with hormones or drugs that control hormone production. Other tumors may be sensitive to some of the new biologic therapies.

Chemotherapy affects both normal and tumor cells: Although chemotherapy drugs have a greater effect on rapidly reproducing cells, such as tumor cells, the drugs cannot always tell the difference between normal cells and tumor cells. The side effects of chemotherapy are really the effects of the chemotherapy drugs on those normal cells.

Chemotherapy drugs affect some normal cells to a greater degree than others. Cells which turn over or regenerate rapidly are also the most vulnerable to side effects. These particularly sensitive areas include the cells which line the mouth and the gastrointestinal tract. For example, some chemotherapy drugs cause mouth sores; those sores are really the shedding of the normal cells lining the mouth. Diarrhea occurs because the rapidly reproducing cells of the gastrointestinal

(GI) tract are also very sensitive to chemotherapy. Good general health prior to starting chemotherapy helps the body heal itself during and after chemotherapy, but this healing takes time.

How is chemotherapy given?

Scientists have developed different ways of getting chemotherapy drugs to the tumor cells. Some of these methods require the drug to spread through the body, via the bloodstream, to the brain—this is called systemic delivery. Other methods focus on placing the drug within or around the tumor—this is called local delivery.

Systemic delivery: Some systemic drugs are given by mouth, also called orally. Lomustine (CCNU) and temozolomide (Temodar) are examples of systemic drugs. They travel through the body via the blood, cross the blood brain barrier, and into the tumor cells. Both CCNU and temozolomide are pills; therefore, they are taken orally.

Some systemic drugs are given by injection. Injection routes may be into an artery, also called intra-arterial (IA) delivery; into a muscle, also called intramuscular (IM) delivery; into a vein, also called intravenous (IV) delivery; and into the skin, also called subcutaneous (SubQ) delivery.

Local delivery: Some drugs can be placed closer to the tumor, or within the areas of tumor growth. The goals of local delivery are to avoid delivering drugs throughout the body, and to increase the concentration of drug at the tumor site. The variations in local delivery are: into the cavity left by tumor removal (intracavitary delivery); into the brain tissue (interstitial delivery): into the space between the meninges (intrathecal delivery); into the tumor by use of gravity or controlled flow (convection enhanced delivery); into the tumor (intratumoral delivery); and into a ventricle (intraventricular delivery).

What type of chemotherapy drugs are used for brain tumors?

Chemotherapy drugs can be generally classified as those that lead to cell death (cytotoxic drugs) or those that prevent cell division or tumor growth (cytostatic drugs).Within those broad categories, chemotherapy drugs are then grouped by the way they work, the effect they have on tumor cells, and the time in the cells' lives during which they are thought to be most effective.

Cytotoxic Drugs

Alkylating agents: These drugs work by forming a molecular bond in the DNA strands inside tumor cells, which prevents them from reproducing. Carboplatin, cisplatin, cyclophosphamide, and temozolomide (Temodar) are examples of alkylating agents. Nitrosoureas are a subclass of alkylating agents. They stop tumor cells from repairing themselves and thus render them unable to reproduce. Carmustine (BCNU) and lomustine (CCNU) are nitrosoureas.

Antimetabolites: These drugs stop tumor cells from making the enzymes needed for new cell growth. Methotrexate (MTX) is an example of an antimetabolite.

Anti-tumor antibiotics: This group of drugs stop the action of enzymes needed for cell growth, and may be able to change the environment around the cell. Rapamycin, for example, is an anti-tumor antibiotic.

Hormones: These substances may be capable of interfering with tumor growth by blocking the production of certain proteins in the tumor cells. For example, tamoxifen is a hormone-based drug also used to treat breast cancer. In studying the way the drug works, researchers observed that tamoxifen may be capable of suppressing some of the proteins involved in the growth of malignant brain tumors. It is a protein kinase C inhibitor.

Mitotic inhibitors: These substances are usually plant-based, natural substances that interfere with the production of the proteins needed to create new cells. Etoposide (VP-16), paclitaxel (Taxol), and vincristine are examples of mitotic inhibitors.

Steroids: These drugs are used to decrease swelling around the tumor. While they are not intended to be cytotoxic therapy, some researchers do believe steroids have some toxic effect on tumor cells. If true, this effect is probably not enough to kill significant numbers of cells. One exception to this, however, is primary central nervous system (CNS) lymphoma, which is particularly sensitive to steroids. Rather than controlling edema, steroids destroy lymphoma tumor cells, but they are not a long-term cure for this tumor.

Cytostatic Agents

Drugs aimed at reducing drug resistance: There are enzymes, found in normal cells in the body, which if occurring in high concentration may be capable of making a tumor resistant to chemotherapy drugs. Drugs are being developed to inhibit these resistance enzymes. O6-benzylguanine (O6-BG), an example of this type of drug, is being tested in clinical trials in the hope of countering this resistance.

Anti-angiogenesis inhibitors: A tumor requires nutrients in order to grow; those nutrients make their way to the tumor via an elaborate system of blood vessels developed by the tumor to maintain an adequate blood supply. The growth of these blood vessels around a tumor is angiogenesis; interference with their growth is angiogenesis inhibition. Thalidomide, interferon, bevacizumab (Avastin), cilengitide (EMD 121974), lenalidomide (Revlimid), AZD 2171 (cediranib), and VEGF Trap are all drugs being tested for their potential in stopping the growth of a tumor's blood supply. Angiogenesis inhibition may be combined with traditional chemotherapy drugs in an effort to increase the effectiveness of both.

Growth factor inhibitors: Normal cell growth relies on a delicate balance of proteins and enzymes in the brain. These growth factors serve as food for brain cells, and are simultaneously capable of controlling the growth of new cells. Inappropriate levels of growth factors, however, may cause the overgrowth of cells and the subsequent development of a brain tumor. Tyrosine kinase inhibitors, such as imatinib mesylate (Gleevec), and drugs that interfere with growth factor receptors such as gefitinib (Iressa), erlotinib (Tarceva), sorafenib (Nexavar), and cediranib (AZD 2171) are being studied.

What type of treatment schedule can I expect?

The doctor who suggests chemotherapy for your tumor will provide you with a treatment plan, or schedule, of the days the drugs will be given. Your schedule will be specific to the type of drug(s) recommended for your tumor, and may be a different schedule than other people you meet who are going through chemotherapy.

A chemotherapy treatment plan may also be based on the purpose of the drug. For example, radiosensitizers are drugs used to make a tumor more sensitive to radiation therapy. They are only used before or during radiation.

Some chemotherapy, such as temozolomide, may be started at the same time as radiation therapy, then used as a maintenance therapy for a while after radiation is completed.

Your treatment schedule may also be impacted by the way your body responds to the drugs and the side effects you may have as a result of the treatment. Common side effects associated with cytotoxic chemotherapy include hair loss, nausea and vomiting, diarrhea or constipation, fatigue, and lowered blood counts. Biologic agents often have side effects that are different than the traditional side effects often associated with chemotherapy. For example, rashes on the hands or face, fatigue or sleepiness, hypertension, skin dryness, or bleeding with a normal platelet count may occur. It is important to talk to your health care team if you are receiving a newer drug, they can tell you what to expect with your particular treatment plan.

Blood tests will be done at regular times during your chemotherapy treatment to monitor the impact on blood counts. Chemotherapy particularly affects white blood cells (which fight infection), red blood cells (which carry oxygen around your body), and platelets (which help the blood to clot). It is not unusual for a person's blood count to be lower during treatment, but this does not necessarily alter your treatment schedule. However, if you have any indication of an infection, such as a fever or abnormal bleeding, notify your doctor immediately. Your next chemotherapy treatment might be postponed until your blood count recovers, but this is ultimately for your benefit.

If your blood cell count begins to drop, ask your nurse at what level you should be concerned. If your blood count reaches that level, ask for tips on protecting your health until those counts again begin to increase. Some simple precautions can help get you back on the road to wellness. Examples include:

- If your white cell count drops to a point that your nurse talks with you about being at increased risk, protect yourself from infection. Eat a well balanced diet, being careful to thoroughly rinse fresh fruits and vegetables, cook meats and poultry until well done, stay away from crowds, and rest.

- If your red cell count drops, you may feel fatigued or tire more quickly than usual. You may also feel dizzy when changing positions. When you first wake up, sit on the side of the bed before standing. Use caution on stairways. Talk with your nurse about ways to manage treatment-related fatigue. Ask your doctor or nurse if iron supplements are appropriate for you.

- If your platelet count drops to a point that your nurse tells you that you are at increased risk of bleeding, you may find that you bleed easier or it takes longer to stop your bleeding. Try to avoid bumping or bruising yourself. Use an electric razor, take precautions in the kitchen, and brush your teeth with a soft foam brush. Call your nurse or doctor immediately if your urine or bowel movements change color or if you have excessive bruising or any bleeding such as from the gums or from the nose.

After your doctor outlines your chemotherapy schedule, talk it over with your family. Planning can help you address the practicalities of being in treatment. Sometimes chemotherapy goes on for a year or more; arranging a new daily schedule for yourself and/or your family can help make the transition a bit easier. Flexible work schedules, part-time or full-time childcare, pre-prepared meals, frequent rest periods, and fewer activities for a couple of days following your treatment can help minimize the impact of the chemotherapy schedule on your life.

What other methods are used to deliver chemotherapy drugs?

The following represent several other approaches to delivering chemotherapy. Not all of these are considered standard methods of delivering drugs, but they do represent innovative ways of bringing drugs closer to the tumor. The use of drugs targeted to specific molecular differences in tumor cells is rapidly moving forward; the American Brain Tumor Association (ABTA) website (www.abta.org) offers updates in drug delivery and targeted drug information.

Blood brain barrier disruption: Treating brain tumors with chemotherapy is different than treating tumors elsewhere in the body. The brain has a natural defense system not present in your other organs. That system, called the blood brain barrier, protects the brain by acting as a filter. This works to our advantage when harmful substances, such as certain chemicals or bacteria, are kept out of the brain. It works to our disadvantage when substances we want to enter the brain, such as chemotherapy drugs, are filtered out.

Some drugs do pass through the blood brain barrier. The drugs called nitrosoureas (such as BCNU and CCNU) are such drugs, as well as procarbazine and temozolomide (Temodar). Studies continue to explore other standard drugs, as well as new drugs, for their ability to penetrate this protective barrier.

Some tumors are behind this barrier. For a drug to be effective in treating these brain tumors, a sufficient quantity must either pass through the blood brain barrier or bypass it entirely. Blood brain barrier disruption is a technique used to temporarily disrupt this barrier in order to allow chemotherapy to flow into the brain. During blood brain barrier disruption, a drug called Mannitol is used to temporarily open the barrier. Very high doses of chemotherapy drugs are then injected into an artery or a vein. The drug travels through the blood, through the blood brain barrier, and into the tumor area. The barrier is restored naturally as the effects of the Mannitol wear off. Researchers are looking into new ways of opening the barrier, and the most effective dose of drug to use once the barrier is open.

Blood-brain barrier disruption has been used mainly to treat primary central nervous system lymphoma and high-grade astrocytoma tumors.

Blood or marrow stem cell transplantation: One of the more common side effects of chemotherapy is damage to the bone marrow—the part of the body that produces new blood cells. The possibility of bone marrow damage limits the amount of drug that can be given.

Doctors can now preserve immature blood cells, called stem cells, and give them back to the patient following their chemotherapy. This procedure is called a stem cell transplant. An autologous transplant means the patient's own stem cells will be used. An allogenic transplant uses stem cells from a donor.

Prior to chemotherapy, stem cells are collected, or harvested, from the donor's circulating blood. They can also be collected from the pelvic bone; however, the use of blood instead of bone marrow is becoming more common. Researchers are also exploring new sources of obtaining stem cells, such as fat cells and skin cells, but this is still experimental.

Following the harvesting of the stem cells or marrow cells, an intensive course of chemotherapy is administered over several days. After therapy is complete, the stem cells are given to the patient through an intravenous solution. During the next ten days, the stem cells begin to mature and reproduce, re-supplying the body with healthy blood cells. Drugs are given to suppress the body's tendency to reject the new cells, and growth factors can be used to boost the growth rate of the new cells.

Because of the possibility of the body rejecting the new stem cells and the risks of intensive chemotherapy, stem cell and bone marrow transplantation is used only in select circumstances. Transplantations should be done at experienced institutions with a multi-disciplinary team. The team can assist with donor matching, supportive counseling, family member housing during treatment, and financial counseling.

Comprehensive resources and information on transplant centers are available from:

Bone Marrow Transplantation (BMT) Network
2310 Skokie Valley Road, Suite 107
Highland Park, IL 60035
Toll-Free: 888-597-7674
Phone: 847-433-3313
Website: http://www.bmtinfonet.org
E-mail: help@bmtinfonet.org

Those seeking a donor, or those wishing to donate stem cells or marrow, can register with:

National Marrow Donor's Registry Program
3001 Broadway St. NE, Suite 100
Minneapolis, MN 55413
Toll-Free: 800-627-7692
Phone: 612-627-8140
Website: http://www.marrow.org
E-mail: patientinfo@nmdp.org

Convection enhanced delivery (CED): One of the newer methods of delivering drugs to a tumor, CED uses the principles of constant pressure to flow or infuse substances through brain tumor tissue. The procedure begins with surgery, during which a catheter (or multiple catheters, depending on the tumor size) is placed into the tumor area. The neurosurgeon then connects a pump-like device to the catheter, filling it with the therapeutic substance to be delivered to the tumor. The fluid flows, by use of pressure and gravity, through the tumor tissue. This bulk flow or convective-delivery method bypasses the blood brain barrier, placing the therapeutic substance in direct contact with tumor tissue.

Clinical trials are exploring the use of CED as a way of placing chemotherapy drugs, immunotoxins, and radioactive monoclonal antibodies at the tumor site.

As this technique is developing, researchers are simultaneously exploring ways to include tracers in the substances flowing into the brain. Those tracers can be viewed on a magnetic resonance imaging (MRI) scan performed during CED, and may allow real-time observations of the movement of therapeutic substances in and around the tumor. Research is also underway to predict the flow pattern that will occur after catheter placement.

High dose chemotherapy: Some scientists believe that higher doses of chemotherapy drugs may cross the blood brain barrier more effectively than lower drug doses spread over a longer treatment period. High-dose chemotherapy involves the administration of massive doses of chemotherapy drug, followed by an antidote which reverses the effect of the drug on normal cells. Methotrexate is the drug most often used for high-dose chemotherapy, and Leucovorin is the most common antidote. This technique has been offered to those with primary central nervous system lymphomas or high-grade astrocytomas. It is sometimes combined with a stem cell transplant.

Intracavity/polymer wafer implants/interstitial therapies: When treatment is delivered into the cavity created by the removal of the tumor, it is known as intracavitary (inside the cavity) therapy. Among these methods are implanted catheters and/or polymer wafer implants placed during surgery. These techniques have the potential advantage of reducing the amount of drug affecting normal cells in the brain and throughout the body, and increasing the amount of drug reaching tumor cells.

Surgery is typically performed to remove as much of the tumor as possible, but because the cells of a malignant tumor may spread into the surrounding brain tissue, additional therapy may be needed. Placing polymer wafer implants soaked in the chemotherapy drug carmustine (BCNU) on the walls of the resection releases the chemotherapy into the local region. The wafer implants, also called Gliadel, limit the amount of BCNU that circulates through the body. Your neurosurgeon will place up to eight wafers into cavity, based on the size of the removed tumor. The wafers are implanted immediately after the tumor is removed, adding only a few additional minutes to the surgical procedure. The neurosurgeon then surgically closes the area, leaving the wafers to gradually dissolve over the next 2–3 week period. As they dissolve, BCNU is released. While the rate that the wafers dissolve varies by patient, studies have found that approximately 70% of the wafers are gone within three weeks of placement at the tumor site. All of the chemotherapy has been released by that time. It is usually not necessary to remove the wafers since they are biodegradable.

Reservoirs and pumps: Chemotherapy can also be delivered directly into the fluid that bathes the brain and spinal cord—the cerebrospinal fluid. This treatment is used for leptomeningeal tumors involving the ventricles or spine, and tumors that tend to seed, or spread, down the spine. A small container system, such as an Ommaya Reservoir, is surgically placed under the scalp. A tube leads from the reservoir into a ventricle of the brain.

Medications are injected via syringe into the reservoir and then the reservoir is flushed with either saline for cerebrospinal fluid. The flushing begins the flow of drug through the ventricles and lining of the spine. Chemotherapy administered this way can be repeated on a regular schedule.

Where is drug research headed?

For years, surgery followed by radiation and/or chemotherapy were the mainstays of brain tumor treatment. Today, however, physicians and scientists are virtually changing the world of brain tumor treatment, most notably through targeted treatments—those aimed at specific parts or functions of tumor cells. The goal is to interfere with and redirect the way those cell functions normally work.

Scientists now know that tumors with the same appearance under a microscope may indeed be different biologically. For example, Tumor A and Tumor B are both glioblastomas per their pathology reports. Biologically, however, Tumor A may be producing more proteins or fewer enzymes than Tumor B. This biologic difference may explain why two people with the same type of tumor (such as glioblastoma) may react differently to treatment, and have very different outcomes. This new knowledge is helping researchers to create therapies that target the biologic markers on the surface of tumor cells or the genetic material inside the tumor cells. As a result, a new world of innovative drugs, immune therapies, and drug delivery systems is emerging. These therapies use altered genes, engineered viruses, and drugs packaged into molecules too small to be seen with microscopes.

Targeted therapies: Some of the newest drugs block the growth and spread of tumor cells by interfering with the proteins that may control tumor growth. Monoclonal antibodies, for example, are proteins that can locate and bind to the surface of tumor cells. There are many types of monoclonal antibodies. Some carry drugs, toxins or radioactive materials directly to tumors. Others interfere with the normal work of the tumor cells, leaving tumor cells incapable of reproducing.

Bevacizumab, also known as Avastin, is a monoclonal antibody that binds to and inhibits vascular endothelial growth factor (VEGF)—a protein capable of controlling the blood supply to a tumor. While Avastin has been successfully used to treat some colorectal and lung cancers, clinical trials show it may slow or stop tumor growth in some glioblastoma patients. Some trials are also exploring Avastin combined with temozolomide, irinotecan (CPT11), or other drugs that may increase the treatment's effectiveness.

Separate research is studying the role of another protein called O6-methylguanine-DNA methyltransferase (MGMT). Scientists are studying this protein as a potential chemosensitivity marker. Other research seeks to learn if a drug called 06 benzylguanine (06BG), given prior to, or with chemotherapy, can interfere with MGMT to make the chemotherapy more effective. Ongoing research also is investigating whether extended treatment with temozolomide (Temodar) chemotherapy, the dose-dense schedule, will reduce MGMT activity and restore chemosensitivity.

In some brain tumors, several cell-growth switches may be simultaneously overactive, thus requiring multiple drugs to stop tumor growth. These switches, formed by molecules called receptor tyrosine kinases (RTK), are often mutated and hyperactive in tumor cells. A number of RTK-blocking drugs are being tested in brain tumors, including imatinib mesylate (Gleevec) and erlotinib (Tarceva).

There are many other targeted drugs now being tested against brain tumors. For help finding a study for your type of tumor, call the National Cancer Institute's Cancer Information Service toll-free at 800-422-6237.

New drug delivery systems: One of the greatest challenges in brain tumor treatment is knowing exactly where the tumor is located, where the borders are, and how to successfully reach the site through surgery and/or drugs. Fortunately, today's therapies are being aided by state-of-the-art drug delivery systems that can pinpoint the exact location of a tumor, and administer precise treatment.

Through nanotechnology, for example, tiny plastic/polymer materials are being developed for use as implants containing anticancer drugs. When the anticancer drug camptothecin (CPT) is linked to the polymer polyethylene glycol (PEG), the drug penetrates more than one centimeter into the drug implant site (ten times deeper than conventional medications).

Studies are being done on nano-bubbles delivering the chemotherapy drug, doxorubicin, directly to cancer cells in mice. When exposed to ultrasound, the bubbles generate an echo allowing the tumor to be imaged. The sound energy from the ultrasound then pops the bubbles and releases the drug.

Treatments of tomorrow: These innovative therapies represent the efforts of thousands of scientists, all focused on finding a cure for brain tumors. In the not too distant future, even more sophisticated scanning will visualize the DNA and ribonucleic acid (RNA) inside tumor cells. We are at the cusp of finding brain tumor treatments specific to the biology of each tumor. Treatment will be personalized not to groups of people, but to your own individual genetic makeup.

What side effects might I experience from chemotherapy?

The side effects of chemotherapy are specific to the drug, or drugs, being used. When your doctor outlines a treatment plan for you, ask for fact sheets or drug sheets about each of the drugs suggested. Following are the more commonly used brain tumor drugs and some of their side effects. Your health care team can talk with you about the chances of these effects occurring based on your treatment plan, and how to care for yourself while taking these drugs.

Bevacizumab (Avastin) alone: Delayed wound healing, high blood pressure, nosebleeds, excessive protein in the urine, and headache. When given in combination with a traditional chemotherapy drug, other symptoms such as decreased immune function, weakness, fatigue, stomach pain, nausea and vomiting, loss of appetite, upper respiratory infection (nose, sinuses, and/or throat), diarrhea, constipation, hair loss, and mouth sores may occur. Bevacizumab may cause the effects of chemotherapy on your blood and bone marrow to be more severe than if the chemotherapy were given alone. Other, less common side effects may include dizziness, shortness of breath, and muscle pain. Rare but serious side effects associated with bevacizumab include: holes in the esophagus and gastrointestinal tract, sudden bleeding at the tumor site, kidney damage, a severe increase in blood pressure possibly leading to a stroke, and heart failure.

Carboplatin: Nausea and vomiting, bleeding, lowered white cell counts, lowered red cell counts, numbness or tingling in the hands and feet, hair loss.

Carmustine given intravenously (BCNU, BiCNU): Fatigue, pain at the injection site, nausea and vomiting, lowered white cell count, lowered red cell count, bleeding, hair loss, diarrhea, confusion, breathing problems, lowered blood pressure, and mouth and throat sores. When administered in polymer wafer implants (Gliadel), side effects may include headache, nausea, and/or fatigue due to temporary increased swelling in the brain. Less common, more serious side effects include seizures, brain edema (swelling), wound infection, partial paralysis (hemiplegia), and language difficulty (aphasia).

Cilengitide (EMD121974): Fatigue, joint pain, nausea, vomiting, drowsiness, loss of appetite, intestinal cramps, mouth sores, altered taste sensations, headache, body ache, vision changes, arm and leg swelling, shortness of breath, coughing, rash, itching, lowered white cell count, lowered platelet count, and kidney damage.

Cisplatin (Platinol): Hearing changes, nausea and vomiting, kidney damage, lowered white cell count, lowered red cell count, bleeding, numbness or tingling in the hands and feet, foot drop, metallic taste to food, and appetite changes.

Etoposide (VP-16): Lowered red cell count, bleeding, lowered white cell count, nausea and vomiting, constipation, decreased blood pressure, hair loss, fatigue, mouth and throat sores, and decreased appetite.

Hydroxyurea (Hydrea): Lowered white cell count, bleeding, lowered red cell count, nausea and vomiting, diarrhea, constipation, rash, itching, fatigue, mouth sores, decreased appetite.

Irinotecan (CPT-11 or Camptosar): Anxiety, diarrhea, changes in stool and urine color, heartburn, indigestion, nausea and vomiting, redness, numbness or tingling sensations in the hands or feet, dizziness, skin rash, drowsiness, low blood counts, hair loss, and sleeplessness.

Lomustine (CCNU): Nausea and vomiting, lowered white cell count, bleeding, mouth sores, hair loss, and lowered red cell count.

Methotrexate (MTX): Mouth sores, lowered white cell count, nausea and vomiting, diarrhea, lowered red cell count, bleeding, fatigue, darkening of the skin, hypersensitivity to sun, liver damage, kidney damage, and decreased appetite.

Procarbazine (Matulane): Nausea and vomiting, confusion, numbness or tingling in the feet and hands, hair loss, depression, nervousness, sleeplessness, appetite changes, lowered white cell count, bleeding, lowered red cell count, muscle aches, fatigue, alcohol intolerance (severe nausea and vomiting if alcoholic beverages are drunk), reactions to food with high-tyramine content (see your doctor for a list of foods to be avoided), and darkened skin color.

Tamoxifen (Nolvadex): Hot flashes, menstrual changes, menopause symptoms, blurred vision, increased fertility (talk with your doctor about this), vaginal discharge, blood clots, temporary memory loss, and increased risk of uterine cancer with long-term use.

Temozolomide (Temodar): Nausea and vomiting, headache, fatigue, seizures, constipation, diarrhea, weakness, bleeding, lowered white cell count, lowered platelet counts, and anemia.

Vincristine (Oncovin): Numbness or tingling of the hands and feet, constipation, nausea and vomiting, vision changes, light sensitivity, depression, drowsiness, confusion, hoarseness, mouth sores, fatigue, hair loss, muscle weakness, problems urinating, and jaw pain.

Are there ways to manage some of the common side effects of chemotherapy?

The nurses on your health care team can give you helpful tips, practical information, and put you in touch with resources to help you feel better through treatment. Following are just a few samples of the type of information available to you as you move through treatment. Reaching out for these resources can help you better control possible treatment effects, and help you feel your best through, and beyond, treatment. Whether you are being treated in a hospital setting, outpatient clinic, or at home, your nurses can help. Just ask.

In addition, the American Brain Tumor Association (ABTA) social workers can help you find wigs, hair accessories, home care services, patient and caregiver support networks. A series of articles, titled "Becoming Well Again," can help you and your family understand the assistance offered to you through rehabilitative medicine programs, memory retraining, physical and occupational therapy services, and much more. ABTA social workers can be reached at 800-886-2282 or by e-mail to socialwork@abta.org.

Vomiting: One of the most feared effects of chemotherapy is vomiting. Remarkable advances have been made in the development of a new generation of drugs called anti-emetics, which control this effect. Prior to starting treatment, ask your health care team if the drug prescribed for you will cause nausea or vomiting. If so, be sure you are provided with an anti-emetic plan specific to the chemotherapy drugs you will be given. There are both preventive drugs that can control vomiting before it starts, and drugs that can be used if you are already nauseated or actively vomiting. Be sure to follow the instructions carefully. Some anti-emetic drugs must be started before the chemotherapy drug is given and continued for two or three days after the chemotherapy. Some anti-emetic drugs are given by mouth, some by injection, and some by suppository (rectally). Be sure you understand how you are to use the drugs, and try not to miss a dose. If you have any questions about your anti-emetic plan, please call the nurse who oversees your chemotherapy drugs or talk with your doctor.

Diarrhea: Chemotherapy-related diarrhea may occur when drugs used to treat the tumor irritate the lining of the gastrointestinal tract. That irritation may cause your intestines to absorb fluids more slowly than they usually would, and thus, diarrhea occurs. While you have diarrhea, avoid high-fiber foods and foods that can irritate the bowel such as bran, whole grain breads, fried foods, fruit juices, milk products, and coffee. Until the diarrhea slows try a diet of bananas, applesauce, toast, and clear liquids. Drink plenty of fluids to prevent becoming dehydrated. Your nurses and doctors can also suggest medications to slow the diarrhea, but do not use over-the-counter medications without first talking with your health care professionals.

Fatigue: The most common side effect of chemotherapy is fatigue; it is experienced by almost everyone undergoing treatment for a brain tumor. This fatigue is different from the fatigue you might have experienced in the past. Treatment-related fatigue is severe, persistent, and does not always follow physical activity. It can be unpredictable and emotionally overwhelming. Most telling, it isn't fully relieved by rest or sleep. If you have already experienced weakness or other neurologic symptoms as a result of the tumor, the fatigue may make these symptoms more severe. The first step in managing fatigue is letting your health care team know the extent of your symptoms. There is a difference between feeling tired and being so exhausted you cannot get out of bed; be sure your nurse or doctor understands the full extent of your symptoms. Your health care team can check to be sure that this is treatment-related fatigue, and verify there are no other underlying medical concerns causing your symptoms. From there, your nurses can talk with you about ways to manage your fatigue and lessen it's impact on your quality of life.

Fertility and fetal injury: For males and females, concerns about fertility and the ability to start a future family must be addressed in advance of your first chemotherapy treatment. The drugs used for chemotherapy may cause damage to an unborn fetus, damage to a child conceived during chemotherapy, or damage to a child conceived within the first two years after chemotherapy (the exact time varies with the drug). Some drugs carry a greater chance of fetal injury than others.

There are many options for saving eggs and sperm, and for other parenthood options, but these must be planned in advance. For information about these options, contact FertileHOPE, a partner of the Lance Armstrong Foundation, at 888-994-4673. They can also be reached via their web site at www.fertilehope.org.

What are the potential benefits of chemotherapy?

The ultimate goal of chemotherapy is to kill tumor cells, or minimally, to stop their growth. Sometimes the intent is to shrink a tumor so that it can be further treated or removed. Chemotherapy may also be used to make a tumor more sensitive to other treatments such as radiation therapy.

There are many benefits that can result from chemotherapy alone, or when combined with other treatments such as surgery or radiation. Your doctor can tell you the goal of your treatment plan. He/she can also help you balance the potential risks of therapy against the benefits, helping you make an informed decision about your care.

What are the potential risks of chemotherapy?

Chemotherapy, like any treatment, carries risks. Some of these are the more common side effects already discussed; others are rarer and do not apply to everyone going through chemotherapy. Those rarer risks include interactions with other drugs, infertility, damage to an unborn fetus, seizures, weakness, balance or coordination difficulties, memory or cognitive problems, brain swelling, damage to other internal organs, stroke, or very rarely, coma or death. Some forms of chemotherapy may possibly prevent your future participation in research studies; your doctor can tell you if the drug or treatment methods suggested for you fall into this area. Ask your doctor and nurses to help you balance the risks against the potential benefits.

How will we know if the chemotherapy is effective?

At periodic intervals, your doctor will order follow-up magnetic resonance imaging (MRI) or computed tomography (CT) scans to be done while you are going through chemotherapy and for a year or two after. It may take a few rounds of chemotherapy, however, before the size of your tumor begins to look smaller on your scans. Sometimes the reduction in tumor size is very dramatic and happens quickly; sometimes it takes a few months. If your tumor size does not reduce as much as your doctor might like, there are other drugs and other treatments that may be chosen as alternatives.

How long will it take me to recover from chemotherapy?

Any treatment is a trauma to your body. Because we each heal at our own pace, some people will recover faster than others. While there is no normal recovery period that applies to all people, your recovery time will depend on the drug(s) used to treat your brain tumor; the method used to deliver the drug/s; and the effect of the drug(s) on your general health.

Ask your doctor to consider your treatment plan and your general medical health then tell you what you can expect as a reasonable recovery time. This will help you set realistic goals for yourself in the weeks following chemotherapy.

The Next Steps

For many people with a brain tumor, chemotherapy follows surgery and radiation therapy. For some, it is the only treatment recommended for their tumor. You may now be moving on to another treatment, or you may be starting a new normal part of your life with brain tumor treatment behind you. Regardless of your prior treatment history, concluding your chemotherapy treatment can be an emotional time. Some people celebrate—others find they are anxious or even depressed. These are all normal responses to a significant change in your life.

Regardless of where you are in your treatment, your task now is becoming well again. Make appointments for your follow-up doctor visits or scans and mark them on your calendar. Seek out support services if you feel they would be of help in this transitional period of your life. See friends. Learn about your tumor. The ABTA website at http://www.abta.org offers extensive brain tumor information, treatment and research updates, and patient/family stories.

Section 10.2

Chemobrain

This section includes excerpts from "Delving into Possible Mechanisms for Chemobrain," National Cancer Institute (NCI), March 24, 2009; and text from "Managing Chemotherapy Side Effects: Memory Changes," NCI, August 2008.

Possible Mechanisms for Chemobrain

Classic symptoms of chemobrain—cognitive changes associated with cancer or cancer treatment—are most often experienced as difficulties with concentration, memory, multi-tasking, and planning ability. These changes usually first become apparent during chemotherapy (hence the name) and, in around 20% of survivors, persist well after treatment has ended. Although chemobrain was first identified and named by breast cancer survivors, research now suggests that the same constellation of symptoms also affects survivors of other cancers. Early studies of patients' cognitive functioning after chemotherapy estimated that the number of survivors with chemotherapy-associated cognitive changes ranged from 17%–75%. When researchers began to measure cancer patients' cognitive functioning both before and after chemotherapy, however, they were surprised to find that before undergoing chemotherapy, 20%–30% of patients had lower cognitive performance than would be expected based on their age and education. Subsequent studies have consistently shown similar findings.

Increased vulnerability: Studies using functional magnetic resonance imaging (fMRI) have identified structural brain abnormalities in patients treated with chemotherapy. In a study using positron emission tomography (PET) imaging, breast cancer survivors who had received chemotherapy in the previous 5–10 years used more of their brains to perform a short-term memory task than control subjects who had never received chemotherapy, a sign that their brains are having to work harder to complete the task.

Dr. Patricia Ganz and her colleagues at University of California–Los Angeles (UCLA) Jonsson Comprehensive Cancer Center suspect that uncontrolled inflammation may be a cause of chemobrain. "Many of the patients in our breast cancer survivorship program who have cognitive complaints also have fatigue, sleep disturbance, or depression," she said. "Our hypothesis is that polymorphisms in genes that regulate the immune system render some patients more vulnerable to this constellation of symptoms."

Many cancer treatments, including surgery, radiation, chemotherapy, and immunotherapy, can increase inflammation, Dr. Ganz added, which may not resolve after treatment ends. "We have found that post-treatment fatigue is associated with specific single nucleotide polymorphisms in genes that code for interleukin-1 and interleukin-6, two cell-signaling molecules associated with both inflammation and cancer-related fatigue," she explained. "Our research is examining whether disruption in immune regulation is also involved in the development of cognitive complaints."

Managing Memory Changes

You or a family member should call your doctor or nurse if you feel confused, very sad, or depressed, or if you have a hard time thinking or remembering things. Your doctor will work to find out what is causing these problems. They may be caused by stress or a medicine you are taking. Or, they may be caused by the cancer, cancer treatment, or other health problems.

Tips for Dealing with Memory Changes

- Plan your day.
- Do things that need the most thinking at the time of day when you feel best.
- Get extra rest.
- Get help to remember things.
- Write down or tape record things you want to remember.
- Write down important dates and information on a calendar.
- Use a pill box or calendar to help keep track of your medicines.
- Ask for help.
- Ask a friend or family member for extra help when you need it.

- Ask your nurse or social worker for help to keep track of medicines and clinic visits.

- If you are very confused, have someone stay with you. Don't stay home alone.

Section 10.3

Questions about Chemotherapy Treatments

Text in this section is excerpted from "Chemotherapy and You,"
National Cancer Institute (NCI), May 2007.

Chemotherapy (also called chemo) is a type of cancer treatment that uses drugs to destroy cancer cells. Chemotherapy works by stopping or slowing the growth of cancer cells, which grow and divide quickly. But it can also harm healthy cells that divide quickly, such as those that line your mouth and intestines or cause your hair to grow. Damage to healthy cells may cause side effects. Often, side effects get better or go away after chemotherapy is over.

What does chemotherapy do?

Depending on your type of cancer and how advanced it is, chemotherapy can cure cancer, control cancer, or ease cancer symptoms.

How is chemotherapy used?

Sometimes, chemotherapy is used as the only cancer treatment. But more often, you will get chemotherapy along with surgery, radiation therapy, or biological therapy. Chemotherapy can make a tumor smaller before surgery or radiation therapy; destroy cancer cells after surgery or radiation therapy; help other therapy to work better; and destroy cancer cells that have returned or spread.

How does my doctor decide which chemotherapy drugs to use?

This choice depends on the type of cancer you have. Some types of chemotherapy drugs are used for many types of cancer. Other drugs are used for just one or two types of cancer. It also depends on whether you have had chemotherapy before; and whether you have other health problems, such as diabetes or heart disease.

How often will I receive chemotherapy?

Treatment schedules for chemotherapy vary widely. How often and how long you get chemotherapy depends on your type of cancer and how advanced it is; the goals of treatment (whether chemotherapy is used to cure your cancer, control its growth, or ease the symptoms); the type of chemotherapy; and how your body reacts to chemotherapy.

You may receive chemotherapy in cycles. A cycle is a period of chemotherapy treatment followed by a period of rest. For instance, you might receive one week of chemotherapy followed by three weeks of rest. These four weeks make up one cycle. The rest period gives your body a chance to build new healthy cells.

Can I miss a dose of chemotherapy?

It is not good to skip a chemotherapy treatment. But sometimes your doctor or nurse may change your chemotherapy schedule. This can be due to side effects you are having. If this happens, your doctor or nurse will explain what to do and when to start treatment again.

How is chemotherapy given?

Chemotherapy may be given in many ways including: injection, intra-arterial (IA), intraperitoneal (IP)—into the area that contains organs such as your intestines, stomach, liver, and ovaries; intravenous (IV); topically; and orally.

Can I work during chemotherapy?

Many people can work during chemotherapy, as long as they match their schedule to how they feel. Whether or not you can work may depend on what kind of work you do. If your job allows, you may want to see if you can work part-time or work from home on days you do not feel well.

Many employers are required by law to change your work schedule to meet your needs during cancer treatment. Talk with your employer about ways to adjust your work during chemotherapy. You can learn more about these laws by talking with a social worker.

Can I take over-the-counter and prescription drugs while I get chemotherapy?

This depends on the type of chemotherapy you get and the other types of drugs you plan to take. Take only drugs that are approved by your doctor or nurse. Tell your doctor or nurse about all the over-the-counter and prescription drugs you take, including laxatives, allergy medicines, cold medicines, pain relievers, aspirin, and ibuprofen. Talk to doctor or nurse before you take any over-the-counter or prescription drugs, vitamins, minerals, dietary supplements, or herbs.

Can I take vitamins, minerals, dietary supplements, or herbs while I get chemotherapy?

Some of these products can change how chemotherapy works. For this reason, it is important to tell your doctor or nurse about all the vitamins, minerals, dietary supplements, and herbs that you take before you start chemotherapy. During chemotherapy, talk with your doctor before you take any of these products.

How will I know if my chemotherapy is working?

Your doctor will give you physical exams and medical tests (such as blood tests and x-rays). He or she will also ask you how you feel. You cannot tell if chemotherapy is working based on its side effects. Some people think that severe side effects mean that chemotherapy is working well. Or that no side effects mean that chemotherapy is not working. The truth is that side effects have nothing to do with how well chemotherapy is fighting your cancer.

Chapter 11

Radiation Therapy

Chapter Contents

Section 11.1

Conventional Radiation Therapy

Why do I need radiation treatments?

The goal of radiation is to destroy or stop brain tumor growth. Radiation success depends on several factors: the type of tumor being treated (some are more sensitive to radiation than others) and the size of the tumor (smaller tumors are usually more treatable than larger ones).

Some tumors are so sensitive to radiation that radiation therapy may be the only necessary treatment. Radiation can be used after a biopsy, or following partial or complete removal of a brain tumor. When a tumor is surgically removed, some microscopic tumor cells may remain. Radiation attempts to destroy these remaining cells.

Radiation is also used to treat inoperable tumors and tumors that have spread to the brain from another part of the body (metastatic brain tumors). Or, radiation may be used to prevent metastatic brain tumors from developing. This type of preventative therapy is called prophylactic radiation, and is most often suggested for people with small-cell lung cancer.

Sometimes the purpose of radiation therapy is to relieve symptoms rather than to eliminate the tumor. This is called palliative radiation.

Before you or your family member begins radiation treatments, you will meet a doctor—a radiation oncologist—who will plan your therapy. A radiation oncologist is a physician with advanced, specialized training in the use of radiation as a treatment for disease. When you meet with the radiation oncologist, ask what the goals are for your treatment plan. This is also your opportunity to ask questions about the treatment itself so you understand the recommendations made by your radiation oncologist.

How does radiation work?

Radiation (also called x-rays, gamma rays, or photons) either kills tumor cells directly or interferes with their ability to grow. Radiation affects both normal cells and tumor cells. However, following standard doses of radiation, healthy cells repair themselves more quickly and completely than tumor cells. As the radiation treatments continue, an increasing number of tumor cells die. The tumor shrinks as the dead cells are broken down and disposed of by the immune system.

Like any organ in the body, normal brain tissue can tolerate only a limited amount of radiation. And different brain tumors require different amounts of radiation to cure or control them. Sometimes a form of local radiation may be used in addition to, or following, conventional radiation. That is called a radiation boost.

Radiation therapy may be given before, during, or after chemotherapy, or with drugs that make tumor cells more sensitive to the radiation (radiosensitizers). In infants and young children, chemotherapy may be used to delay radiation therapy until the developing brain is more mature.

What happens before treatment begins?

First, the radiation oncologist will review your medical records including the operative reports, pathology reports, and imaging studies such as computed tomography (CT) or magnetic resonance imaging (MRI) scans. The type and location of the tumor is determined from your records. The radiation oncologist then decides on the radiation target area and the amount of radiation that area should receive.

The area to be radiated usually includes the tumor and an area surrounding the tumor. This is because some brain tumors have roots that extend out into surrounding normal brain tissue. For those with a metastatic tumor, radiation may be given to the entire brain. If the tumor has spread to the spinal cord, or if there is a high risk of this type of spread, the spine might be radiated as well.

To maximize the amount of radiation the tumor receives, and to avoid as much healthy tissue as possible, the radiation may be directed from several different angles. Computers are used to help shape and direct the radiation beams. The radiation oncologist will usually require a CT or MRI to assist with the treatment planning process and to confirm the target area.

Once the decision to proceed with radiation has been made, one or two planning sessions (called simulations) are required. Each session will last between thirty minutes and two hours. Special marks will be placed on your skin, or you may be fitted for a face mask designed to help hold your head still. The marks and face mask help insure the accurate position of your head for the radiation treatment.

You also will have the opportunity to meet with the radiation oncologist before your treatments begin. Use that time to ask any questions you still have. You might want to discuss the benefits and risks of the treatment. Managing potential side effects during or after treatment is another common area of concern. Make sure you have a clear idea of who to call, the number, and when that call should be made if something unusual occurs between treatment sessions.

Before starting your treatments, be sure to let the radiation oncologist know about all the medications you are taking. Also, if you are using antioxidant vitamins or herbal supplements, bring the bottle(s) with you so the doctor can see the products and the amounts you are taking. He or she will give you instructions about using them during radiation therapy.

Once your radiation oncologist has planned the treatment, certified radiation technologists called radiation therapists will actually operate the treatment equipment. They administer the prescribed treatments under the doctor's supervision.

What happens during treatment?

Radiation therapy is usually given on an outpatient basis. Unless radiation is to be delivered to the spine, you won't have to remove or change your clothes for treatment. The total procedure—checking into the radiation department, waiting your turn, and receiving treatment—should take between ten and twenty minutes. The treatment itself takes just a few minutes.

The session takes place in a specially designed room which houses the treatment machinery (a linear accelerator, or linac). The radiation equipment is very large. The therapist will help you onto the table used for the treatment and position you. The radiation machine will then be directed to rest above, below, or to the side of you.

Your therapist will leave the room prior to the actual treatment (just as the dentist does when x-raying your teeth). Don't worry—you'll be seen and heard on a closed-circuit television monitor. Even though you seem to be alone, you're still in close contact. If you need help, just speak up.

Radiation treatments are painless and feel no different than getting a chest x-ray. You will not feel, see, or hear anything. During the treatment, a few people notice an unusual smell or see flashes of light even when their eyes are closed. That is normal. You will need to remain perfectly still until the session is over. Special equipment or medication can help infants and young children stay still. During the treatment you may hear a gentle humming noise which is made by the treatment machine. Sometimes, the therapist will come in and out of the treatment room, usually to reposition you or the treatment equipment.

A typical schedule for radiation therapy consists of one treatment per day, five days a week for two to seven weeks. However, treatment schedules may vary. Your doctor will explain your individualized schedule to you.

You are not radioactive during or after this type of radiation therapy. The radiation is active only while the machine is on. There is no need to take any special precautions for the safety of others.

When will I see the results of therapy?

Tumor cells damaged by radiation cannot reproduce normally. Tumor cells that are unable to reproduce die over a period of weeks to months. During that time, the brain works to clear away those dead or dying tumor cells. This may cause swelling in the area of the tumor.

The best way to measure the effects of radiation is by a CT or MRI scan. An initial follow-up scan is usually planned for one to three months following treatment unless there is some reason to perform one sooner. Scans taken during this time can be confusing because the dying or dead cells are often accompanied by brain swelling, resulting in the mass appearing larger than the original tumor when scanned. And, that mass may cause symptoms similar to the original tumor.

If your post-treatment scans do not show shrinkage immediately, don't be disappointed. It often takes several months or more before your scans show the real results of treatment, and sometimes the scan does not look improved because the tumor is replaced by scar tissue.

Your symptoms may fade as your tumor shrinks. Sometimes they disappear completely. But some effects may continue even if your brain tumor is cured. Some symptoms, whether related to the tumor or its treatments, may not resolve. Your doctor can discuss this possibility with you.

What are some of the common side effects?

Most people have some side effects from radiation therapy. The immediate or short-term effects tend to be manageable discomforts rather than pain or serious problems. Knowing about these in advance can help you plan for some temporary, but necessary, flexibility in your schedule.

149

Fatigue: The most common side-effect of radiation therapy is extreme fatigue (tiredness). Fatigue is temporary. You may begin to feel unusually tired a few weeks into treatment, and this may last weeks or even several months after treatment has ended.

Make a plan to conserve your energy, but don't become inactive. Do what you must at the time of day you feel best. Ask family and neighbors to help with routine jobs such as laundry, grocery shopping, or car pools. Can you work shorter hours while you are in treatment? Can you do some of your work at home? Plan easy meals using prepared foods or rely on frequent, nutritious snacks.

Also, a small amount of exercise (if approved by your doctor) may actually increase your energy level. Once you finish treatment, you'll probably begin feeling better, but be patient. It can be a long time (as long as six months or more) before you feel normal again.

Hair loss: About two weeks into treatment you may start to lose the hair in the path of radiation beams. Hair loss is related to the amount of radiation, the area radiated, and the use of other treatments such as chemotherapy. Your doctor can tell you if you will experience this effect, and if it is likely to be permanent or temporary.

If the loss is temporary, hair regrowth usually begins about 2–3 months following treatment, but may take six months to a year for maximum regrowth. A change of texture and/or change in the color of the regrowth may occur. Attractive scarves (some even have bangs sewn onto them) or caps can help.

Skin changes: You may notice changes in your skin over the area being treated. It may be reddened, darkened, itchy, or appear sunburned. It's important not to scratch or rub these spots. If your ears are in the path of the radiation beams, they may become sore and reddened inside and out. You may have difficulty with your hearing, due to fluid collecting in your middle ear. Do not treat any of these symptoms by yourself. Ask your doctor or radiation therapist for advice. Over-the-counter lotions can make the situation worse; use only products your doctors or nurses suggest. Avoid anything that causes irritation to the area being radiated. Do not use heating pads or ice packs during this time. Stay out of the direct sun, or keep your head covered if you have any skin problems or are taking a radiosensitizing drug.

Swelling/edema: Edema (brain swelling) is another common, usually temporary side effect of radiation therapy. The edema can cause an increase in your brain tumor symptoms. Steroids are medications used to help reduce that swelling. The medications may be given to you during and for a while after your treatments.

Be sure to follow your doctor's exact instructions for taking the steroids. Never abruptly discontinue steroid medications. When they are no longer needed, your doctor will give you instructions for tapering or slowly reducing the steroids. This process allows your body time to slowly begin making its own natural steroids again.

Often, your doctor will prescribe a medicine to prevent the stomach irritation which may occur with steroid use. Taking the steroids with meals can also help reduce this side-effect. Some people who take steroids experience a markedly increased appetite, along with weight gain which often is most apparent in the face and abdomen. Your facial appearance and body shape will return to baseline once the steroids are discontinued, but it will take several months.

Nervousness or difficulty sleeping can be a side effect of steroids. Your doctor may prescribe a medication to calm you or help you sleep. Some people who take steroids develop a yeast infection in their mouth. If this occurs, you'll notice a sore mouth or throat, possibly with fruity smelling breath. Yeast infections are easily treated with medication. People with (or prone toward) diabetes might experience an increase in their blood sugar level. If you begin to have excessive thirst with frequent urination—common symptoms of diabetes—let your doctor know immediately. Also, people who take steroids for more than a month may notice a weakness in their legs. This may be noticed when they try to stand from a sitting position, or when they get up from the bed or the toilet. This symptom will disappear once the steroids are discontinued, although it may take several weeks to months for one's strength to completely return.

Nausea: Sometimes, people feel sick to their stomach following their radiation treatment especially if they are receiving chemotherapy at the same time. There are medications, called antiemetics, which help control nausea. These medicines are generally taken prior to, and sometimes after, your treatments. It's important to let your doctor or nurse know if you feel nauseated so they can help you manage this symptom. If for any reason the first antiemetic medication does not work, call your nurses to let them know. Other medications or medication combinations can be tried until a treatment is found that works best for you.

While you are gong through treatment, your body needs extra protein and calories to keep your immune system healthy and to heal the effects of radiation. Ask your doctor for a referral to the dietician or nutritionist at the hospital. She or he can determine your personal nutrition needs, and help you with personalized dietary counseling. If you choose to look for nutrition services outside of the hospital, be sure to seek a licensed and registered professional.

Sexual effects: Your desire for sexual activity may be lowered now. Again, this is a normal—and temporary—side effect of therapy. The fatigue of treatment, as well as the conscious and unconscious stress associated with having a brain tumor, can cause this effect in both men and women. For now, try non-sexual closeness. Sexual desires often return to normal after treatment. (Also, don't be surprised if one of the side effects of steroid treatments is an increase in sexual interests.)

Blood clots: For reasons that are not well understood, as many as one in three people with a brain tumor may develop a blood clot. Most often, the clot develops in one leg, causing swelling of the foot, ankle and/or calf, usually with pain in the calf or behind the knee. If you develop these symptoms, call your doctor immediately. A special test called a Doppler study can be performed. If a clot is seen, blood thinners can be prescribed to dissolve the clot and prevent it from travelling into the lungs.

Because people who have a brain tumor tend to have blood clots more often than people who do not have a brain tumor, it is important that your doctor be aware of all the medications you are using. This includes over-the-counter drugs, herbs, vitamin supplements, and complementary or alternative therapies. Filling your prescriptions at one pharmacy can also help avoid drug interactions that can make clotting problems worse.

Other effects: Radiation therapy may have intermediate and long-term effects. Information about those effects should be obtained from your doctor who can help you weigh the benefits of the treatment against the risks involved. If you have any questions, or notice any changes you think are important or worrisome, call your doctor or the radiation department at the hospital.

When the Treatments Are Over

Most people feel an unexpected sense of depression when their treatments end. The frequent appointments for therapy stop and appointments for follow-up care become further apart. The pace slows, and another period of adjustment begins. It is a time when it becomes difficult to do nothing after having done so much.

Your task now is becoming well again. Make appointments for your follow-up doctor visits or scans and mark them on your calendar. Begin to rebuild your life. Exercise and eat well, within the guidelines set by your health care team. Get out—go to the movies, visit museums. Find a support group if you'd like to meet others with brain tumors. See friends. Be very good to yourself! You deserve it. But be patient—getting well takes time.

Section 11.2

Stereotactic Radiosurgery

"Stereotactic Radiosurgery," © 2007 American Brain Tumor Association (www.abta.org). Reprinted with permission.

What is stereotactic radiosurgery?

Stereotactic radiosurgery is a special form of radiation therapy—it is not surgery. Stereotactic radiosurgery allows precisely focused, high dose x-ray beams to be delivered to a small, localized area of the brain. It is used to treat small brain and spinal cord tumors (both benign and malignant); blood vessel abnormalities in the brain; defined areas of cancer; certain small tumors in the lungs and liver; and neurologic problems such as movement disorders. In this section, we address radiosurgery only as used for brain tumors.

What is radiation therapy?

The radiation treatments used for brain tumors are very similar to the radiation you know as a treatment for cancer in other parts of the body. When radiation is used to treat brain tumors, the goal is to slow or arrest the tumor growth. Radiation either kills tumor cells directly or it interferes with their ability to grow. Radiation is not completely selective, however. It can affect both normal cells and tumor cells. Because of this, scientists worked to develop a special type of radiation that focuses the high-dose zone of radiation just on the target area. This focused form of radiation is called radiosurgery.

Radiosurgery Is Different from Conventional Radiation Therapy

Conventional external beam radiation therapy—the most common form of radiation therapy—delivers full dose radiation to the tumor and some of the surrounding brain tissue. For several reasons, the target area for conventional radiation deliberately includes a border (called a margin) of normal brain around the tumor. These reasons include uneven tumor borders, the risk of invisible spread of the tumor into the surrounding tissue, a larger tumor size, or the presence of multiple tumors. This larger zone of full-dose radiation includes the borders of the tumor where microscopic tumor cells may be located.

Since normal brain tissue is included in the full-dose region, conventional radiation is broken down into small daily doses so the normal brain tissue can tolerate it. As a result, reaching the desired dose of radiation takes several weeks of daily treatment.

Radiosurgery focuses radiation beams more closely to the tumor than conventional external beam radiation. This is possible through the use of highly sophisticated computer-assisted equipment. A head frame or face mask used for this treatment allows very precise set up, localization and treatment of the tumor. Using advanced computer planning, radiosurgery minimizes the amount of radiation received by normal brain tissue and focuses radiation in the area to be treated.

Since conventional radiation therapy covers more normal tissue, it can often be given only once. Radiosurgery, however, may be considered for re-irradiation due to its precision and the possibility of avoiding previously treated areas.

Types of Radiosurgery Equipment

There are three general types of equipment used to deliver radiosurgery: a system with fixed radioactive source, such as the Gamma Knife; linear accelerators; and cyclotrons.

Gamma knife: The Gamma Knife is a dedicated radiosurgery unit containing two hundred and one cobalt-60 radiation sources which can all be computer-focused onto a single area of the brain.

Linear accelerators: Linear accelerators are the machines used to deliver conventional external beam radiation therapy. A linear accelerator can be modified to deliver a single high-energy computer-shaped beam to the tumor, or the liner accelerator may have been manufactured specifically for use in radiosurgery.

Proton beam radiosurgery: Cyclotrons are nuclear reactors capable of smashing atoms to release proton, neutron and helium ion beams that can be harnessed for radiosurgery purposes. There are only a few of these machines in use.

Names of Radiosurgery Equipment

Several companies manufacture radiosurgery equipment and software for computer-based systems. Each company gives their radiosurgery system a brand name, much in the same way an automobile manufacturer names their cars. For example, GE, Radionics, Accuray and BrainLab are companies that manufacture linear accelerator-based radiosurgery systems or software. Each manufacturer names their equipment: the X-Knife, Stealth Station, CyberKnife, and Novalis System are some of the brand names of linear-accelerator-based radiosurgery systems or software.

Each system has some inherent differences in the way the planning is done or the radiation is delivered, each with its own advantages and disadvantages. At this time, there is no definitive proof that one system is better than another.

The Gamma Knife is a radiosurgery system with a fixed source of energy. In this system, the radioactive cobalt-60 sources used to produce the radiation beams remain in one place while the patient is moved on a sliding couch toward the source of the radiation.

STAR (Stereotactic Alignment for Radiosurgery), Conforma 3000, and PROBEAT are systems used to deliver proton beam radiosurgery. Proton beams are created by a cyclotron (a nuclear reactor) which smashes atoms, releasing the protons used in this therapy.

You may have also heard the term stereotactic radiotherapy. Stereotactic radiosurgery is given in a single session. If given in multiple sessions, the treatment may be called stereotactic radiotherapy or fractionated stereotactic radiotherapy.

Frameless radiosurgery refers to radiosurgery that does not use a metal frame to immobilize the head during treatment. Rather, markers able to be viewed on a scan are placed on the scalp, or a face mask is used to help hold the head steady. The treatment equipment is then aligned with the markers or with the face mask.

The Goals of Radiosurgery

In general, the purpose of any form of radiation therapy is to shrink and destroy tumor cells. Some tumors can be cured by radiation therapy, while others may be controlled. There are situations where a tumor does not shrink in response to radiosurgery but is still cured. This is a common circumstance for patients with certain benign brain tumors.

Because radiosurgery is a highly-focused treatment, this form of radiation therapy is useful in situations where the tumor is small and contained in a localized area. Although the definition of small may vary slightly from institution to institution, small tumors are generally considered to be those three centimeters (cm) (or about 1.18 inches) or less in diameter.

Radiosurgery can be used for tumors in the brain or in the spinal cord. It may be used to treat multiple tumors if the tumors are small and there are a limited number. Sometimes, radiosurgery is used to treat tumors that cannot be removed, or those that can be only partially removed. Also, radiosurgery may be used as a local boost at the end of conventional external beam radiation therapy.

How is radiosurgery given?

There are several techniques used to deliver radiosurgery. In the paragraphs that follow, we describe a typical day of treatment using the more common types of radiosurgery equipment. Although the equipment or method you see may vary, the goal of the treatment is the same.

Your first contact with the radiosurgery unit will likely be with one of the members of the radiosurgery team. Radiosurgery requires a team of specialists. That team may include a neurosurgeon, radiation oncologist, radiologist, radiation physicist, neurologist, anesthesiologist, specially trained nurses, technologists, and the unit support staff. Members of the team first review your medical records to decide if radiosurgery would be of benefit to you. If it is determined that radiosurgery is an option and you consent to treatment, the next step will be obtaining the records and scans needed to plan your personalized treatment. Your recent magnetic resonance imaging (MRI) scans, a current scan or additional images, biopsy or surgical reports, pathology reports, and specially designed planning software are used to precisely determine the plan for treating your tumor. The radiosurgery team calibrates the equipment to match your personalized treatment plan, including the area to be treated and the dose of radiation to be given.

In general, the area radiated includes the abnormal area with a tiny margin of surrounding normal tissue. The dose of radiation is centered over the entire volume of the target area. The radiation dose decreases rapidly as the distance away from the target area increases.

Before the treatment, your team may prescribe medications such as steroids (which prevent brain swelling) or anti-seizure drugs (which control seizures). The staff at the radiosurgery unit will also provide you with specific instructions to follow in preparation for your treatment. Be sure to tell them—in advance—about all of the medications you are using including prescription drugs, over-the-counter medications, vitamins, dietary supplements, or herbal preparations. They will tell you which drugs to continue, and which to stop prior to treatment. You will also receive information about your diet the day prior to the treatment, any special shampoo instructions for the evening before, the time and location of your appointment, and transportation guidelines. Plan to bring someone with you to drive you home.

When you arrive at the radiosurgery unit for your treatment, you may have an IV (intravenous) line started to help prevent dehydration. If you have questions, remember to ask them before any relaxing medication is given to you. This will allow you to better understand the answers.

Most forms of radiosurgery require placement of a lightweight head frame, also called a halo. The head frame has two functions. It helps your doctor define the exact location of the tumor, and it will keep your head immobilized so that there is no movement during treatment. The head frame is attached the day of your treatment. Your doctor will first inject a local anesthetic into your scalp at the places where the pins will be placed. This anesthetic is a freezing medication similar to that used by your dentist. Once the scalp is numbed, screws or pins are positioned. Those pins will hold the head frame in place during the treatment planning and actual treatment. Placing the pins and positioning your head frame can take several hours, depending on the technique used. If your treatment will be given in more than one session, computerized markers may be used to exactly match the previous pin locations. Or, the head frame may be attached to your head with a mouthpiece that is custom made for you, and allows exact reproduction of the position of the frame during each session.

Those being treated with proton beam radiosurgery may be fitted with a molded plastic face mask, which serves the same purpose as a head frame. If your radiosurgery is to be done with a frameless system, you may also be fitted for a face mask. Low-dose x-ray images will be taken to continually track your position during treatment.

Once the head frame or face mask is in position, magnetic resonance imaging (MRI) and/or computed tomography (CT) scans will be done with the head frame on. You will then be able to rest while the treatment plan is calculated by the radiosurgery team. Your physician may give you a mild sedative to help you relax during this planning time and the subsequent treatment. For gamma knife treatment, you will be placed on a couch, and then a large, oversized helmet will be attached over your head frame. Open holes in the helmet allow computer-programmed beams to match the shape of your tumor. The entire couch (with you securely on it) is then slid into a doughnut hole shaped piece of equipment called a gantry through which the radiation beams are delivered.

If you are treated with a linear accelerator, you will be positioned on a sliding bed around which the linear accelerator circles. There are two common techniques by which linear accelerators deliver radiosurgery. One is by directing many arcs of photon beams at the target area. The pattern of the arc is computer-matched to the shape of your tumor. The second technique is to deliver the radiosurgery by a series of shaped fixed fields and not arcs. In some cases the radiation dose pattern is shaped by varying the intensity of radiation through these fields. This technique of varying the intensity is known as intensity modulated radiation therapy (IMRT).

For proton beam-based radiosurgery, you will usually be positioned on a table with your head in a fitted face mask or a frame. As the nuclear reactor smashes atoms, the released protons are directed toward the tumor through beam-shaping blocks. The beams are computer-programmed to match the shape of your tumor.

The actual treatment time for any of these techniques generally ranges from fifteen minutes to about two hours. After you receive your treatment, the head frame is removed. Generally, you return home the same day or you may be kept overnight for observation. The radiosurgery team will provide you with instructions for caring for yourself in the next few days, and for your followup visit with your own physician. Most people feel able to resume their usual activities within a day or two.

If you are to receive multiple treatments, these will be done on an outpatient basis. You will be given a schedule of appointments, and your head frame or mask will be repositioned each time you receive treatment.

After you complete your treatments, you should feel free to contact the radiosurgery team with any questions or concerns. Unless your team instructs you differently, the doctor coordinating your usual brain tumor care is the doctor with whom you make your followup appointments. A scan will be done in a few months to evaluate the initial effect of the treatment, but it may take a year (sometimes longer) to truly evaluate the full effect of the treatment.

Side Effects of Treatment

When your treatment planning is first done, your radiosurgery team can talk with you about the potential effects of the treatment specifically planned for you. Some people have few or no side effects from this type of radiation therapy. Once they have rested following the treatment and have resumed their regular activities, tenderness at the pin sites may be their only side effect. Your doctor can suggest pain medications if needed, or perhaps a topical gel to help numb the pin site until it heals. Other people have reactions which vary from early side effects to delayed reactions.

Early symptoms are often due to brain edema (swelling) caused by the radiation. These symptoms can include nausea, vomiting, dizziness, and headaches. Your doctor can prescribe steroids, anti-nausea drugs or pain relievers to control these symptoms, which are usually temporary. Once the swelling resolves, these symptoms usually resolve.

Two to three weeks after treatment, you may experience hair loss in the area radiated, but this does not occur in everyone. Hair loss depends on the dose of radiation received by portions of the scalp and the ability of the radiated hair follicles to heal. Regrowth usually begins in 3–4 months, and may be a slightly different color or texture than before. Your scalp may also become temporarily irritated. Since some lotions cause further irritation, do not treat this yourself. Call your radiosurgery team for advice.

Some patients may experience delayed reactions weeks or months after treatment. These reactions can include necrosis or cell death in the high radiation dose region due to swelling in reaction to the radiation effect on the target region. These symptoms are mainly due to swelling or death of brain tissue in the treated area. They may mimic the symptoms of tumor regrowth or stroke. Treatment will be based on the type of side effect that occurred. Other effects depend on the location of the tumor. All treatments, even those claiming to be natural therapies, have the potential for serious or life-threatening effects. When your doctor discusses the possible side effects of the treatment planned for you, ask her or him to help you weigh the benefits of the treatment against the risks.

Chapter 12

Brain Surgery

Alternative names: Craniotomy; surgery-brain; neurosurgery; craniectomy; stereotactic craniotomy; stereotactic brain biopsy; endoscopic craniotomy

Definition: Brain surgery treats problems in the brain and the structures around it through an opening (craniotomy) in the skull (cranium).

Description

The hair on part of the scalp is shaved. The scalp is cleansed and prepared for surgery. An incision is made through the scalp. The incision may be made behind the hairline and in front of your ear, at the hairline near your neck, or elsewhere, based on where the problem in your brain is located.

- The scalp is pulled up. A hole is created in the skull. A piece of the skull (a bone flap) is removed. Most of the time, this flap will be placed back after the surgery is over.

- Through this hole, your surgeon may clip off an aneurysm to cut off the blood flow, biopsy or remove a tumor, remove an abnormal part of your brain, or drain blood or an infection.

- Your surgeon may use a special microscope to perform the procedure. Monitors to check pressure may also be used.

- If possible, the surgeon will make a smaller hole and insert a tube with a light and camera on the end (endoscope). The surgery will be done with tools placed through the endoscope.

The surgeon may use computers to help find the exact spot that needs to be treated (magnetic resonance imaging [MRI] or computed tomography [CT] scans). The bone is usually replaced and secured in place using small metal plates, sutures, or wires. The bone flap may not be put back if your surgery involved a tumor or an infection, or if the brain was swollen. (This is called a craniectomy.) The time it takes for the surgery varies based on the type of problem that is being treated.

Why the Procedure Is Performed

Brain surgery may be needed to treat or remove:

- brain tumors,
- bleeding (hemorrhage) or blood clots (hematomas) from injuries (subdural hematoma or epidural hematomas),
- weaknesses in blood vessels (cerebral aneurysms),
- abnormal blood vessels (arteriovenous malformations [AVM]),
- damage to tissues covering the brain (dura),
- infections in the brain (brain abscesses),
- severe nerve or facial pain (such as trigeminal neuralgia or tic douloureux),
- skull fractures,
- pressure in the brain after an injury or stroke,
- some forms of seizure disorders (epilepsy),
- certain brain diseases (such as Parkinson disease) that may be helped with an implanted electronic device.

Risks

Risks for any anesthesia are reactions to medications and problems breathing. Possible risks of brain surgery are:

- surgery on any one area may cause problems with speech, memory, muscle weakness, balance, vision, coordination, and other functions (these problems may last a short while or they may not go away);

- blood clot or bleeding in the brain;
- seizures;
- stroke;
- coma;
- infection in the brain, in the wound, or in the skull;
- brain swelling.

Before the Procedure

You will have a thorough physical exam. Your doctor may perform many laboratory and x-ray tests. Always tell your doctor or nurse:

- if you could be pregnant;
- what drugs you are taking, even drugs, supplements, vitamins, or herbs you bought without a prescription; and
- if you have been drinking a lot of alcohol.

During the days before the surgery:

- you may be asked to stop taking aspirin, ibuprofen, warfarin (Coumadin), and any other drugs that make it hard for your blood to clot;
- ask your doctor which drugs you should still take on the day of the surgery;
- always try to stop smoking (ask your doctor for help);
- your doctor or nurse may ask you to wash your hair with a special shampoo the night before surgery.

On the day of the surgery:

- you will usually be asked not to drink or eat anything for 8–12 hours before the surgery;
- take the drugs your doctor told you to take with a small sip of water;
- your doctor or nurse will tell you when to arrive at the hospital.

After the Procedure

After surgery, you'll be closely watched in the intensive care unit (ICU). When you are stable, you will then go to a room where a doctor or nurse will monitor you closely to make sure your brain functions are working well. They may ask you questions, shine a light in your eyes, and ask you to do simple tasks. You may need oxygen for a few days.

The head of your bed will be kept higher to help reduce swelling of your face or head, which is normal.

You may have pain after surgery while you are in the hospital. Your doctor or nurse will give you medicines to help with this.

You will usually stay in the hospital for 3–7 days. You may need physical therapy (rehabilitation) while you are in the hospital or after you leave the hospital.

Outlook (Prognosis)

The results depend on the disease or problem being treated, your general health, which part of the brain is involved, what procedure is being done, and the surgical techniques used.

References

Ortiz-Cardona J, Bendo AA. Perioperative pain management in the neurosurgical patient. *Anesthesiol Clin.* 2007 Sep 01;25(3):655-74, xi.

Patterson JT, Hanbali F, Franklin RL, Nauta HJW. Neurosurgey. In: Townsend CM, Beauchamp RD, Evers BM, Mattox KL, eds. *Sabiston Textbook of Surgery.* 18th ed. Philadelphia, Pa: Saunders Elsevier; 2007:chap 72.

Chapter 13

Restoring Consciousness: Aiding Recovery from Coma

Theresa Pape's work made headlines in the fall of 2008 when she reported how a study participant spoke his first words since suffering a severe brain injury in a car crash almost a year earlier. Joshua Villa, age 26 when injured, had been in a vegetative state for nearly ten months when his mother agreed to have him take part in Pape's research on transcranial magnetic stimulation (TMS). The treatment involves holding an electromagnetic coil over specific areas of the skull to excite the brain cells beneath the coil.

It was after the 15th treatment—out of a total of 30 sessions over six weeks—that Pape noticed a spike in Villa's responses on a measure called the Disorders of Consciousness Scale. The instrument, developed by Pape, measures an unconscious person's responses to sensory stimuli. "I couldn't believe that the gains were that dramatic and significant," recalls Pape. "I must have done the analyses ten times to make sure there wasn't a mistake."

Three sessions later, Villa uttered his first words. Pape reported: "There must have been about half a dozen of us in the room, and our mouths just hung open. We all looked at each other thinking, 'Did he just say that?'" A couple of days later, when his mother was with him, Villa said "Mom" and "Help me."

Pape is a researcher at the Edward Hines Veteran's Administration (VA) Hospital near Chicago. She also collaborates with staff at several

"Restoring Consciousness," *VA Research Currents*, January 2009, U.S. Department of Veterans Affairs.

rehabilitation hospitals in the area. Her study involving Villa is available online in the journal *Brain Stimulation.*

TMS, developed in Europe in the 1980s, has been used successfully to treat depression, schizophrenia, and other mental disorders. Pape is among the first to explore its usefulness in promoting recovery from coma. In depression, doctors apply the magnetic coil to an area of the brain called the left dorsolateral prefrontal cortex. Pape's theory is that the same area on the opposite side might be best for those in coma or other unconscious states due to traumatic brain injury. "My challenge is finding the optimal dose at the optimal site," she says. "I'm trying to maximize efficacy and minimize the potential for adverse events while optimizing the site on the brain. I chose the dose according to safety data from healthy controls and efficacy data from patients with mental illness, but that doesn't mean it's the optimal dose for traumatic brain injury. Likewise, I chose the site according to neurological theory, but that doesn't mean it's the most optimal site."

Only a handful of other researchers in the United States are exploring the same general topic: how to promote recovery from coma. So Pape has reached out to other countries, such as Denmark, for collaborators. Her vision is that different groups of researchers will explore different TMS doses and apply the magnetic coils to different sites on the brain. That would speed the research process. "I would love it if someone chose a different site or dose and studied it," she says.

Familiar Voices May Stir Brain Response

Pape plans additional research on TMS, but she is also exploring other treatments to help people in comas or vegetative states due to brain injury. One example is familiar vocal stimulation. This treatment works like this: Family members tell stories about events they took part in with their loved one. Transcripts are written, and the families then recite the stories into digital recorders, as if talking to their loved one. Pape offers an example of how the monologues might sound: "Oh, do you remember we went to this wedding and I wore that red dress, and you thought I looked fantastic?"

The therapy is low-cost and as noninvasive as they come, although patients will undergo a brain scan called functional magnetic resonance imaging (fMRI) as they listen to the audio. That will allow researchers to check for responses in the form of more blood flow to different parts of the brain. Pape expects to activate those areas that normally process familiar voices, such as the temporal lobes and hippocampus. Her team uses professional audio-editing programs to ensure the right quality and volume—even amid the clanging of the MRI machine. "We're talking about them hearing a tone in a person's voice, an attitude—all the pragmatic cues mediated in healthy people by the right side of the brain. These are the verbal cues that let someone know who's talking to them without them seeing the person.

The study will include 45 patients. One group will listen to their families' stories for four 10-minute sessions daily, for six weeks. A second group will listen to familiar voices less frequently. A third group will receive only "sham" treatment—in this case, the presence of a compact disk (CD) player but no sound. "Everybody's getting a similar process," says Pape.

Families Find Hope through Research

TMS and familiar vocal stimulation might work together, says Pape. TMS would first induce "brain plasticity" by exciting neurons. Over time, TMS could boost the function of axons—the fibers nerve cells use to talk with each other. Dormant neurons could be revived, and new neural networks created. Vocal stimulation could then "shape and guide that plasticity" and help in the recovery of auditory skills.

The other focus of her research, the Disorders of Consciousness Scale, provides a reliable, accurate way to track the effects of various therapies. It may also yield data to help identify factors linked to recovery from coma. Why some patients recover from serious brain injuries while others linger in a coma for many years is still largely an enigma.

Pape's work has taken on special significance for U.S. Department of Veterans Affairs (VA), as some 20% of troops injured in combat in Iraq or Afghanistan have a brain injury. Most of the injuries are considered mild, and only a relatively small percentage result in long-term loss of consciousness. But for those patients who do remain unconscious, any new hope is welcome.

Stimulating the Brain

TMS is one of several therapies being studied that use electrical current to stimulate the brain. It is among the least invasive. Other methods include:

Deep brain stimulation: Electrodes are implanted in the brain to stimulate specific brain regions.

Electroconvulsive therapy: The process involves inducing a seizure in an anesthetized patient by applying electric current to the brain. It has been found safe and effective for depression and other conditions when drugs don't work.

Chapter 14

Brain Rehabilitation

Chapter Contents

Section 14.1

Rehabilitation Therapies

Note: Although the information in this section refers specifically to brain surgery rehabilitation, these therapies are used for brain rehabilitation in general.

For many patients, surgery is not the end of the process. Some will require rehabilitation to recover from their deficits or even the surgery itself. Your doctor or surgeon may or may not discuss this with you prior to surgery as it will depend on your condition afterwards. Patients are often discouraged to hear that they might need rehabilitation, even though it can really be a very positive thing since it can greatly accelerate the patient's recovery. It is difficult to provide a single description of brain surgery rehab since it will vary greatly from patient to patient. In this section we will attempt to give an overview of rehab and some of the issues that patients and families might experience.

The deficits each person will experience after a bleed or after surgery vary greatly based upon: the location in the brain, the condition going into surgery, as well as the success of the surgery. Even patients with seemingly similar angiomas report different types and severity of deficits. If a patient is left with a deficit that would restrict their quality of life or their ability to care for themselves or to work, they will likely be provided with rehabilitation. Rehab can take many forms but generally there are four ways that it can be delivered.

During the Hospital Stay

Most hospitals today have rehab specialists on staff. Often, this will be limited to the basic rehab disciplines of physical therapy (PT), occupational therapy (OT), respiratory therapy, and speech therapy. Although some hospitals share their therapists between inpatient and outpatient practices, therapists on staff with hospitals typically are very strong at dealing with those first few days or weeks of a patient's recovery because this is what they see most. They will often come to a patient's room and perform an evaluation shortly after surgery to determine if any therapy is required. If so, they will visit the patient's room on a regular schedule to help the patient begin the process of therapy. Because this type of session is most often one on one, the amount of time the therapist can spend with each patient will likely be limited to less than an hour per day. Hospitals are simply not set up for longer term (and more intense) therapy. Once a patient does not require hospital care they are typically either sent home or to a dedicated rehabilitation facility.

Inpatient Rehabilitation Facility

If the patient recovers to the point that they no longer need the level of care provided by a hospital but they are still not capable of living unassisted, they will often be sent to an inpatient rehabilitation facility. These rehabs offer rooms that are often similar to a hospital room and many times are connected to a hospital, but they are geared completely towards rehab. Because the level of medical care is typically not as robust as a hospital, they are lower cost and therefore offer the opportunity for longer-term rehabilitation than the average hospital where beds are at a premium. Various rehab facilities specialize in different types of recovery so it is fair to ask what options are available and to understand which would be best suited to working with brain surgery recovery. Often, a good indicator is a facility that deals with stroke recovery since it is more common than brain surgery but requires many of the same skills. At an inpatient rehabilitation facility, the patient will typically get a much more rigorous schedule with several group classes and individual sessions per day. Because of this and because the therapists here are likely to be very experienced, rapid progress can be made in a good inpatient setting. Patients will wear their own clothes: sweat pants and t-shirts or sweat shirts during the day because of the gym-like atmosphere.

During the stay at an inpatient rehabilitation facility, the physician that is in charge of patient care is often a physiatrist. A physiatrist is a physician that specializes in physical medicine and rehabilitation. Their focus is on restoring function to patients. Some common areas of specialty for a physiatrist are sports medicine, pediatrics, geriatric medicine, and brain injury. The physiatrist may treat the patient directly, such as prescribing any needed medication, or may lead an interdisciplinary team that is treating the patient. The physiatrist may meet with all of the different types of therapists that are treating the patient at periodic intervals such as once a week, to determine the patient's progress, and to assess continuing and evolving needs. This group, led by the physiatrist, will make recommendations as to how to treat the patient as well as when to release the patient from rehab.

Outpatient Rehabilitation

Once the patient has recovered enough to go home from either the hospital or the inpatient rehab facility, they will often be given some amount of outpatient rehabilitation. This is most often provided at a rehabilitation facility that the patient will travel to a few times a week but it can also be in the home. The trade-off between the two is that although in-home is more convenient, often insurance will cover more visits at a rehab facility due to lower cost and the rehab facility will often have better equipment and skills than in-home care. One advantage that opens up to a patient once they reach outpatient care is that there will often be a wider variety of types of rehab than might be within a given hospital or rehab facility. The patient might seek out specialists in balance therapy, vision therapy and other "boutique" rehabs that could be especially useful to the patient.

Ongoing Maintenance

Insurance normally will pay for a limited amount of therapy. It is often governed by progress reports from the therapist which indicate that the patient is still making progress. At the end of that therapy, it is not unusual for the patient to be left with some exercises that can be done on his or her own for long-term maintenance. If the patient's deficit is with walking for instance, there might be trunk and leg strengthening exercises that the patient can do that will help them maintain the strength to overcome their deficit.

There are too many types of rehab to list here, but some common types of therapy include the following:

Physical therapy (PT): This is a very broad category of therapy that involves most strengthening and coordination work designed to overcome any physical weakness that the patient is left with after surgery. Physical therapists, for example, work with patients who have had hip or knee replacements to increase their strength and flexibility so that they can walk again.

Although brain surgery does not directly affect the muscles and joints in the same way that a hip replacement does, it can require much of the same recovery for two reasons. First, anytime a patient is immobilized in a hospital bed for some time they lose strength. If that immobilization is extended the patient may need some PT to get strong enough to safely go home. More common for brain surgery is that the control of some muscle or set of muscles is weakened for neurological reasons. Put simply, the muscle is healthy but the neural pathway (the nerves or areas of the brain that control the nerves) are damaged in some way. It is likely that a neural pathway can be damaged but not destroyed; therefore, the muscles affected seem to be dramatically weakened. This can be thought of as the brain just not being able to "get enough of a signal" to the muscle to fully activate it. In these cases, therapy can be very effective at exercising that pathway and helping it to become more useful. This is the same process that a stroke patient will go through. In many cases PT will also include balance, coordination, gait training, and overall strengthening. It is very broad by definition.

Occupational therapy (OT): OT will focus very specifically on the needs of the patient to be able to work as well as daily living tasks such as personal grooming and household care. If a patient had a weakness in the fingers for example, an occupational therapist will evaluate the ways in which this patient needs to use those fingers in their daily life and work and will help them to adapt. OT is a combination of rebuilding the deficits and finding ways to work around deficits to allow the patient to continue to perform the needed task. An occupational therapist might prescribe adaptations to the patient's home or work environment such as handrails, modified shower, lowered counters, and so forth. Typical inpatient facilities have kitchens, bathrooms, and work environments in which they help the patient practice the life skills that they will need.

Speech and swallowing therapy: If there is a weakness or deficit with the mouth or throat, it can manifest itself as a lack of clear speech or a slow or weakened swallow. Speech therapists specialize in these oral deficits and provide exercises that will strengthen the specific muscles that are slow or weak. Speech and swallowing are amazingly complex activities that require a great deal of coordination between the oral muscles. Speech therapists can use a combination of observation and imaging diagnostics such as moving x-ray that allow them to understand and treat these conditions.

Balance therapy: Brain surgery has the potential to affect a patient's balance. Some PTs specialize in balance or what is often called

173

vestibular rehabilitation. Balance therapists are skilled at retraining the brains ability to interpret and react to the balance related signals that it gets from the inner ear, eyes, and feet. It is physical therapy focused on the patent's balance. Some patients will have a problem with vertigo as well as balance. Balance therapy will address these issues.

Respiratory therapy: Since the brain controls breathing and since surgery carries with it some risk of respiratory complications, it is likely that a patient will at least be evaluated by respiratory therapists during their recovery.

Neuropsychology: Deals with cognitive processes of the brain including, but not limited to, short- and long-term memory, concentration, attention, problem solving, and abstract reasoning. Don't confuse this with psychotherapy—neuropsychology is not counseling. Neuropsychologists will give a battery of standardized tests to determine the presence and extent of any neurological deficiencies. Note that these tests cannot take into account the patient's cognitive level prior to surgery. However, testing may determine the patient is functioning below average in specific cognitive categories and help them to understand and improve on their deficiencies. Also, this information may be very important in determining the patient's ability to return to work and/or if the patient qualifies for disability.

Vision therapy: For your eyes, just like physical therapy is for your body. When a body part isn't functioning correctly, health professionals attempt to bring it back into full use with exercise and retraining. In the case of a turned eye or an eye lacking in mobility, vision therapy can help:

• strengthen the muscles controlling the eyes;

• speed the time it takes for the eye to return to the regular position;

• teach the eyes to work as a team again (just because an eye goes back to its proper position, doesn't mean the eyes will automatically work together as a team again).

With a turned eye, the use of prism glasses, with slowly decreasing prescriptions (lessoned every six weeks or so to make the eye work back to its proper location), along with vision therapy can be a helpful combination to keep the patient using the problem eye (rather than turning it off and only seeing with one eye). It is important to start vision therapy as quickly as possible so the muscles in the affected eye stay strong.

Thoughts on Therapy

Physical demands: Rehab can be extremely hard work. This is particularly important to remember given that the patient has just had major surgery and is trying to recover from the surgery itself. The added challenge of overcoming any deficits is a difficult one in some cases. Inpatient rehabilitation in particular can be extremely demanding physically and mentally.

Preconditioning: Surgery is a physically draining process so if it is elective and time and ability permits, it is recommended that you build your strength and stamina prior to the operation. You would be surprised how quickly your stamina can diminish when you are in a hospital bed, so it is always a benefit to get in the best shape possible prior to starting this process and not knowing exactly the outcome.

Mental and emotional aspects: Rehab can be very difficult emotionally. A patient undergoing brain surgery will understandably be focused on the surgery as the major event. When the surgery is over, it can be very draining to find that there is still a great deal of hard work to do in rehab. It is like running a marathon then at the finish line finding out that there are a few more miles to go. It is possible for progress to seem slow and this can lead to depression. In the movies, characters will knuckle down and rebuild themselves, but in real life you don't get to fast forward. It is not unusual to have some temporary additional deficits right after surgery that will go away in a few days or weeks, but overall the brain makes a slow but steady recovery. The downside is that it can seem excruciatingly slow at times, but the good news is that the brain can continue to make gradual improvements for years. This slow progress can be very frustrating at times.

Another emotional factor is simply the loss of independence. Regardless of how minimal the deficits are after surgery, the patient will no doubt be dependent on other people to help them as they recover. This loss of independence can be very frustrating for the patient. The corollary to this is that when the patient regains their independence, if this time has been long, it can be stressful for them to be on their own again after getting used to the constant support of friends, family, doctors, and nurses.

How hard to push: For each person, the decision on how much the support person can or should push the patient in their recovery will be a difficult and individual one.

Visitors: While visitors can be a tremendous boost for the patient, they can also be so draining that it is actually a detriment to the patient's recovery process. This is particularly true in the hospital and inpatient rehabilitation settings. If the patient is not able to make these decisions, the caregiver must assist with this and may need to limit visitors to less busy times or days depending on the needs of the patient. Especially in the inpatient rehab setting the 15 minute rest or nap between therapies may be more beneficial to the patient than using that energy to talk to visitors. This again will depend upon each individual situation and will vary greatly.

Insurance: Insurance will qualify for a number of sessions or until a certain level is achieved. Most therapies have measurements to determine where the person is in their recovery and this information is relayed to the insurance provider.

The role of surgeons in rehab: It is natural to have great respect for a brain surgeon, especially if they have just completed your operation. It is important to remember that although the surgeon has immense knowledge about your surgery, they are likely to have little practical experience with rehabilitation. Your surgeon may not be able to clearly answer your questions about the rehabilitation process. However, rehabilitation therapists often are an enormous source for information about recovery beyond the hospital. As good as surgeons are at surgery, they do not have the experience that therapists have of spending their days watching and helping patients recover. If you have deficits after your surgery, you should search for the most qualified rehab people you can find because they can make a huge difference in how quickly you recover.

Duration of rehab and recovery: This is often first question people ask. The length of rehab and recovery are specific to each individual. A patient may bounce right back or may be left with a long-term deficit. The bad news is that it possible to have a deficit for a long time because the brain heals slowly; the good news is that the brain continues to heal for a long time. The important thing is to not give up hope—research has shown that motivation and a positive attitude are the things that differentiate those who continue to improve versus those who reach a plateau and do not move past it.

Section 14.2

Cognitive Rehabilitation

Help for Attention, Memory, and Other Problems with Thinking: Or, Why Can't I Remember to Pick Up Bread on the Way Home?

Brain injury of any sort, including that from cavernous malformations, can cause a variety of cognitive impairments. For example, after a bleed or surgery, individuals often complain of difficulty with attention, short-term memory, and multitasking even if they have no visible physical deficits. Neuropsychology is the discipline that is designed to assess and treat these cognitive problems. It's surprising how infrequently patients are referred for neuropsychological evaluation and treatment—it's certainly something to request if you believe that you can benefit. Most major United States (U.S.) insurance companies will cover the cost of an evaluation and of follow-up treatment.

What is a neuropsychological evaluation?

A neuropsychological evaluation involves testing that is sensitive to problems in brain functioning. Unlike computed tomography (CT) or magnetic resonance imaging (MRI) scans, which show what the structure of the brain looks like, neuropsychological testing examines how well the brain is working when it performs certain functions (for example, remembering). The types of tests that you will take depend upon the questions you and your doctor have. The tests may assess the following areas: attention and memory, reasoning and problem-solving, visual-spatial functions, language functions, sensory-perceptual functions, motor functions, academic skills, and emotional functioning. The tests are not invasive; that is, they do not involve attaching you to machines or using x-rays. Most of the tests will involve questions and answers, or working with materials on a table. Some tests may use a computer. The testing may be performed by the neuropsychologist or by a trained staff member. The neuropsychologist or a staff member will also spend some time talking with you about your medical, personal, and school history. The total time involved in your evaluation will depend upon the questions you and your doctor have.

What is a neuropsychologist?

A neuropsychologist is a licensed psychologist specializing in the area of brain-behavior relationships. Although a neuropsychologist has a doctoral degree in psychology, he or she does not just focus on emotional or psychological problems. The neuropsychologist has additional training in the specialty field of clinical neuropsychology. That means a neuropsychologist is educated in brain anatomy, brain function, and brain injury or disease. The neuropsychologist also has specialized training in administering and interpreting the specific kinds of tests included in your neuropsychological evaluation. As a part of the required education, a neuropsychologist also has years of practical experience working with people who have had problems involving the brain.

Cognitive Rehabilitation

Treatment for cognitive impairments is called cognitive rehabilitation. The neuropsychological test battery can feel very long, but it is important for the neuropsychologist to have as much information as possible about your functioning before he or she develops a cognitive rehabilitation plan. Like any rehabilitation therapy, cognitive therapy has two parts: 1) improving your ability to perform the impaired function through therapy techniques and at home practice; and 2) developing strategies for compensating for any residual deficits. Also, like other rehabilitation therapies, neuropsychological assessment and cognitive rehabilitation break down functions into their individual components so that the broken links can be found and addressed. In physical therapy, walking is assessed by looking at a variety of factors including muscle strength, range of motion, and balance. It doesn't make sense to focus on strength when the real issue is balance. This is also true for cognitive rehabilitation.

Let's take apart some of the common cognitive functions and see how neuropsychologists understand and address them.

Attention

What is attention? Do any of the following apply to you?

- "I try to watch television but I just drift off. I can't seem to stay focused on anything even when I'm relaxed and there are no distractions."

- "I can't cook while there is noisy construction work happening next door. I get too distracted."

- "I can't listen to the lecture and take notes at the same time. I can't switch back and forth quickly enough."

- "I can't brush my daughter's hair while I talk on the phone. I can't do two things at once anymore."

For the neuropsychologist, all of these are problems with attention, but the kind of attention required varies from task to task. As a result, the rehabilitation exercises vary depending on the problem.

Sustained attention: "I try to watch television, but I just drift off. I can't seem to stay focused on anything even when I'm relaxed and there are no distractions." Drifting off is a problem with focused or sustained attention. Although it can happen on occasion to anyone, this is most often a continuing problem for those with brainstem bleeds or surgeries.

Cognitive rehabilitation offers several types of exercises to address this issue. For the most basic exercises, you would listen to a tape and hear a series of numbers. You are asked to push a button every time you hear a specific number, for example "4." You practice increasing the amount of time that you can continue the task without errors. The task can be made much more difficult by changing the rules for responding. For example, you could be asked to press the button every time you see a number that is two less than the number that came before it (* = push button): 10, 12, 8, 6*, 4*, 9, 7.* The task could use letters or words rather than numbers as well. In a second type of task, you are asked to count backwards from 100 by 3s, 4s, and so forth. This also can be made more difficult by adding more rules. For example, counting backward by 3s then adding 1: 100, 97, 98, 95, 96, and so forth.

Selective attention: "I can't cook while there is noisy construction work happening next door. I get too distracted." Getting distracted by background noise is an issue of selective attention. Selective attention is the ability to focus on the important or relevant stimuli in the presence of distracting stimuli.

To treat selective attention, you would perform exercises like those mentioned, but add background noise, often on tape. Ideally, the background noise should be the same type as that which is a problem for you in your real life. Many individuals are distracted by internal stimuli such as thoughts or worries. For this, neuropsychologists may encourage writing down thoughts and worries before beginning the task. Being distracted by internal stimuli also can be a sign of depression or an anxiety disorder. Therapy or medication to treat these underlying causes may be in order.

Alternating attention: "I can't listen to the lecture and take notes at the same time. I can't switch back and forth quickly enough." Not being able to switch back and forth is a problem of alternating attention. Alternating attention is required for any two tasks that require thought and that are performed at the same time.

Several types of exercises can begin to treat this. In one, you are presented with a list of numbers. You would cross out odd numbers until the therapist says "change." You would then begin to cross out even numbers. The task becomes more difficult as the length of time between changes shortens. Alternately, you could be presented with pairs of numbers and be asked to change back and forth between adding and subtracting when cued. Finally, you may look at words that are printed differently from the meaning of the word: BIG little LITTLE BIG LITTLE big little LITTLE. You would be asked first to read the words and then to say the size of each word. In this example, the response should be "big little little big little big little little" and then the size of each word "big little big big big little little big." There are many other exercises that work along this same principle. These types of exercises are very difficult even for most people without any type of brain injury.

Divided attention: "I can't brush my daughter's hair while I talk on the phone. I can't do two things at once anymore." Not being able to do two things at once is a problem with divided attention. In divided attention, an individual is being asked to perform two tasks at once, but one task should be something that a person can do without thinking or with very little thought. In the example of brushing a child's hair while talking on the phone, brushing hair should be an automatic task performed with some attention but little thought. To address this issue, you may be asked to perform the task of pushing a buzzer in response to a specific number as in the sustained attention example earlier. The difference here is that you will both hear numbers through a headset and see number flashed individually on a screen. They will not be the same numbers. You must push the buzzer if either tape or screen has the specific number. Alternately, you may be asked to perform sorting exercises. For example, you may be presented with a deck of cards and asked to sort the cards by suit. During the sorting, you also are supposed to turn over any card that contains a specific letter, such as the letter "n" (one, seven, nine, ten, queen, king). Again, this is quite a challenge, even for those without a cavernous angioma or other brain injury.

Processing speed: Reduced processing speed, how long it takes to move through a task, is often a problem for those with cavernous angiomas. All of the exercises mentioned are designed to address this issue as well. Individuals can try to increase their speed at performing each task with practice.

Stages of Memory

Memory is a multi-step process and a problem can occur at any step along the way. It is helpful for a neuropsychologist to explore where in the process your memory is being affected, particularly since what seem like memory issues may instead be problems with attention or with visual or auditory processing. For problems that are caused directly by memory deficits, the most common and most effective way to manage the situation is to develop compensatory techniques, things outside of you that can help you stay organized and remember. Let's look at the stages of memory.

Attention and memory: This is the first stage. You can't process something and store it if you haven't paid attention to it in the first place. All of the exercises mentioned are intended to address this part of the memory process.

Encoding: In encoding, a person links information to something that is already known. In other words, a piece of information is categorized. How well you are able to do this plays a large role in whether you are able to store information. For example, suppose you are just learning what a pot is. It is much more effective to categorize it as cookware than as something that rhymes with spot. Problems in encoding can arise in several ways. It may not be a categorization problem, but

181

could be the result of a problem with the language center of the brain or with visual or auditory processing areas. In this case, addressing those other issues may help with encoding. Damage to the frontal lobes or in the dorsomedial thalamus can result directly in problems with categorization and organization. Some ideas for treating these and other memory stage issues follow.

Storage: Individuals, particularly those with hippocampal damage and associated mesial temporal lobe damage can be left with a limited ability to store new information. Encoded information does make it to long-term memory, but the memory deteriorates quickly and the information can't be retrieved. You may have categorized a pot correctly as cookware and have stored this information, but your brain just isn't able to keep the information for long. The next time you see a pot, you won't remember what it is.

Consolidation: Consolidation happens when you integrate your new knowledge—a pot is cookware—with more detailed information that you already know. For example, when you have consolidated, you have figured out how it fits into the class of cookware: that a pot is different from a pan, that you can use it to boil water, and so forth.

Retrieval: The ability to get information out of memory without cues. Retrieval problems can be the result of damage to a language area (aphasia), or can occur directly with damage to many different areas of the brain. A person with a retrieval problem often has the tip of the tongue phenomena: "Dorothy came from….oh, the name of the town is on the tip of my tongue. Just name a few towns in Kansas. I'll recognize it when I hear it." If the memory problem happens before the retrieval stage, a person will not be able to recognize the right name from a list.

Treatment for Memory Problems

There are many ideas about the most effective methods for improving memory after brain injury. A couple of methods by McKay Moore Sohlberg and Catherine Mateer are listed.

A common complaint among folks with memory problems is difficulty remembering to do things they were supposed to do. In one exercise, you are given a task to perform, but are asked to wait a specific period of time before doing it. During the wait time, the exercise can be set up so that you either just sit or you perform an alternate activity (a distracter task). You do have access to a clock. The exercise becomes more difficult by increasing the amount of time between being assigned the task and having to perform it.

Another way in which memory problems are treated is through the development of a memory notebook system with very detailed instruction and a great deal of practice in using it. A memory notebook is a binder or planner filled with forms and divided by categories. It is much like a Daytimer® but with sections tailored to address the individual's memory deficit. Possible sections could include:

Orientation: A script that you can use to give people pertinent information about yourself, your medical history, and any other relevant information.

Memory log: Forms for charting information about what you have done. You are asked to make a note every time you change your activity during the day. On average, you will be making a note hourly. As time consuming as this may seem, the memory log is usually part of everyone's memory notebook. Keeping the log helps memory by forcing you to think about what you have done for that period of time. Writing it down further increases the likelihood that you will remember what you have done later. And, if your memory does fail, you have a reference to look at.

Calendar: The calendar should have dates and times that you can use for scheduling appointments and other activities.

Things to do: This section has forms for listing errands and other future tasks. It would also contain a space for the due date and completion date.

Transportation: If you have trouble remembering how to get places, this may contain maps and/or bus information to get you to the places you most commonly go.

Feelings log: This section has forms to record your feelings about events, and so forth.

Names: Contains forms to record names and identifying information of new people.

Today at work: These are forms that are adapted for your specific job that allow you to record all the necessary information you need to perform your work.

As you are using the memory notebook in real life, you will find that some things that occur will fall into multiple sections. For example, if you are invited to a potluck on Sunday night and asked to bring an entrée, you will need to put a note on both the calendar and in the Things to Do section (make an entrée). You may also need to note receiving the invitation in your Memory log, put directions in the Transportation section, or put the host's information in the Names section. Although this can be somewhat complicated, with practice it will become second nature. The memory notebook itself is a way of developing better categorization and organization skills that will lead to better encoding even without the notebook.

Executive Functions

Executive functions are those things we do that require a variety of processes, for example, planning or time management. Often, these activities become difficult for individuals who have had a bleed or a surgery. Following, we'll look at a few of these and talk about ways in which they may be addressed in cognitive rehabilitation.

Planning: We all carry out activities every day that require planning, even if we are not aware of it. Grocery shopping, paying bills, planting a garden, getting ready for work all include an element of planning. Some individuals have difficulty developing, organizing, and executing plans after a bleed or surgery.

The planning process can be broken down into six steps that can be addressed by cognitive rehabilitation.

1. Knowing the steps needed to complete a plan: To address this, a therapist would give you a task that requires planning skills such as applying for a credit card, preparing a meal, or finding a job, and ask you to list all of the steps involved in the process in any order. You would be graded on how complete your list is.

2. Putting the steps in order (sequencing): You would be asked to take the list you developed above and put the items in sequential order.

3. Initiate the plan: Taking the first step can be difficult for individuals with some types of brain injury. To improve this, a person must first become aware of the problem and then practice initiating in many different settings. For example, you could be asked to initiate a conversation, sit down with the checkbook, or write a paragraph on a topic you know well.

4. Carrying out the plan: Carrying out a plan often requires performing many steps and some may have multiple components. It may require higher level organizational skills to keep the plan moving along, and it can be easy to become overwhelmed. To practice, a therapist could develop a list of errands to run and ask you to do them. The errands would be arranged from least to most complex. Happily, you'd be able to use your memory notebook if you have one, and there should be someone to come along with you.

5. Repair: Many times plans need to be changed because an obstacle develops that makes the original plan impossible to complete. A therapist can develop hypothetical situations that require you to think about how you would change a plan. For example, what if you needed Shitake mushrooms to complete a meal you were preparing for a special dinner party, but the grocery store was out of them? Alternately, what if you needed to get to an appointment, but you walked out of your house and saw that you had a flat tire? Working out hypothetical situations can make coping with obstacles in real life easier.

6. Speed of response: This means that you accomplish your goal in a reasonable amount of time. Practicing planning and carrying out plans should improve your efficiency over time.

Time management: Brain injuries can result in difficulties with time management. It may become harder to judge time and to estimate how long it will take to perform a task. Good time management involves several steps.

1. Time estimation: Individuals with bleeds or surgery in the frontal lobe may have difficulty judging how much time has passed. You may start an activity and look up to discover that an hour has passed without your noticing. To improve this, a therapist may ask you to tell her when a certain amount of time has passed, for example one minute, five minutes, or fifteen minutes. Sometimes you may just sit and wait for the time to pass or you may have a distracting activity in the interim. The task gets harder as the length of time increases.

2. Creating a time schedule: It's important to be able to estimate how long it is going to take to complete tasks. You may practice creating realistic time schedules with a therapist for activities like getting ready in the morning (shower, dressing, breakfast,

and so forth), cleaning the house, running errands, or performing work-related tasks. This requires both time management and planning skills.

3. Carrying out activities in the amount of time scheduled. Next, you may be asked to carry out the activities on your time schedule to see if your estimates were reasonable for you. To do this, you need to keep track of how long it actually took to complete the items on your schedule and compare this to your estimates. You may also need to look at whether you got stuck in an activity and kept at it too long without thinking about when your next task was supposed to start. For example, perhaps you needed to assemble a bike in the morning and then get to a doctor's appointment in the early afternoon. If the bike assembly doesn't go well, you'll need to track the time and recognize that it may need to be left incomplete in order to make it to the appointment on time.

4. Repairing the schedule: Finally, it is important to be able to revise a schedule if it's not working. This can be done in the middle of a schedule by revising the time estimates for all of the subsequent activities. Or, it can be done once the entire schedule is completed.

Self-regulation: Self-awareness is the ability to use internal and external feedback to control and change your behavior. Often with frontal lobe damage, this ability may be compromised.

Becoming self-aware requires three primary skills:

1. Awareness: This means that you are able to make statements about your own behavior that indicates you understand what you are doing and the impact it has on others.

2. Ability to respond to this feedback: This means being able to change your behavior, if needed, in response to your awareness.

3. Impulse control: Self-regulation also requires impulse control. This means that you are able to think before acting. Having good impulse control helps in controlling inappropriate behavior.

The key to addressing these issues is improving awareness. A therapist may design an exercise in which you are asked to put a hash mark on a piece of paper every time you do a behavior, such as interrupting another person while they are talking. The therapist will give you a specific period of time during which you observe yourself, and the therapist will track the behavior as well. At the end of the time, you and the therapist will compare notes. The behavior doesn't have to be something you need to change—the point of the exercise is simply to become aware of what you do. Increasing awareness is often the best way to change a behavior over time, and can go a long way toward improving self-control.

Treatment using compensation: Some people continue to have executive function impairments even after a great deal of cognitive rehabilitation. For these individuals, developing a very set schedule and routine may help in compensating for the deficit. The individual may need to change professions to a job with more structure, less responsibility, and reduced social interaction in order to function more successfully.

Other areas addressed by cognitive rehabilitation: Cognitive rehabilitation can be used to address other types of cognitive impairment as well. For example, a therapist may be able to help with visual processing. The work would focus on how you understand what you see and how you respond to what you see. This is different from a vision therapist or ophthalmologist who would concentrate on the actual muscles and nerves of your eye.

A therapist may address the use of language. Unlike speech therapy, the focus of cognitive rehabilitation is to learn how to use the right language at the right time. For example, after a bleed or surgery, a person may experience increased difficulty initiating a conversation and knowing how to make small talk. Or, a person may not think about asking for help when needed. Cognitive rehabilitation therapists work on the practical use of everyday speech.

A therapist may address directly issues of problem solving. Some problem solving is involved in planning, time management, and self-regulation training, but it can become the focus of the treatment if needed.

Finally, a cognitive rehabilitation therapist may address abstract reasoning. Some types of reasoning include creative reasoning, logical reasoning, and social reasoning. A typical example of logical thinking is the dinner party exercise in which you are asked to design a seating chart for a dinner party but have many identified guests who have special seating needs, for example, Jane won't sit next to Sandy, Sandy must sit to the right of Ben, and so forth. The challenge is to figure out how to arrange the seats so that everyone is happy. An example of creative reasoning is brainstorming—generating as many ideas on a topic as you can. For example, you could be asked to come up with as many ways of using a piece of paper as possible (for example, write on it, use it as a fan, make a paper airplane, start a fire, line your birdcage, and so forth). Finally, social reasoning involves understanding why some behaviors are or are not appropriate. For example, what are two good reasons why most people call ahead before visiting an out-of-town friend? Or, when would it be a good idea to send flowers to someone? When would it be a bad idea?

Cognitive rehabilitation can be enormously helpful in regaining some of the mental abilities you had before your bleed or surgery. The easiest way to find a neuropsychologist in your area is to ask your neurologist. If this doesn't work, call a local rehabilitation hospital with a stroke and brain injury unit or your state's psychological association for a referral.

References

Cigna Health Corporation. "Cigna Healthcare Coverage Position: Cognitive Rehabilitation," July 15, 2005.

National Academy of Neuropsychology. "What is a Neuropsychological Evaluation?" Brochure, 2001.

Sohlberg, M. and Mateer, C. *Introduction to Cognitive Rehabilitation: Theory and Practice*. New York: Guilford Press, 2001.

Section 14.3

Scales and Measurements of Brain Functioning

This section begins with an excerpt from "Traumatic Brain Injury: Hope through Research," National Institute of Neurological Disorders and Stroke (NINDS), updated December 21, 2009; and continues with excerpts from "Traumatic Brain Injury in the United States: Available Measures for Assessing Outcomes of TBI in Children and Youth," Centers for Disease Control and Prevention (CDC), September 19, 2006.

Medical Care for the Traumatic Brain Injury Patient

Medical care usually begins when paramedics or emergency medical technicians arrive on the scene of an accident or when a traumatic brain injury (TBI) patient arrives at the emergency department of a hospital. Because little can be done to reverse the initial brain damage caused by trauma, medical personnel try to stabilize the patient and focus on preventing further injury. Primary concerns include insuring proper oxygen supply to the brain and the rest of the body, maintaining adequate blood flow, and controlling blood pressure. Emergency medical personnel may have to open the patient's airway or perform other procedures to make sure the patient is breathing. They may also perform cardiopulmonary resuscitation (CPR) to help the heart pump blood to the body, and they may treat other injuries to control or stop bleeding. Because many head-injured patients may also have spinal cord injuries, medical professionals take great care in moving and transporting the patient. Ideally, the patient is placed on a backboard and in a neck restraint. These devices immobilize the patient and prevent further injury to the head and spinal cord.

As soon as medical personnel have stabilized the head-injured patient, they assess the patient's condition by measuring vital signs and reflexes and by performing a neurological examination. They check the patient's temperature, blood pressure, pulse, breathing rate, and pupil size in response to light. They assess the patient's level of consciousness and neurological functioning using the Glasgow Coma Scale, a standardized, 15-point test that uses three measures—eye opening, best verbal response, and best motor response—to determine the severity of the patient's brain injury.

Glasgow Coma Scale

Eye opening: The eye opening part of the Glasgow Coma Scale has four scores:

- 4 indicates that the patient can open his eyes spontaneously.
- 3 is given if the patient can open his eyes on verbal command.
- 2 indicates that the patient opens his eyes only in response to painful stimuli.
- 1 is given if the patient does not open his eyes in response to any stimulus.

Verbal response: The best verbal response part of the test has five scores:

- 5 is given if the patient is oriented and can speak coherently.
- 4 indicates that the patient is disoriented but can speak coherently.
- 3 means the patient uses inappropriate words or incoherent language.
- 2 is given if the patient makes incomprehensible sounds.
- 1 indicates that the patient gives no verbal response at all.

Motor response: The best motor response test has six scores:

- 6 means the patient can move his arms and legs in response to verbal commands.
- A score between 5 and 2 is given if the patient shows movement in response to a variety of stimuli, including pain.
- 1 indicates that the patient shows no movement in response to stimuli.

The results of the three tests are added up to determine the patient's overall condition. A total score of 3–8 indicates a severe head injury, 9–12 indicates a moderate head injury, and 13–15 indicates a mild head injury.

Measures for Assessing Outcomes of TBI in Children and Youth

Many more measures for assessing TBI outcomes have been developed for use with school-aged children and youth than for very young children. The majority of measures developed for children aged five years or younger are developmental measures not specifically designed for children with TBI. Longitudinal research that applies the appropriate measures at each developmental level, but that also tracks important milestones and late emerging deficits from early childhood through older ages, will be especially challenging.

Specific measures: A wide range of child health and other measures are available. However, not all of these measures are useful or appropriate for studying children and youth with TBI.

Child Health Questionnaire (CHQ)

This summary was presented by Jeanne Landgraf, who developed the CHQ measure.

Characteristics

- Serves as a generic quality-of-life instrument.

- Assesses physical and psychosocial well being.

- Is appropriate for ages 5–17 years; version for ages less than five years is under development.

- Measures 14 health concepts.

- Includes 28- or 50-item parent-completed forms.

- Includes 87-item child-completed form (a short form is currently being developed).

- Probes for information about the family.

- Includes normative data and has been used in studies of a wide range of other conditions; thus, it can be used to help estimate the burden of TBI compared to other conditions.

Strengths

- Is specifically developed for children and youth. Provides high reliability.

- Scores can be compared to available norms and benchmarks.

- Allows for parallel reporting of parents and children.

Weaknesses

- The majority of studies to date using the CHQ have used a cross-sectional design.

- Limited data about sensitivity to change over time are available.

- No published studies used it with children with TBI/cognitive impairment, but some work is currently planned or being conducted (reported by Keith Yeates and Melissa McCarthy).

- CHQ may not be as sensitive as condition-specific instruments.

- Paper and pencil version have normative data; the telephone interview version is scripted, but normative data are not available.

Pediatric Evaluation of Disability Inventory (PEDI)

This summary was presented by Stephen Haley, who developed the PEDI measure.

Original PEDI

- Serves as a functional assessment instrument.

- Is designed for children in active rehabilitation programs or children with severe problems.

- Is standardized for children between ages 6 months–7.5 years.

- Can also be used in inpatient and outpatient rehabilitation settings with older children who are functioning at lower levels.

New Version of PEDI

- Is based on the World Health Organization (WHO) model of disability.

- Is being developed for children with brain injury.

- Is designed for children and youth aged 1–18 years.

- Has an activity scale that extends beyond basic functional skills; intended to examine recovery of basic skills needed for return to the community.

- Includes a participation scale that emphasizes life roles and assesses levels of participation in the community and school environments.

- Is designed to be completed by parents or providers; a child-administered form is not available.

- Is designed for use in the rehabilitation setting.

- Will allow risk-adjustment to account for variability across institutions.

- Can be adapted for use in follow-up studies, although not originally developed for such studies.

Selected Clinical Measures

A wide range of clinical measures is available for assessing outcomes of TBI some of which were originally developed for use with adults.

Glasgow Coma Scale (GCS)

- Is a useful indicator of severity, but not for children younger than age five.

- Scores for the same patient vary depending on when they were collected, for example, GCS scores collected by emergency medical technicians (EMTs) before admission are not as reliable as those collected in the emergency department (ED) or hospital. Centers for Disease Control and Prevention (CDC) TBI surveillance guidelines recommend use of the first GCS after admission to ED or hospital.

Children's Coma Score

- A modification of the Glasgow Coma Score designed to be used in children aged three years and younger.

- Eye opening and motor response sub-scales are identical to the GCS, but the verbal response subscale rates behavior/affect in preverbal populations. (Multilingual Resources Assessment Tools. Available at: www.multilingualresources.com/ assessment.html. Accessed January 9, 2001).

- Is unclear how widely this score is being used or whether the score represents a significant improvement in the GCS for use with children.

Abbreviated Injury Score/Injury Severity Score (AIS/ISS)

- Used routinely in the clinical setting.

- Most recent version (AIS 98) is better than previous versions for assessing children.

- Because of the variability within AIS levels, researchers should consider supplementing AIS/ISS with Therapeutic Intensity Level, which is used in some clinical settings to determine severity based on the intensity of treatment required by the patient.

- The AIS score for the head is highly correlated with GCS and is a useful measure of TBI severity.

Loss of Consciousness (LOC)

- Measures the length of time between injury and when the patient regains consciousness.

- Is strongly correlated with outcomes in children and adults and is a key piece of information that should be collected.

Length of Post-Traumatic Amnesia (PTA)

- Measures the time from when a patient emerges from coma until he or she is no longer disoriented.

- Appears to be strongly correlated with outcome; however, it is difficult to document consistently and accurately within a hospital protocol.

- Inter-rater reliability is low; that is, different people report different lengths of PTA.

- Despite limitations, PTA should be collected and reported as accurately as possible.

Rancho Los Amigos Scale

- Is a 7-level scale for assessing early recovery in the brain injury rehabilitation setting.

- Rates behavior, cognitive functioning, and response to the environment.

- Levels range from no response (Level I) through purposeful-appropriate responses (Level VII). (Multilingual Resources

Assessment Tools. Available at: www.multilingualresources.com/assessment.html)

- May be useful for research on outcomes but to date has not been used widely or evaluated for that purpose.

Pediatric Trauma Score (PTS)

- Is a composite injury score in which the injured child receives a score of -1 (severely injured), +1 (moderately injured), or +2 (slightly injured or not injured) in each of six areas—body weight or size, airway, blood pressure, central nervous system activity, open wounds and skeletal injuries.

- Score is not useful for TBI research because it does not separate head injury from injury to other body regions/functions.

Neuropsychological / Psychiatric Tests

- These detailed tests of cognitive and psychological functioning are frequently conducted by trained professionals.

- Results from these tests are important, particularly to document more subtle deficits, but they must be done in a clinical setting.

School Performance Assessments

Assessments of school performance include achievement tests, which measure students' academic performance, and school function assessments, which assess students' ability to behave appropriately in the classroom.

Achievement Tests

- These tests of academic achievement are not sensitive to TBI-related problems.

- Thinking and reasoning are not assessed.

- Bright students may do well based on previous learning, thus masking TBI-related problems.

- Scores may improve even as behavior worsens.

- Achievement test results, if available for review, might provide some useful information about previous performance; however, meeting participants did not strongly recommend including them in studies assessing longer term outcomes of TBI.

School Function Assessments

- These checklists are specifically designed to assess functioning in the classroom setting.

- They are helpful in detecting problems specific to the classroom, including awareness of hygiene and behavior regulation.

- Meeting participants recommended including at least some key items from school function assessments in studies of outcomes of TBI in children and youth.

Section 14.4

Types of Services for People with Brain Disorders

"Rehabilitation Services," © National Association of State Head Injury Administrators (www.nashia.org). Reprinted with permission.

As has been well documented in the literature, individuals with brain injury and their families seek an array of services and supports from a variety of state agencies. While there may be limitations on services or other requirements imposed by individual states, the definitions below do not reflect any limitations.

Assessment/evaluation: Refers to the use of a test or scale or battery of tests or scales, observation(s), and may include physical assessment to determine: (1) the extent of injury and prognosis for recovery; (2) deficits as the result of the injury as opposed to preinjury conditions that contribute to functional status; (3) strengths in cognitive, psychosocial, vocational and other skills; (4) specific treatment/rehabilitation or support needs and objectives; (5) objectively-based prognosis for return to work, school, and other activities of daily living; and (6) the basis for determining other needs in planning for lifelong care.

Assisted living: An assisted living program is a congregate residential setting that provides housing, supportive services, personalized assistance, 24-hour care supervision, and health care assistance designed to meet the individual's needs on a daily basis. These needs may include assistance with bathing, dressing, balancing a checkbook, and medication. Residents live in rooms, suites, or apartments, or they may share their quarters with their spouses or roommates.

Assistive technology devices: Refer to any item, piece of equipment, or product system, whether acquired commercially off the shelf, modified, or customized, that is used to increase, maintain, or improve functional capabilities of an individual with a disability, including an individual with a TBI.

Behavioral programs and services: An individually-designed strategy or approach intended to improve an individual's adaptive social behavior and to decrease any maladaptive behaviors that interfere with the individual's ability to remain in the community. This may include, but is not limited to the following: clinical redirection, token economies, reinforcement, extinction, modeling, and over-learning. This service may include: (1) a complete assessment of behavior; (2) development of a structured behavior intervention plan; (3) implementation of the behavior plan; (4) ongoing training and supervision to caregivers and others; and (5) periodic reassessment of the plan. Behavioral programs and services may be provided in a structured residential program specifically designed to address behavior issues, a rehabilitation setting or by a professional or team of professionals assisting the individual with a TBI, and/or family, caregiver, employer or others in order for the individual to live in the community.

Case management and service coordination: Designed to assist the individual with a TBI in maximizing services and resources in order to achieve the highest level of functioning. Case management/ service coordination services may include: (1) information, education, and referral; (2) assessment of the individual's needs and goals; (3) identification of programs, services, resources, and funding options; (4) coordination and monitoring of services; (5) ongoing evaluation of current and future needs; and (6) advocacy. The case manager/service coordinator collaborates with an interdisciplinary treatment/ rehabilitation team and external entities and providers to assess, coordinate, implement, and evaluate all services required to meet the individual's needs.

Community and family education: This service offers training and education to instruct a parent, spouse, another family member, or primary caregiver about treatment/rehabilitation regimens, as well as use of adaptive equipment. Training generally consists of assisting and improving the caregiver's ability to give care (for example, instruction, behavioral intervention strategies, community integration, and stress management).

Companion and homemaker services: Companion services are non-medical supervision and socialization services designed to assist an individual in maintaining community living. A companion may assist the person with such tasks as meal preparation, laundry and shopping, but does not perform these activities as discrete services. A companion may also perform light housekeeping tasks that are incidental to the care and supervision of the individual and also may accompany the individual into the community. Homemaker services are provided by a trained homemaker when the individual with a TBI, family member(s), or primary caregiver regularly responsible for these activities is temporarily absent, or unable to manage the home and care for himself/herself or others in the home. Homemaker services are generally directed toward enabling an individual to remain in the community and thus avoid institutionalization. Homemaker services include meal preparation, routine household care, shopping and errands, assisting with daily activities, arranging transportation, providing emotional support and social stimulation, and monitoring safety and well being.

Comprehensive facility-based acute rehabilitation: A highly intensive skilled service delivered in the hospital setting during the inpatient admission to optimize the individual's medical condition and to improve functional status. Focus of therapies is usually on development of bowel and bladder control, communication, mobility, basic hygiene, orientation, and learning.

Comprehensive facility-based post-acute rehabilitation: Advanced rehabilitation services provided through an interdisciplinary team approach that assesses and coordinates a rehabilitation plan to assist the individual in returning to the community, school, and/or work. Services are based on an assessment of the individual's cognitive, physical, and emotional deficits and may include cognitive rehabilitation services, behavior management, and the development of coping skills and compensatory strategies Post-acute rehabilitation services are generally provided by a rehabilitation agency or in a rehabilitation setting within a hospital staffed by an array of professionals. These services include psychologists or neuropsychologists, therapists (for example, speech/language, physical and occupational), special educators, social workers, and counselors. These services are offered once the individual is medically stable and ready for community integration. The individual usually participates in two to four types of therapy, three to five times per week, generally from three months to six months.

Day services (medical model): Refers to a nonresidential or outpatient program intended to improve the functional ability of the individual through therapeutic interventions and supervised activities to facilitate successful community integration. The program is generally designed to assist an individual in maximizing functional skills and addresses psychological and behavioral adjustment and vocational rehabilitation needs. Professional staff, which may include nursing staff to administer or assist with medications, administer the program.

Day services (social model): Refers to a structured community-based program that offers services in a group setting to improve and maintain the individual's community living skills. The program is designed to meet the needs of adults who are not employed full-time by providing health, social, recreational, and therapeutic activities; supervision; support services; and personal care.

Environmental modifications: These include physical adaptations to an individual's home which are necessary to ensure the health, welfare, and safety of the individual; to help that individual function with greater independence in his or her own home; and which are necessary to accommodate medical equipment and supplies that may be required for the individual's welfare. Such adaptations may include, but are not limited to, the installation of ramps and grab-bars and widening of doorways.

Facility-based subacute care: A hospital-based or skilled nursing-based residential program that focuses on providing comprehensive medical assessment, nursing care, rehabilitation, and therapeutic activities to individuals who are medically stable or who have complex nursing needs. The facility offers nursing care and related services to individuals seriously injured, including those who are ventilator dependent, or who have had a tracheotomy and require tube feeding.

Housing supplements and subsidies: Provide the individual or family with financial assistance to either supplement or pay for full cost of living in one's own home or apartment, including money for rent or mortgage, rental deposits, utilities, utility deposits, housing maintenance, or other items associated with maintaining a home.

Independent living skills training: Provides training and assistance to an individual with a TBI for activities related to daily living and maintenance of a household. These skills are taught either in an environment that most closely resembles an individual's home, or in the environment in which he or she will use these skills. Instruction and training may also be provided to the family to assist the individual in the learning process and to reinforce the learned skills in the natural environment. Examples of training activities include: directing personal care, performing household management chores, menu planning, grocery shopping, meal preparation, budgeting, auto and lawn care, creating and maintaining a weekly schedule, arranging and accessing public transportation, and scheduling and keeping appointments with social service agencies, attorneys, physicians, and so forth.

In-home nursing: Professional services provided by licensed staff relevant to the medical needs of the individual with TBI. Such services are provided through direct intervention or consultation. Services are generally designed to protect the individual's well being; restore, rehabilitate and maintain maximum level of health and independence; and prevent hospitalization. Nursing services include direct interventions that are within the scope of professional practice of the registered nurse (RN) and are generally provided face-to-face. These services may include medication management, nutrition and feeding, ventilator care, tracheotomy care and suctioning, bowel and bladder care, hygiene, assessing skin integrity, and immobility management. Nursing services may be provided by a home health care agency or individually by a licensed nurse.

Long-term residential services: Generally provided in a nursing facility, residential care facility, or other structured residential program that provides either skilled nursing care and related services, or supervision and related services, to individuals who are unable to live independently in the community with or without supports.

Personal care assistance: Personal care services include assistance with eating, bathing, dressing, personal hygiene, and activities of daily living. This service may also include meal preparation and such housekeeping chores as bed making, dusting, and vacuuming, which are incidental to the care provided and essential to the health and welfare of the person. These services may be provided by an individual or agency, such as a home health care agency, depending on the individual's needs and desires. Self-directed personal care services allow the individual with a TBI to direct his or her own care, hire and fire the personal care assistant, train the personal care assistant, and to decide the level and intensity of care that will be provided.

Personal emergency response system: Provides immediate assistance in case of physical, emotional, or environmental emergency through a community-based electronic communications device. This service provides a direct link to health professionals to secure immediate assistance by the activation of an electronic unit in the individual's home. The unit is connected to the telephone line and is programmed to send an electronic message to a community-based, 24-hour emergency response center. There is also a personal "help" button that can be either carried or worn by the subscriber.

Pre-vocational services: These prepare an individual for paid or unpaid employment by teaching such concepts as compliance, attendance, task completion, problem solving, and safety. This service uses actual work experience to promote the individual's use of behavioral and cognitive compensatory strategies in a facility-based or community site work setting. Specific target goals are identified for intervention such as production rate, inappropriate social behavior, or fatigue. These goals are intended to address the individual's identified barriers to direct vocational placement or entry into vocational rehabilitation services. These services are generally not covered under the Rehabilitation Act of 1973 as amended.

Recreation: Programs or services offer opportunities for individuals with TBI to participate in social and recreational activities and the development of recreation skills. The service may include assessment of leisure function; therapeutic recreation service; recreation programs in community agency; and leisure education. These services may be segregated services that offer a structured recreational or social opportunity specifically for individuals with brain injury; or, the service may provide an opportunity to participate in recreational and social opportunities that may be available to the public at large.

Respite services: Provide time-limited and temporary relief for emergency situations or from the ongoing responsibilities of caregiving by the family or other primary caregiver. These services may be offered in a structured setting where the individual with a TBI may leave his or her home to stay or may be provided by someone staying in the home to allow that individual to remain at home.

Specialized medical equipment and supplies: Items that are of direct medical or remedial benefit to an individual with a TBI.

Substance abuse services: May be provided in a structured day program or through individual treatment to help the individual to reduce or eliminate substance abuse. Substance abuse services may offer: (1) prevention services to motivate a person to choose not to use, or resume use, following brain injury; (2) intervention activities that facilitate the acceptance of professional help for a substance use problem; and (3) treatment to motivate a person with a substance use problem to consider, achieve, and maintain abstinence. Follow-along or follow-up services may be provided to support the individual after he or she returns to work, home, and community.

Support groups: Help individuals, family members, and friends cope with and become more educated about issues related to brain injury. Support group members may provide emotional support, information, resources, and an opportunity to network and learn what other people have done in similar situations.

Supported employment: Refers to the training, placement, and follow-up or extended services necessary for the individual to remain employed. Supported employment services provide supervision and training to an individual with a TBI in a competitive work setting or in a non-competitive, integrated setting which focuses on skills that lead to competitive work. Individuals in competitive employment must earn at least the minimum wage. To achieve successful employment placements, short-term vocational rehabilitation services provided by the state vocational rehabilitation agency, are augmented with ongoing support provided by other public or nonprofit agencies or organizations (extended services). State vocational rehabilitation agencies provide time-limited services for a period not to exceed 18 months, unless a longer period to achieve job stabilization has been established in the individualized plan for employment. Once this period has ended, the vocational rehabilitation agency must arrange for extended services provided by other appropriate state agencies, private nonprofit organizations, or other sources for the duration of that employment.

Alternative therapy (individual): Alternative or complementary therapies are therapies that are outside the field of traditional Western medicine. They are used as an adjunct to traditional medical treatment and include such practices as yoga, tai chi, acupressure, and acupuncture. Other examples include therapeutic massage, meditation, biofeedback, and homeopathic treatment (for example, natural pharmaceuticals derived from plants, minerals, and animals).

Cognitive therapy (individual): Cognitive therapy assists an individual in the management of specific problems in perception, memory, thinking, and problem solving. The purpose of cognitive therapy is to enhance an individual's functional competence in real-world situations. The process includes direct retraining, use of compensatory strategies, and use of cognitive tools. Skills are practiced and strategies are taught to help improve function and compensate for remaining deficits. The interventions are based on an assessment and understanding of the person's brain-behavior deficits and services are provided by qualified practitioners.

Occupational therapy (individual): Occupational therapy is provided by a qualified occupational therapist to improve, develop, or restore functions impaired or lost through injury. It is a skilled service designed to treat upper extremity motor dysfunction and cognitive dysfunction that affect performance of activities of daily living. The service includes evaluation, identification of adaptive equipment and energy conservation strategies that facilitate performance of daily living tasks, task analysis to facilitate planning and organization, and therapeutic activities directed toward instrumental activities of daily living. Therapeutic activities may be conducted in a variety of settings.

Physical therapy (individual): Physical therapy is provided by a qualified physical therapist to assist the individuals to return to the highest possible degree of personal independence. The physical therapist plans and administers individualized treatment programs that are designed to restore functional movement, relieve pain, promote healing and recovery, and when necessary, help individuals with TBI adapt to permanent disability. The service includes evaluation through tests, observations, and interviews that provide vital information about an individual's strength, reflexes, sensory perception, posture, gait, cardiopulmonary endurance, and daily living activities. Treatment includes various forms of exercise and physical modalities including heat, cold, ultrasound, electricity, and hands-on manual techniques.

Speech, hearing, and language therapy (individual): Speech and language services are provided by a qualified speech therapist or pathologist to maximize an individual's language, pragmatic, and cognitive skills. The therapist evaluates and treats disorders of speech and language that affect the individual's ability for functional communication. These therapeutic services are to improve the individual's ability to use verbal or non-verbal commands, improve receptive and expressive language functions, and improve or correct deficits in voice, articulation, rate, and rhythm.

Transportation services: Assists individuals with brain injury in getting to and from medical and health care appointments, specific rehabilitation and community programs, or to conduct business errands, essential shopping, and socialization activities. The service may be provided by a program provider as a part of its service package, an authorized transportation service, or through financial reimbursement for purposes of purchasing private transportation (taxi) or for reimbursing a family member, care provider, or non-professional (neighbor or friend) to transport an individual with a brain injury as needed.

Vehicle modification(s): Allows the individual to be able to transport himself or herself, or the family or caregiver to transport the individual. Such modifications may include wheelchair lifts, adapted seating, installing hand-controlled gears, and wheelchair securing devices.

Vocational services: Offer employment-related services that go beyond those found in routine job training programs. These services may include vocational evaluation, occupational skill training, job counseling, medical and therapeutic services, work adjustment, job training, job placement, job coaching, sheltered and supported employment, and job clubs. These services may also include assessment for and provision of assistive technology such as customized computer interfaces for persons with physical or sensory disabilities. These services are often provided by community vocational agencies that specialize in job training and placement, as well as other professionals who conduct assessment or other services as needed for vocational training.

Section 14.5

Finding Rehabilitation Facilities

"Rehab Checklist," © 2008 Brain Injury Resource Center
(www.headinjury.com). Reprinted with permission.

Finding Rehabilitation Facilities

Instructions: These questions are designed to collect and analyze
information on programs and treatments for brain injury rehabilitation. A high number of "yes" responses in each section will mean a
higher probability that the program will be of good quality, provide cost
effective services, and meet the needs of the patient and family.

Program and Procedures

1. Is the program accredited by the Commission of Accreditation
   of Rehab Facilities (CARF) and/or the Joint commission on Accreditation of Healthcare Organizations (JCAHO)?

2. What sources of funding does the program accept?

3. When was the program founded, and what is its guiding philosophy?

4. Has the facility been operational for at least five years?

5. Is the program viewed favorably by the medical and rehabilitation professional community outside the program, such as
   awards or citations?

6. Are programs custom-tailored to meet individual client needs?

7. Does the program provide a daily schedule? What role do
   patients have in directing the schedule and selecting the program components?

8. Can client's family members live with the client during his or
   her program when desired or appropriate?

9. Does the program have provisions to address behavioral concerns?

10. May I expect to receive timely progress reports that accurately account for services rendered?

11. How do you make decisions about who to admit into the program?

12. Are admission decisions made by clinical versus marketing staff?

13. Will pre-admission evaluations include a thorough review of past medical and rehabilitative care and treatment?

14. Will evaluators spend time with me and my and family to truly understand our needs and rehab goals?

15. May I have a copy of your policy concerning the rights and responsibilities of participants in this program? Will you discuss it with me and my family?

16. If I choose this program, what do you need to do prior to admission? How long will that take? What do you need me to do?

17. Will I be allowed to spend a day or so observing the program?

18. Will you arrange for me and my family to speak with former patients?

19. What forms or contracts am I expected to sign prior to admission? Will you give me a copy of each to read thoroughly before I sign?

20. May I count on frequent communication after admission?

21. If I choose this program, will you get previous medical and other important (school) records and other information you may need in order to decide?

22. Will the evaluation include a detailed projection of program cost and outcome goals?

23. Will the evaluation include objective, quantifiable goals for the program to be evaluated against?

24. Will progress reports be individualized, with objective quantifiable goals in all disciplines?

25. Is the program responsive to the requests of the case manager? Does it solicit programing input from patient and family?

26. Will the evaluation specify the length of time the program would take to accomplish the goals stated in the evaluation?

27. Will the evaluation include an assessment of special needs upon discharge such as housing, job coach, vocational rehab, recreational, attendant care, social services, nursing home, parent's home?

28. Are the progress reports, charts, medical records, and therapy documentation accessible upon request?

29. What is the average length of stay?

30. Will you provide me with a proposed service or treatment plan before I decide?

31. Will you coordinate with the program or service I am in now to facilitate a smooth admission and transition?

32. What is your understanding of the role of funding source in the decision-making process about the program I select?

33. What is your understanding of my role in the decision-making process about the program I select?

34. What is your program's greatest strength?

35. What distinguishes your program from its nearest competitor?

36. What is your program's worst failing?

37. In an ideal world, what would you change about the program?

38. What is your program's greatest success story?

39. How many of your patients realize their rehab goals?

40. What is your program's worst failing?

41. What is the average outcome?

42. What is the average length of treatment?

43. What type of follow-up programs and services do you offer?

44. What is your staff to patient ratio?

The Rehab Team

1. What are the qualifications of the members of the rehab team that would be assigned to my case? Does it employ the following?

   - Neuropsychology staff

   - Clinical psychology staff

   - Vocational rehabilitation counseling staff

   - Registered or licensed vocational staff

   - Practical nursing staff

   - Recreational therapy staff

   - Physical therapy staff

   - Occupational therapy staff

   - Speech or language pathology staff

   - Educational therapy staff

   - Social services staff, case management staff

2. Do the licensed professionals provide more than half the treatments for his or her discipline?

3. Does the program have a core of senior therapeutic and clinical management staff with more than five years treatment experience?

4. Does the mentioned staff hold professional licensure? If so, are these licenses available for review?

5. Is the majority of therapy conducted on a one-to-one basis?

6. Is senior management and treating staff readily available for consultation or to answer your questions?

7. Does the program employ rather than use contract therapy and medical staff?

8. Does the program regularly obtain medical consultation for client health issues?

9. Does the program have a medical director?

10. Will my personal physician be included in providing medical services while I am in the program?

11. How does the program handle medical emergencies?

12. Will your doctors monitor medications and medication interactions?

Insurance Matters and Program Costs

1. What agreement does the program have with my funding source?

2. What is the daily cost of the program?

3. What does this include (room and board, medications, physician services, therapy, transportation, and so forth)?

4. What is billed extra (special diet, telephone, internet, laundry, bed hold fees)?

5. How are charges calculated (per diem, per unit)?

6. Who is billed for services my funding source will not pay for?

The Rehab Setting

1. Does the facility have an outpatient program?

2. Do you provide follow up services in the home, the school, and the job?

3. Is therapy performed in a residential or clinical setting? What are the differences between the two models, and why do you believe one is more effective over the other?

4. Is therapy conducted in community settings, such as field trips, work and school settings, shopping malls?

5. Is the program designed to prepare the client for the intended discharge setting, for example, return to home, school, and work?

6. How is a person's ability to get around and to use community services and resources evaluated and addressed?

7. What local resources are used by the program to address the needs of the individual?

8. What do people generally do during unscheduled times?

9. How is the need for specialized adaptive equipment identified? How is the equipment provided and paid for?

Family and Friends

1. Does your program involve family members and friends?

2. Are family members and friends involved in team meetings?

3. What kind of family training, support groups, and therapy is offered? Is there a charge for participation?

4. What is your policy about visitors?

5. How does your program address changes in sexual functioning and intimacy?

Home

1. Will I receive a written plan upon discharge that addresses issues, such as housing, job coach, vocational rehab and counseling, recreational, social services, nursing home, parent's home?

2. Once we return to home, work, or school, what type of personal and attendant services will be necessary?

3. How are the services provided and paid for?

4. What type of adaptive equipment will be necessary?

5. How is the equipment provided and paid for?

6. What type of home modifications will be necessary?

7. How are the home modifications provided and paid?

8. Once we return to home, work, or school, what type of special accommodations will be necessary?

9. Does your program provide for respite services?

10. Does your program provide resources and services for caregivers?

11. Will your doctors continue to monitor my medications following discharge?

12. Will your team work with my schools, employers, and social service agencies?

13. Will your program provide periodic post-program follow-up sessions to reinforce the stage of compensatory mechanisms?

14. Will your team assist us with the transition to the home environment including behavioral and mood problems?

Overall Impressions

1. Did the evaluation provide you with more information than you had before the evaluation?

2. How did the program rate in areas of your primary concerns?

3. What are your greatest reservations concerning this program and how will you resolve them?

4. Total "yes" answers:

5. Total "no" answers:

6. Overall impressions:

   - Admission process

   - Program—relative to rehab goals

   - Rehab team—expertise, philosophy, and compatibility

   - Administration and client assistance features

   - Rehab setting—appearance, accommodations, and location

   - Involvement of patient, friends, and family

Part Three

Genetic and Congenital Brain Disorders

Chapter 15

Adrenoleukodystrophy

X-linked adrenoleukodystrophy is a disorder that occurs most often in males. It mainly affects the nervous system and the adrenal glands, which are small glands located on top of each kidney. People with this disorder often have progressive destruction of the fatty covering (myelin) that insulates nerves in the brain and spinal cord. They may also have a shortage of certain hormones caused by damage to the outer layer of the adrenal glands (adrenal cortex). This hormonal deficiency is known as adrenocortical insufficiency. There are three distinct types of X-linked adrenoleukodystrophy: a childhood cerebral form, an adrenomyeloneuropathy type, and a type called Addison disease only.

Children with the cerebral form of X-linked adrenoleukodystrophy experience learning and behavioral problems that usually appear by the age of ten. Over time the symptoms worsen, and these children may have difficulty reading, writing, understanding speech, and comprehending written material. Additional signs and symptoms of the cerebral form include aggressive behavior, vision problems, and impaired adrenal gland function. The rate at which this disorder progresses is variable; however, total disability within several years is not uncommon.

Signs and symptoms of the adrenomyeloneuropathy type appear between early adulthood and middle age. Affected individuals develop

Text in this chapter is excerpted from "X-Linked Adrenoleukodystrophy," Genetics Home Reference, U.S. Library of Medicine, September 2008.

progressive stiffness and weakness in their legs (paraparesis), experience urinary and genital tract disorders, and often show some degree of brain dysfunction. Most people with the adrenomyeloneuropathy type also have adrenocortical insufficiency.

When adrenocortical insufficiency occurs without any other symptoms, it is sometimes called Addison disease. People with X-linked adrenoleukodystrophy whose only symptom is adrenocortical insufficiency are said to have the Addison disease only form. Adrenocortical insufficiency may cause weakness, weight loss, skin changes, vomiting, and coma. Most people initially diagnosed with the Addison disease only form of X-linked adrenoleukodystrophy eventually develop all the signs of adrenomyeloneuropathy by the time they reach middle age.

For reasons that are unclear, different types of X-linked adrenoleukodystrophy can be seen in affected individuals within the same family. The prevalence of X-linked adrenoleukodystrophy is approximately one in 20,000 individuals worldwide. This condition occurs with a similar frequency in all populations.

Genes related to X-linked adrenoleukodystrophy: Mutations in the ABCD1 gene cause X-linked adrenoleukodystrophy. The ABCD1 gene provides instructions for producing the adrenoleukodystrophy protein (ALDP), which is involved in transporting molecules into peroxisomes. ABCD1 gene mutations result in a shortage (deficiency) of ALDP. When this protein is lacking, the breakdown of very long-chain fatty acids is disrupted, causing abnormally high levels of these fats in the body. The accumulation of very long-chain fatty acids may be toxic to the adrenal cortex and the myelin membranes that surround many of the nerves in the brain and spinal cord.

X-linked adrenoleukodystrophy inheritance: This condition is inherited in an X-linked pattern. A condition is considered X-linked if the mutated gene that causes the disorder is located on the X chromosome, one of the two sex chromosomes in each cell. In males (who have only one X chromosome), one altered copy of the gene in each cell is sufficient to cause the condition. Because females have two copies of the X chromosome, one altered copy of the gene in each cell usually leads to less severe symptoms in females than in males, or may cause no symptoms at all.

Many females who carry one altered copy of the ABCD1 gene do not have any features of X-linked adrenoleukodystrophy; however, some females with one altered copy of the gene have medical problems associated with this disorder. The signs and symptoms of X-linked adrenoleukodystrophy tend to appear at a later age in females than in males. In affected women, the disorder is usually similar to the adrenomyeloneuropathy type, although it may occasionally impair adrenal gland function. Less commonly, affected females have signs of the childhood cerebral form of this condition.

Chapter 16

Batten Disease (Neuronal Ceroid Lipofuscinoses)

Batten disease is a fatal, inherited disorder of the nervous system that begins in childhood. Early symptoms of this disorder usually appear between the ages of five and ten years, when parents or physicians may notice a previously normal child has begun to develop vision problems or seizures. In some cases, the early signs are subtle taking the form of personality and behavior changes, slow learning, clumsiness, or stumbling. Over time, affected children suffer mental impairment, worsening seizures, and progressive loss of sight and motor skills. Eventually, children with Batten disease become blind, bedridden, and demented. Batten disease is often fatal by the late teens or twenties.

Batten disease is named after the British pediatrician who first described it in 1903. Also known as Spielmeyer-Vogt-Sjogren-Batten disease, it is the most common form of a group of disorders called neuronal ceroid lipofuscinoses (NCL). Although Batten disease is usually regarded as the juvenile form of NCL, some physicians use the term Batten disease to describe all forms of NCL.

There are three other main types of NCL, including two forms that begin earlier in childhood and a very rare form that strikes adults. The symptoms of these three types are similar to those caused by Batten disease, but they become apparent at different ages and progress at different rates.

Excerpted from "Batten Disease Fact Sheet," National Institute of Neurological Disorders and Stroke (NINDS), updated October 23, 2009.

219

- Infantile NCL (Santavuori-Haltia disease) begins between about six months and two years of age and progresses rapidly. Affected children fail to thrive and have abnormally small heads (microcephaly). Also typical are short, sharp muscle contractions called myoclonic jerks. Patients usually die before age 5, although some have survived in a vegetative state a few years longer.

- Late infantile NCL (Jansky-Bielschowsky disease) begins between ages two and four years. The typical early signs are loss of muscle coordination (ataxia) and seizures that do not respond to drugs. This form progresses rapidly and ends in death between ages eight and twelve years.

- Adult NCL (Kufs disease or Parry's disease) generally begins before the age of 40, causes milder symptoms that progress slowly, and does not cause blindness. Although age of death is variable among affected individuals, this form does shorten life expectancy.

Batten disease and other forms of NCL are relatively rare, occurring in an estimated 2–4 of every 100,000 live births in the United States. These disorders appear to be more common in Finland, Sweden, other parts of northern Europe, and Newfoundland, Canada. Although NCLs are classified as rare diseases, they often strike more than one person in families that carry the defective genes.

How are NCLs inherited?

Childhood NCLs are autosomal recessive disorders; that is, they occur only when a child inherits two copies of the defective gene, one from each parent. When both parents carry one defective gene, each of their children faces a one in four chance of developing NCL. At the same time, each child also faces a one in two chance of inheriting just one copy of the defective gene. Individuals who have only one defective gene are known as carriers, meaning they do not develop the disease, but they can pass the gene on to their own children. Because the mutated genes that are involved in certain forms of Batten disease are known, carrier detection is possible in some instances.

Adult NCL may be inherited as an autosomal recessive, or less often, as an autosomal dominant disorder. In autosomal dominant inheritance, all people who inherit a single copy of the disease gene develop the disease. As a result, there are no unaffected carriers of the gene.

What causes these diseases?

Symptoms of Batten disease and other NCLs are linked to a buildup of substances called lipofuscins (lipo-pigments) in the body's tissues. These lipo-pigments are made up of fats and proteins. Their name comes from the technical word lipo, which is short for lipid or fat, and from the term pigment, used because they take on a greenish-yellow color when viewed under an ultraviolet light microscope. The lipo-pigments build up in cells of the brain and the eye as well as in skin, muscle, and many other tissues. Inside the cells, these pigments form deposits with distinctive shapes that can be seen under an electron microscope. Some look like half-moons, others like fingerprints. These deposits are what doctors look for when they examine a skin sample to diagnose Batten disease.

The biochemical defects that underlie several NCL have recently been discovered. An enzyme called palmityl-protein thioesterase has been shown to be insufficiently active in the infantile form of Batten disease (this condition is now referred to as CLN1). In the late infantile form (CLN2), a deficiency of an acid protease, an enzyme that hydrolyzes proteins, has been found as the cause of this condition. A mutated gene has been identified in juvenile Batten disease (CLN3), but the protein for which this gene codes has not been identified.

How are these disorders diagnosed?

Because vision loss is often an early sign, Batten disease may be first suspected during an eye exam. An eye doctor can detect a loss of cells within the eye that occurs in the three childhood forms of NCL. However, because such cell loss occurs in other eye diseases, the disorder cannot be diagnosed by this sign alone. Often, an eye specialist or other physician who suspects NCL may refer the child to a neurologist, a doctor who specializes in diseases of the brain and nervous system.

In order to diagnose NCL, the neurologist needs the patient's medical history and information from various laboratory tests. Diagnostic tests used for NCLs include the following:

- Blood or urine tests

- Skin or tissue sampling

- Electroencephalogram (EEG)

- Electrical studies of the eyes

- Brain scans

- Measurement of enzyme activity

- Deoxyribonucleic acid (DNA) analysis (In families where the mutation in the gene for CLN3 is known, DNA analysis can be used to confirm the diagnosis or for the prenatal diagnosis of this form of Batten disease. When the mutation is known, DNA analysis can also be used to detect unaffected carriers of this condition for genetic counseling.)

Is there any treatment?

As yet, no specific treatment is known that can halt or reverse the symptoms of Batten disease or other NCLs. However, seizures can sometimes be reduced or controlled with anticonvulsant drugs, and other medical problems can be treated appropriately as they arise. At the same time, physical and occupational therapy may help patients retain function as long as possible.

Some reports have described a slowing of the disease in children with Batten disease who were treated with vitamins C and E and with diets low in vitamin A. However, these treatments did not prevent the fatal outcome of the disease.

Support and encouragement can help patients and families cope with the profound disability and dementia caused by NCLs. Often, support groups enable affected children, adults, and families to share common concerns and experiences. Meanwhile, scientists pursue medical research that could someday yield an effective treatment.

Chapter 17

Cerebral Autosomal Dominant Arteriopathy with Subcortical Infarcts and Leukoencephalopathy (CADASIL)

Before we go into detail about CADASIL, let's break down its complex name so that we understand what it means. Although complex the name is self-explanatory and gives an exact medical description regarding the location, mode of inheritance, causative factors, and the pathological outcome.

Cerebral: Relating to the brain; thus implying that other systems in the body are relatively unaffected.

Autosomal dominant: A method of inheritance, whereby a single abnormal copy of a gene causes disease, despite the fact that the other good copy of the gene is present.

Arteriopathy: Disease of the arteries, usually medium to small size arteries.

Subcortical: Relating to the portion of the brain immediately below the cerebral cortex. White matter and the deep gray structures constitute the subcortical region. They play an important part in most higher functions such as sensation, voluntary muscle movement, thought, reasoning, memory, and so forth.

Infarcts: Areas of tissue that have undergone a type of cell death (called necrosis), as a result of loss of blood supply.

Leukoencephalopathy: A disease of the brain caused by damage to the white matter.

What is the cause of CADASIL?

CADASIL is a inherited disorder caused by mutations in a gene called Notch3, which is a protein that is involved in determining cell fate during fetal development. For example, it might determine whether a particular cell will ultimately be a smooth muscle cell in the wall of a blood vessel, or if it will be a liver cell. Post-developmental function of Notch3 includes maintaining the integrity of the arterial vessel wall.

Mutation in Notch3 causes the arterial wall to disintegrate, which leads to a loss of blood supply in the region supplied by that blood vessel. The abnormal Notch3 protein accumulates in blood vessels of the brain as well as in other parts of the body. The white matter and deeper parts of the brain are predominantly affected leading to infarcts.

CADASIL is an autosomal dominant disease, which means that a single abnormal copy of the Notch3 gene overrides the other "good" copy, producing disease. This means that if a parent is affected, every child of that parent has a 50% chance of having the disorder as well. If the child receives the abnormal copy, the child has a 100% chance of developing CADASIL.

What are the symptoms of CADASIL?

Initial symptoms of CADASIL, in the twenties or thirties, include migraine (a type of headache) and mood disorders, which may occur in 30%–40% of patients. Magnetic resonance imaging (MRI) abnormalities can be seen in the twenties and thirties as well. Strokes occur in the 40s and 50s. Over the next few decades as the disease advances, strokes and dementia are common symptoms. Death generally occurs 10–20 years after the onset of strokes and dementia.

The most common symptoms of CADASIL include the following:

- Migraine with aura: A migraine is a vascular headache resulting from changes in the sizes of the arteries in the brain. An aura refers to an abnormal sensation that the migraine is going to occur.

- Psychiatric disturbance: Any number of mood disorders can occur as a result of CADASIL, including depression.

- Ischemic episodes: Loss of blood flow to the brain, causing symptoms similar to those of a stroke.

- Cognitive deficits: These might include deficits in memory, attention, multi-tasking, and personality; the cognitive abilities generally decline as the disease worsens.

- Progressive memory loss and dementia.

- Multiple strokes leading to hemiparesis (paralysis of one side of the body), walking difficulty, and visual impairment.

- Rarely, epileptic seizures.

How can CADASIL be diagnosed?

Currently, the most reliable method of diagnosis is sequencing the Notch3 gene. This method can diagnose greater than 95% of cases of CADASIL with certainty. The method involves a blood test sent to a specialized laboratory. Availability of the test result makes diagnosis of other family members relatively easy.

Prior to availability of the gene tests, skin biopsy was used to diagnose CADASIL. A technique called electron microscopy was used to look for the characteristic accumulations of granular material (called granular osmiophilic material, or GOM) commonly seen in CADASIL. Presence of the material can positively diagnose CADASIL, though a negative result does not necessarily mean that the disease is not present. Additionally, a skin biopsy tissue can be tested for the accumulation of Notch3, using a molecule that specifically detects this protein. The accumulation occurs well before any symptoms, and therefore, it can be used to diagnose other family members. At this time, skin biopsy may be used to confirm doubtful cases.

Magnetic resonance imaging (MRI) may show characteristic alterations in the brain, but the alterations do not appear to be specific only to CADASIL. Therefore, brain MRI should not be considered as a single diagnostic tool.

How is CADASIL treated?

In a CADSAIL patient, migraine should be treated like most other patients of migraine, except the use of a group of medications called triptans (for example, Imitrex) is usually contraindicated due to increased risk of stroke.

Several medications are used to prevent migraine in patients who have frequent or severe migraine attacks and these should be used as recommended by the neurologist. Some examples of preventative medications are valproic acid, topiramate, gabapentin, propranolol, and tricyclic anti-depressants. Acetazolamide has been used in the past due to its property of dilating blood vessels.

Most neurologists agree to use of low dose daily aspirin in patients with CADASIL. Aspirin is used in patients who have other risk factors for stroke such as diabetes and heart disease as a prophylactic (preventative) medication.

In the event of an acute stroke-like episode, patients with CADASIL should not be treated with a thrombolytic agent (clot dissolving medication). This medication is usually used in patients with acute stroke within the first three hours. Patients with CADASIL have an increased risk of bleeding in the brain. Therefore, the current consensus is that this type of medication should be avoided.

Smoking and use of birth control pills are risk factors for stroke. We encourage patients with CADASIL to limit their use. Healthy lifestyle with adequate exercise and control of other risk factors for stroke such as high blood pressure, diabetes, and high cholesterol are highly recommended.

Recently, a randomized trial that tested Donepezil (Aricept), a drug recommended for Alzheimer disease, did not find it to be effective in CADASIL. However, some patients may benefit in terms of improved concentration and attention.

Other forms of supportive therapies such as physical therapy and speech therapy are instituted for rehabilitation from stroke.

Other clinical names for CADASIL include:

- hereditary multi-infarct dementia,

- chronic familial vascular encephalopathy,

- familial disorder with subcortical ischemic strokes,

- agnogenic medial arteriopathy, and

- familial Binswanger disease.

Chapter 18

Mental Health Disorders Rooted in Genetic Brain Disorders

Genomics and neuroscience, two areas of science fundamental to psychiatry, have undergone revolutionary changes in the past 20 years. Yet methods of diagnosis and treatment for patients with mental disorders have remained relatively unchanged. Indeed, during the same time, the public health burden of mental disorders has grown alarmingly. Mental disorders are now among the largest sources of medical disability worldwide and, like acquired immunodeficiency syndrome (AIDS) and cancer, they are urgent and deadly.

In this chapter, we argue that psychiatry's impact on public health will require that mental disorders be understood and treated as brain disorders. In the past, mental disorders were defined by the absence of a so-called organic lesion. Mental disorders became neurological disorders at the moment a lesion was found. With the advent of functional neuroimaging, patterns of regional brain activity associated with normal and pathological mental experience can be visualized, including detection of abnormal activity in brain circuits in the absence of an identifiable structural lesion. If mental disorders are brain disorders, then the basic sciences of psychiatry must include neuroscience and genomics and the training of psychiatrists in the future needs to be profoundly different from what it has been in the past.

Excerpted from "Psychiatry as a Clinical Neuroscience Discipline," National Institute of Mental Health (NIMH), February 27, 2009. The complete document including references is available at http://www.nimh.nih.gov/about/director/publications/psychiatry-as-a-clinical-neuroscience-discipline.shtml.

Mental Disorders as Complex Genetic Disorders

Mental disorders are considered genetically complex, similar to hypertension, diabetes, and cancer. This means they are not the result of a single causative mutation as in cystic fibrosis; rather, several common genetic variations likely contribute to risk. Scores of genes will likely be involved in risk for schizophrenia, autism, bipolar disorder, and even the vulnerability to addiction, but, as we have seen in hypertension and certain types of cancer, their function may aggregate around key intracellular pathways. In the past few months, the map of human haplotypes has been added to the map of the human genome (http://www.hapmap.org). This new map provides a guide to individual variation, a critical tool for identifying the vulnerability genes for genetically complex disorders. Defining the risk architecture of the major psychiatric disorders appears now limited only by being able to identify the phenotypes and endo-phenotypes of the illnesses, having access to deoxyribonucleic acid (DNA) from enough patients and their relatives, and learning to detect critical gene-environment interactions.

It is also important to recognize the limitations of genetics for complex illnesses, such as schizophrenia. Although identifying the alleles associated with psychopathology may indicate risk, it is not clear that genetics research will yield a binary diagnostic test for most of the psychiatric disorders. Nevertheless, identifying genetic variations associated with disease should provide a gateway into pathophysiology, revealing new targets for treatment. Genomics should also yield an approach to understanding risk and thus possible strategies for preventive interventions.

Gene-Environment Interactions

Twin studies and genetic epidemiological research indicate that the environment, in both a social and physical sense, interacts with genetic vulnerability to exert a powerful influence on the development of mental disorders. Psychiatry has spent much of the last century investigating the infantile roots of adult psychopathology. The current era is extending this investigation to molecular mechanisms, asking how environmental factors during critical intervals of development exert long-term effects on gene expression. Exploring the mechanisms of gene-environment interactions for depression is not substantially different from understanding how environmental toxins contribute to cancer or how diet influences cardiovascular diseases. However, for mental disorders the trigger may be psychosocial experiences, the exposure may only have an impact at specific stages of development, and the effects may be limited to a narrow range of cells in the brain.

New Approaches to Neural Regulation

One of the major insights from the Human Genome Project has been the discovery of the number of human genes: roughly 23,000 with perhaps 50% of these expressed in the brain. It is likely that, until very recently, 99% of the literature on the neurochemistry of mental disorders has focused on less than 1% of the genome. Most genes code for many proteins, so the number of proteins in the brain undoubtedly exceeds 100,000. Theories of mental disorders based on a few mono-amines, such as serotonin and dopamine, while helpful, will no doubt appear naive as research reveals vast numbers of new proteins found in the brain. In a sense, neuroscience is in a discovery phase, often called neurogenomics, with a goal of understanding where and when all of the genes in the brain are expressed.

Neurogenomics will provide maps of ribonucleic acid (RNA) in the brain and should alter our understanding of neuroanatomy, but is un-likely to yield a biomarker for any mental disorder. Newer approaches, proteomics and metabolomics, attempt to measure all of the available proteins or metabolic pathways to detect potential biomarkers asso-ciated with major mental disorders. It seems likely that among the vast sea of RNAs or proteins, some unique patterns will be associated with specific mental disorders, providing either a trait or state marker that will permit a finer grain of diagnosis than has been possible with clinical observation. These may come from cerebrospinal fluid, central nervous system cells, or peripheral cells grown in culture, but the sig-nificances of these results may be limited by our inability to sample cells in the relevant brain circuits. Early results in schizophrenia, posttraumatic stress disorder, and autism are just emerging.

Although the number of DNA variations, RNA expression patterns, or protein changes that have been linked to mental disorders remain limited, molecular and cellular neuroscience studies are already pointing to critical principles of neural regulation. For example, the increasing recognition of neurogenesis in the adult brain has led to a novel hypothesis of the pathophysiology and treatment of depres-sion. Clinical imaging studies have reported decreased hippocampal volume in people with major depressive disorder. Although it is not clear that depression is associated with reduced neurogenesis and changes in hippocampal volume have yet to be shown to be part of the pathophysiology of depression, animal studies have demonstrated that stress reduces neurogenesis in these regions and several classes of antidepressants increase the rate of neurogenesis in the hippocampus. In one study, a selective blockade of a drug's effect on neurogenesis also reduced the behavioral effect of the antidepressant. The resulting hypothesis is that chronic stress reduces the rate of neurogenesis in a critical pool of forebrain neurons, leading to a depressive episode in genetically vulnerable individuals. The importance of this hypothesis is that it introduces a long roster of known molecular mechanisms for neurogenesis as novel targets for developing new classes of pharmacological and behavioral treatments.

Revealing Brain Systems as Biomarkers

Ultimately, biomarkers for mental disorders may not be proteins or neurotransmitters but may emerge from neuroimaging (functional magnetic resonance imaging, single-photon emission computed tomography). Logically, if these are disorders of brain systems, then the visualization of abnormal patterns of brain activity should detect the pathology of these illnesses. One can imagine studies in which patterns of brain activation following stimulation may be diagnostic, just as cardiac imaging during a stress test is now used to diagnose coronary artery disease.

Multiple approaches to identifying abnormal functional activity in the brain already are emerging, from functional magnetic resonance imaging to *in vivo* neurochemistry and studies of brain receptors. One approach uses functional imaging to identify differences in regional activity. For instance, evidence from several different approaches implicates circuitry involving ventral, medial prefrontal cortex (Area 25) with major depressive disorder. In addition to structural studies reporting decreased gray matter volume in this region, positron emission tomographic studies comparing responders and non-responders to selective serotonin reuptake inhibitors, treatment with selective serotonin reuptake inhibitors and cognitive behavior therapy, and even placebo responders with non-responders have all shown that recovery from depression is associated with a decrease in activity in this region. This region has nearly the highest serotonergic innervation in the human forebrain as measured by the expression of the serotonin transporter. Individuals with the short allele of the serotonin transporter gene have reduced expression of the transporter and appear to be at a higher risk for developing depression following stressful life events. Recently, this short allele has been shown to be associated with reduced gray matter volume of Area 25 and uncoupling of an anterior cingulate-amygdala circuit necessary for extinction of negative affect, providing a model for linking genetic risk and environmental stress to a specific neural circuit implicated in depression. Studies of this circuit might soon be used to predict response to treatment, just as imaging is used to predict treatment response in other areas of medicine.

As another approach, imaging of receptors may reveal regional abnormalities that could serve as a biomarker or diagnostic test. However, only a few applications to date are promising for patient care. Although there is a recent report of reduced serotonin 1a receptor binding in the cingulate cortex of patients with panic disorder and there are remarkable reports of enduring changes in striatal dopamine D2 receptors following psychostimulant abuse, no receptor studies exist for the diagnosis or treatment of major mental disorders. Unfortunately, relatively few radioligands for membrane-bound receptors have been identified, and the technique may fail to detect small, localized changes or intracellular changes distal to the receptor. Despite these shortcomings, it seems likely that imaging receptors or cell signaling pathways could allow a quantitative approach to biodiagnosis of mental disorders in the coming decade.

Training in clinical neuroscience: The recognition that mental disorders are brain disorders suggests that psychiatrists of the future will need to be educated as brain scientists. Indeed, psychiatrists and neurologists may be best considered clinical neuroscientists, applying the revolutionary insights from neuroscience to the care of those with brain disorders. The recent scientific recognition of the importance of effective treatments of mental illnesses in cardiovascular disease and diabetes mandates the incorporation of psychiatry into truly integrated and effective treatment teams.

Future treatment: Currently, patients with mental disorders are treated episodically with medications that are focused on symptoms and not on the core pathology. The available treatments are slow, incomplete, and can be limited by adverse effects. In mental disorders, just as in the rest of medicine, better understanding of pathophysiology should yield diagnosis based on biomarkers and treatments based on rational designs targeting the pathophysiology. It is critical to realize that clinical neuroscience does not entail designing exotic technologies for a few privileged patients. The ultimate goal is personalized or individualized care for a broad spectrum of patients with mental disorders. Recently a better understanding of pathophysiology has led to a strategy for individualizing treatment of cancer. Currently in psychiatry, specific treatments for any given patient are largely developed empirically. With more knowledge about the pathophysiology of mental disorders, treatments should become more specific, more effective, and ultimately more accessible.

Clinical neuroscience can now look forward to an era of translation with more accurate diagnoses and better treatments as well as very early detection and prevention. Early detection will require a thorough understanding of risk, based on a comprehensive understanding of genetics and experience. For example, preventive interventions might be available to prevent a first psychotic episode in an adolescent at high risk for schizophrenia.

Chapter 19

Other Inherited Neurological Disorders

Aicardi Syndrome

Aicardi syndrome is a rare genetic disorder that primarily affects newborn girls. The condition is sporadic, meaning it is not known to pass from parent to child. (An exception is a report of two sisters and a pair of identical twins, all of whom were affected.) The mutation that causes Aicardi syndrome has not been identified. Scientists believe that the gene associated with the condition is located on the X chromosome because nearly all affected individuals are female and the only reports of boys having Aicardi syndrome are in boys born with an extra X chromosome. (Females have two X chromosomes, while males normally have an X and a Y chromosome.) Girls with Aicardi syndrome often develop seizures prior to three months and most before one year of age.

Originally, Aicardi syndrome was characterized by three main features: 1) partial or complete absence of the structure (corpus callosum) that links the two halves of the brain; 2) complex seizures, generally starting as infantile spasms; and, 3) retinal lacunae, lesions on the

---

This chapter includes excerpts from the following National Institute of Neurological Disorders and Stroke (NINDS) documents: "Aicardi Syndrome Information Page," updated January 24, 2010; "Alpers Disease Information Page," July 2, 2008; "Gerstmann-Sträussler-Scheinker Disease Information Page," February 13, 2007; "Infantile Neuroaxonal Dystrophy Information Page, February 14, 2007; and "Leigh Disease Information Page," October 8, 2008.

retina that look like yellowish spots. However, Aicardi syndrome is now known to have a much broader spectrum of abnormalities than was initially described. Not all girls with the condition have the three features described above and many girls have additional features.

Typical findings in the brain of girls with Aicardi syndrome include heterotopias, which are groups of brain cells that, during development, migrated to the wrong area of brain; polymicrogyria or pachygyria, which are numerous small, or too few, brain folds; and cysts, (fluid filled cavities) in the brain. Girls with Aicardi syndrome have varying degrees of mental retardation and developmental delay. Many girls also have developmental abnormalities of their optic nerves and some have microphthalmia (small eyes). Skeletal problems such as absent or abnormal ribs and abnormalities of vertebrae in the spinal column (including hemivertebrae and butterfly vertebrae) have also been reported. Some girls also have skin problems, facial asymmetry, or other characteristic facial features.

Treatment: There is no cure for Aicardi syndrome nor is there a standard course of treatment. Treatment generally involves medical management of seizures and programs to help parents and children cope with developmental delays. Long-term management by a pediatric neurologist with expertise in the management of infantile spasms is recommended.

Prognosis: The prognosis for girls with Aicardi syndrome varies according to the severity of their symptoms. There is an increased risk for death in childhood and adolescence, but survivors into adulthood have been described.

Alpers Disease

Alpers disease is a rare, genetically determined disease of the brain that causes progressive degeneration of grey matter in the cerebrum. The first sign of the disease usually begins early in life with convulsions. Other symptoms are developmental delay, progressive mental retardation, hypotonia (low muscle tone), spasticity (stiffness of the limbs), dementia, and liver conditions such as jaundice and cirrhosis that can lead to liver failure. Optic atrophy may also occur, often causing blindness. Researchers believe that Alpers disease is caused by an underlying metabolic defect. A number of individuals with Alpers disease have mutations in the polymerase-gamma gene, which results in the depletion of mitochondrial deoxyribonucleic acid (DNA).

Researchers suspect that Alpers disease is sometimes misdiagnosed as childhood jaundice or liver failure, since the only method of making a definitive diagnosis is by autopsy or brain biopsy after death.

Treatment: There is no cure for Alpers disease and no way to slow its progression. Treatment is symptomatic and supportive. Anticonvulsants may be used to treat the seizures. Valproate should be used with caution since it can increase the risk of liver failure. Physical therapy may help to relieve spasticity and maintain or increase muscle tone.

Prognosis: The prognosis for individuals with Alpers disease is poor. Those with the disease usually die within their first decade of life. Continuous, unrelenting seizures often lead to death. Liver failure and cardiorespiratory failure may also occur.

Gerstmann-Sträussler-Scheinker Disease

Gerstmann-Sträussler-Scheinker disease (GSS) is an extremely rare, neurodegenerative brain disorder. It is almost always inherited and is found in only a few families around the world. Onset of the disease usually occurs between the ages of 35 and 55. In the early stages, patients may experience varying levels of ataxia (lack of muscle coordination), including clumsiness, unsteadiness, and difficulty walking. As the disease progresses, the ataxia becomes more pronounced and most patients develop dementia. Other symptoms may include dysarthria (slurring of speech), nystagmus (involuntary movements of the eyes), spasticity (rigid muscle tone), and visual disturbances, sometimes leading to blindness. Deafness also can occur. In some families, parkinsonian features are present. GSS belongs to a family of human and animal diseases known as the transmissible spongiform encephalopathies (TSEs). Other TSEs include Creutzfeldt-Jakob disease, kuru, and fatal familial insomnia.

Treatment: There is no cure for GSS, nor are there any known treatments to slow progression of the disease. Current therapies are aimed at alleviating symptoms and making the patient as comfortable as possible.

Prognosis: GSS is a slowly progressive condition usually lasting from two to ten years. The disease ultimately causes severe disability and finally death, often after the patient goes into a coma or has a secondary infection such as aspiration pneumonia due to an impaired ability to swallow.

Infantile Neuroaxonal Dystrophy

Infantile neuroaxonal dystrophy (INAD) is a rare inherited neurological disorder. It affects axons, the part of a nerve cell that carries messages from the brain to other parts of the body, and causes progressive loss of vision, muscular control, and mental skills. While the basic genetic and metabolic causes are unknown, INAD is the result of an abnormal build-up of toxic substances in nerves that communicate with muscles, skin, and the conjunctive tissue around the eyes. Symptoms usually begin within the first two years of life, with the loss of head control and the ability to sit, crawl, or walk, accompanied by deterioration in vision and speech. Some children may have seizures. Distinctive facial deformities may be present at birth, including a prominent forehead, crossed eyes, an unusually small nose or jaw, and large, low-set ears. INAD is an autosomal recessive disorder, which means that both parents must be carriers of the defective gene that causes INAD to pass it on to their child. Electrophysiology (nerve conduction velocities) may be helpful for diagnosis, although diagnosis is usually confirmed by tissue biopsy of skin, rectum, nerve, or conjunctive tissue to confirm the presence of characteristic swellings (spheroid bodies) in the nerve axons.

Treatment: There is no cure for INAD and no treatment that can stop the progress of the disease. Treatment is symptomatic and supportive. Doctors can prescribe medications for pain relief and sedation. Physiotherapists and other physical therapists can teach parents and caregivers how to position and seat their child, and to exercise arms and legs to maintain comfort.

Prognosis: INAD is a progressive disease. Once symptoms begin, they will worsen over time. Generally, a baby's development starts to slow down between the ages of six months to three years. The first symptoms may be slowing of motor and mental development, followed by loss or regression of previously acquired skills. Rapid, wobbly eye movements and squints may be the first symptoms, followed by floppiness in the body and legs (more than in the arms). For the first few years, a baby with INAD will be alert and responsive, despite being increasingly physically impaired. Eventually, because of deterioration in vision, speech, and mental skills, the child will lose touch with its surroundings. Death usually occurs between the ages of five to ten years.

Leigh Disease

Leigh disease is a rare inherited neurometabolic disorder that affects the central nervous system. This progressive disorder begins in infants between the ages of three months and two years. Rarely, it occurs in teenagers and adults. Leigh disease can be caused by mutations in mitochondrial DNA or by deficiencies of an enzyme called pyruvate dehydrogenase. Symptoms of Leigh disease usually progress rapidly. The earliest signs may be poor sucking ability, and the loss of head control and motor skills. These symptoms may be accompanied by loss of appetite, vomiting, irritability, continuous crying, and seizures. As the disorder progresses, symptoms may also include generalized weakness, lack of muscle tone, and episodes of lactic acidosis, which can lead to impairment of respiratory and kidney function.

In Leigh disease, genetic mutations in mitochondrial DNA interfere with the energy sources that run cells in an area of the brain that plays a role in motor movements. The primary function of mitochondria is to convert the energy in glucose and fatty acids into a substance called adenosine triphosphate (ATP). The energy in ATP drives virtually all of a cell's metabolic functions. Genetic mutations in mitochondrial DNA, therefore, result in a chronic lack of energy in these cells, which in turn affects the central nervous system and causes progressive degeneration of motor functions.

There is also a form of Leigh disease (called X-linked Leigh disease) which is the result of mutations in a gene that produces another group of substances that are important for cell metabolism. This gene is only found on the X chromosome.

Treatment: The most common treatment for Leigh disease is thiamine or Vitamin B1. Oral sodium bicarbonate or sodium citrate may also be prescribed to manage lactic acidosis. Researchers are currently testing dichloroacetate to establish its effectiveness in treating lactic acidosis. In individuals who have the X-linked form of Leigh disease, a high-fat, low-carbohydrate diet may be recommended.

Prognosis: The prognosis for individuals with Leigh disease is poor. Individuals who lack mitochondrial complex IV activity and those with pyruvate dehydrogenase deficiency tend to have the worst prognosis and die within a few years. Those with partial deficiencies have a better prognosis, and may live to be six or seven years of age. Some have survived to their mid-teenage years.

Chapter 20

Birth Defects That Affect the Brain

Chapter Contents

Section 20.1

Agenesis of the Corpus Callosum

Text in this section is from "Agenesis of the Corpus Callosum
Information Page," National Institute of Neurological Disorders and
Stroke (NINDS), October 1, 2007.

Agenesis of the corpus callosum (ACC) is a birth defect in which
the structure that connects the two hemispheres of the brain (the
corpus callosum) is partially or completely absent. ACC can occur
as an isolated condition or in combination with other cerebral abnormalities, including Arnold-Chiari malformation, Dandy-Walker
syndrome, Andermann syndrome, schizencephaly (clefts or deep divi-
sions in brain tissue), and holoprosencephaly (failure of the forebrain
to divide into lobes). Girls may have a gender-specific condition called
Aicardi syndrome, which causes severe mental retardation, seizures,
abnormalities in the vertebra of the spine, and lesions on the retina of
the eye. ACC can also be associated with malformations in other parts
of the body, such as midline facial defects. The effects of the disorder
range from subtle or mild to severe, depending on associated brain
abnormalities. Intelligence may be normal with mild compromise of
skills requiring matching of visual patterns. But children with the
most severe brain malformations may have intellectual retardation,
seizures, hydrocephalus, and spasticity.

Treatment: There is no standard course of treatment for ACC.
Treatment usually involves management of symptoms and seizures
if they occur.

Prognosis: Depends on the extent and severity of malformations.
ACC does not cause death in the majority of children. Mental retardation does not worsen. Although many children with the disorder have
average intelligence and lead normal lives, neuropsychological testing reveals subtle differences in higher cortical function compared to
individuals of the same age and education without ACC.

Section 20.2

Arteriovenous Malformations and Other Vascular Lesions

Excerpted from "Arteriovenous Malformations and Other Vascular Lesions of the Central Nervous System," National Institute of Neurological Disorders and Stroke (NINDS), December 18, 2009.

Arteriovenous malformations (AVMs) are defects of the circulatory system that are generally believed to arise during embryonic or fetal development or soon after birth. They are comprised of snarled tangles of arteries and veins. Arteries carry oxygen-rich blood away from the heart to the body's cells; veins return oxygen-depleted blood to the lungs and heart. The absence of capillaries—small blood vessels that connect arteries to veins—creates a short-cut for blood to pass directly from arteries to veins. The presence of an AVM disrupts this vital cyclical process. Although AVMs can develop in many different sites, those located in the brain or spinal cord—the two parts of the central nervous system—can have especially widespread effects on the body.

AVMs of the brain or spinal cord (neurological AVMs) are believed to affect approximately 300,000 Americans. They occur in males and females of all racial or ethnic backgrounds at roughly equal rates.

Symptoms: Most people with neurological AVMs experience few, if any, significant symptoms, and the malformations tend to be discovered only incidentally, usually either at autopsy or during treatment for an unrelated disorder. But for about 12% of the affected population (about 36,000 of the estimated 300,000 Americans with AVMs), these abnormalities cause symptoms that vary greatly in severity. For a small fraction of the individuals within this group, such symptoms are severe enough to become debilitating or even life-threatening. Each year about 1% of those with AVMs will die as a direct result of the AVM.

Seizures and headaches are the most generalized symptoms of AVMs, but no particular type of seizure or headache pattern has been identified. AVMs also can cause a wide range of more specific neurological symptoms that vary from person to person, depending primarily upon the location of the AVM. Such symptoms may include muscle

241

weakness or paralysis in one part of the body; a loss of coordination (ataxia) that can lead to such problems as gait disturbances; apraxia, or difficulties carrying out tasks that require planning; dizziness; visual disturbances such as a loss of part of the visual field; an inability to control eye movement; papilledema (swelling of a part of the optic nerve known as the optic disk); various problems using or understanding language (aphasia); abnormal sensations such as numbness, tingling, or spontaneous pain (paresthesia or dysesthesia); memory deficits; and mental confusion, hallucinations, or dementia. Researchers have recently uncovered evidence that AVMs may also cause subtle learning or behavioral disorders in some people during their childhood or adolescence, long before more obvious symptoms become evident.

One of the more distinctive signs indicating the presence of an AVM is an auditory phenomenon called a bruit, coined from the French word meaning noise. (A sign is a physical effect observable by a physician, but not by a patient.) Doctors use this term to describe the rhythmic, whooshing sound caused by excessively rapid blood flow through the arteries and veins of an AVM.

Symptoms caused by AVMs can appear at any age, but because these abnormalities tend to result from a slow buildup of neurological damage over time they are most often noticed when people are in their twenties, thirties, or forties. If AVMs do not become symptomatic by the time people reach their late forties or early fifties, they tend to remain stable and rarely produce symptoms. In women, pregnancy sometimes causes a sudden onset or worsening of symptoms, due to accompanying cardiovascular changes, especially increases in blood volume and blood pressure.

In contrast to the vast majority of neurological AVMs, one especially severe type causes symptoms to appear at, or very soon after, birth. Called a vein of Galen defect after the major blood vessel involved, this lesion is located deep inside the brain. It is frequently associated with hydrocephalus (an accumulation of fluid within certain spaces in the brain, often with visible enlargement of the head), swollen veins visible on the scalp, seizures, failure to thrive, and congestive heart failure. Children born with this condition who survive past infancy often remain developmentally impaired.

How do AVMs damage the brain and spinal cord?

AVMs become symptomatic only when the damage they cause to the brain or spinal cord reaches a critical level. This is one of the reasons why a relatively small fraction of people with these lesions experiences significant health problems related to the condition. AVMs damage the brain or spinal cord through three basic mechanisms: by reducing the amount of oxygen reaching neurological tissues; by causing bleeding (hemorrhage) into surrounding tissues; and by compressing or displacing parts of the brain or spinal cord.

Where do neurological AVMs tend to form?

AVMs can form virtually anywhere in the brain or spinal cord—wherever arteries and veins exist. Some are formed from blood vessels located in the dura mater or in the pia mater, the outermost and innermost, respectively, of the three membranes surrounding the brain and spinal cord. (The third membrane, called the arachnoid, lacks blood vessels.)

Dural and pial AVMs can appear anywhere on the surface of the brain. Those located on the surface of the cerebral hemispheres—the uppermost portions of the brain—exert pressure on the cerebral cortex, the brain's gray matter. Depending on their location, these AVMs may damage portions of the cerebral cortex involved with thinking, speaking, understanding language, hearing, taste, touch, or initiating and controlling voluntary movements. AVMs located on the frontal lobe close to the optic nerve or on the occipital lobe, the rear portion of the cerebrum where images are processed, may cause a variety of visual disturbances.

AVMs also can form from blood vessels located deep inside the interior of the cerebrum. These AVMs may compromise the functions of three vital structures: the thalamus, which transmits nerve signals between the spinal cord and upper regions of the brain; the basal ganglia surrounding the thalamus, which coordinate complex movements; and the hippocampus, which plays a major role in memory.

AVMs can affect other parts of the brain besides the cerebrum. The hindbrain is formed from two major structures: the cerebellum, which is nestled under the rear portion of the cerebrum, and the brainstem, which serves as the bridge linking the upper portions of the brain with the spinal cord. These structures control finely coordinated movements, maintain balance, and regulate some functions of internal organs, including those of the heart and lungs. AVM damage to these parts of the hindbrain can result in dizziness, giddiness, vomiting, a loss of the ability to coordinate complex movements such as walking, or uncontrollable muscle tremors.

What are the health consequences of AVMs?

The greatest potential danger posed by AVMs is hemorrhage. Researchers believe that each year between 2%–4% of all AVMs hemorrhage. Most episodes of bleeding remain undetected at the time they occur because they are not severe enough to cause significant neurological damage. But massive, even fatal, bleeding episodes do occur. The present state of knowledge does not permit doctors to predict whether or not any particular person with an AVM will suffer an extensive hemorrhage. The lesions can remain stable or can suddenly begin to grow. In a few cases, they have been observed to regress spontaneously. Whenever an AVM is detected, the individual should be carefully and consistently monitored for any signs of instability that may indicate an increased risk of hemorrhage.

A few physical characteristics appear to indicate a greater-than-usual likelihood of clinically significant hemorrhage. Smaller AVMs have a greater likelihood of bleeding than do larger ones. Impaired drainage by unusually narrow or deeply situated veins also increases the chances of hemorrhage. Pregnancy also appears to increase the likelihood of clinically significant hemorrhage, mainly because of increases in blood pressure and blood volume. Finally, AVMs that have hemorrhaged once are about nine times more likely to bleed again during the first year after the initial hemorrhage than are lesions that have never bled.

The damaging effects of a hemorrhage are related to lesion location. Bleeding from AVMs located deep inside the interior tissues, or parenchyma, of the brain typically causes more severe neurological damage than does hemorrhage by lesions that have formed in the dural or pial membranes or on the surface of the brain or spinal cord. (Deeply located bleeding is usually referred to as an intracerebral or parenchymal hemorrhage; bleeding within the membranes or on the surface of the brain is known as subdural or subarachnoid hemorrhage.) Thus, location is an important factor to consider when weighing the relative risks of surgical versus non-surgical treatment of AVMs.

What other types of vascular lesions affect the central nervous system?

Besides AVMs, three other main types of vascular lesion can arise in the brain or spinal cord: cavernous malformations, capillary telangiectases, and venous malformations. These lesions may form virtually anywhere within the central nervous system, but unlike AVMs, they are not caused by high-velocity blood flow from arteries into veins. In contrast, cavernous malformations, telangiectases, and venous malformations are all low-flow lesions. Instead of a combination of arteries and veins, each one involves only one type of blood vessel. These lesions are less unstable than AVMs and do not pose the same relatively high risk of significant hemorrhage. In general, low-flow lesions tend to cause fewer troubling neurological symptoms and require less aggressive treatment than do AVMs.

What causes vascular lesions?

Although the cause of these vascular anomalies of the central nervous system is not yet well understood, scientists believe that they most often result from mistakes that occur during embryonic or fetal development. These mistakes may be linked to genetic mutations in some cases. A few types of vascular malformations are known to be hereditary and thus are known to have a genetic basis. Some evidence also suggests that at least some of these lesions are acquired later in life as a result of injury to the central nervous system.

Researchers have recently identified changes in the chemical structures of various angiogenic factors in some people who have AVMs or other vascular abnormalities of the central nervous system. However, it is not yet clear how these chemical changes actually cause changes in blood vessel structure.

By studying patterns of familial occurrence, researchers have established that one type of cavernous malformation involving multiple lesion formation is caused by a genetic mutation in chromosome 7. This genetic mutation appears in many ethnic groups, but it is especially frequent in a large population of Hispanic Americans living in the Southwest; these individuals share a common ancestor in whom the genetic change occurred

How are AVMs and other vascular lesions detected?

Physicians now use an array of traditional and new imaging technologies to uncover the presence of AVMs. Angiography provides the most accurate pictures of blood vessel structure in AVMs. The technique requires injecting a special water-soluble dye, called a contrast agent, into an artery. The dye highlights the structure of blood vessels so that it can be recorded on conventional x-rays. Although angiography can record fine details of vascular lesions, the procedure is somewhat invasive and carries a slight risk of causing a stroke. Its safety, however, has recently been improved through the development of more precise techniques for delivering dye to the site of an AVM.

Two of the most frequently employed noninvasive imaging technologies used to detect AVMs are computed tomography (CT) and magnetic resonance imaging (MRI) scans. CT scans use x-rays to create a series of cross-sectional images of the head, brain, or spinal cord and are especially useful in revealing the presence of hemorrhage. MRI imaging, however, offers superior diagnostic information by using magnetic fields to detect subtle changes in neurological tissues. A recently developed application of MRI technology—magnetic resonance angiography (MRA)—can record the pattern and velocity of blood flow through vascular lesions as well as the flow of cerebrospinal fluid throughout the brain and spinal cord. CT, MRI, and MRA can provide three-dimensional representations of AVMs by taking images from multiple angles.

How can AVMs and other vascular lesions be treated?

Medication can often alleviate general symptoms such as headache, back pain, and seizures caused by AVMs and other vascular lesions. However, the definitive treatment for AVMs is either surgery or focused irradiation therapy. Venous malformations and capillary telangiectases rarely require surgery; moreover, their structures are diffuse and usually not suitable for surgical correction and they usually do not require treatment anyway. Cavernous malformations are usually well defined enough for surgical removal, but surgery on these lesions is less common than for AVMs because they do not pose the same risk of hemorrhage.

The decision to perform surgery on any individual with an AVM requires a careful consideration of possible benefits versus risks. The natural history of an individual AVM is difficult to predict; however, left untreated, they have the potential of causing significant hemorrhage, which may result in serious neurological deficits or death.

Today, three surgical options exist for the treatment of AVMs: conventional surgery, endovascular embolization, and radiosurgery. The choice of treatment depends largely on the size and location of an AVM. Because so many variables are involved in treating AVMs, doctors must assess the danger posed to individuals largely on a case-by-case basis.

Section 20.3

Moebius Syndrome

Excerpted from "Moebius Syndrome Information Page,"
National Institute of Neurological Disorders (NINDS),
September 16, 2008.

Moebius syndrome is a rare birth defect caused by the absence or underdevelopment of the 6th and 7th cranial nerves, which control eye movements and facial expression. Many of the other cranial nerves may also be affected, including the 3rd, 5th, 8th, 9th, 11th, and 12th. The first symptom, present at birth, is an inability to suck. Other symptoms can include: feeding, swallowing, and choking problems; excessive drooling; crossed eyes; lack of facial expression; inability to smile; eye sensitivity; motor delays; high or cleft palate; hearing problems; and speech difficulties. Children with Moebius syndrome are unable to move their eyes back and forth. Decreased numbers of muscle fibers have been reported. Deformities of the tongue, jaw, and limbs, such as clubfoot and missing or webbed fingers, may also occur. As children get older, lack of facial expression and inability to smile become the dominant visible symptoms. Approximately 30%–40% of children with Moebius syndrome have some degree of autism.

There are four recognized categories of Moebius syndrome:

• Group I, characterized by small or absent brain stem nuclei that control the cranial nerves;

• Group II, characterized by loss and degeneration of neurons in the facial peripheral nerve;

• Group III, characterized by loss and degeneration of neurons and other brain cells, microscopic areas of damage, and hardened tissue in the brainstem nuclei; and

• Group IV, characterized by muscular symptoms in spite of a lack of lesions in the cranial nerve.

Treatment: There is no specific course of treatment for Moebius syndrome. Treatment is supportive and in accordance with symptoms.

Infants may require feeding tubes or special bottles to maintain sufficient nutrition. Surgery may correct crossed eyes and improve limb and jaw deformities. Physical and speech therapy often improves motor skills and coordination, and leads to better control of speaking and eating abilities. Plastic reconstructive surgery may be beneficial in some individuals. Nerve and muscle transfers to the corners of the mouth have been performed to provide limited ability to smile.

Prognosis: There is no cure for Moebius syndrome. In spite of the impairments that characterize the disorder, proper care and treatment give many individuals a normal life expectancy.

Section 20.4

Neuronal Migration Disorders

Excerpted from "Neuronal Migration Disorders Information Page," National Institute of Neurological Disorders and Stroke (NINDS), February 14, 2007.

Neuronal migration disorders (NMDs) are a group of birth defects caused by the abnormal migration of neurons in the developing brain and nervous system. In the developing brain, neurons must migrate from the areas where they are born to the areas where they will settle into their proper neural circuits. Neuronal migration, which occurs as early as the second month of gestation, is controlled by a complex assortment of chemical guides and signals. When these signals are absent or incorrect, neurons do not end up where they belong. This can result in structurally abnormal or missing areas of the brain in the cerebral hemispheres, cerebellum, brainstem, or hippocampus. The structural abnormalities found in NMDs include schizencephaly, porencephaly, lissencephaly, agyria, macrogyria, pachygyria, microgyria, micropolygyria, neuronal heterotopias (including band heterotopia), agenesis of the corpus callosum, and agenesis of the cranial nerves. Symptoms vary according to the abnormality, but often feature poor muscle tone and motor function, seizures, developmental delays, mental retardation, failure to grow and thrive, difficulties with feeding, swelling in the extremities, and a smaller than normal head. Most infants with an NMD appear normal, but some disorders have characteristic facial or skull features that can be recognized by a neurologist. Several genetic abnormalities in children with NMDs have been identified. Defects in genes that are involved in neuronal migration have been associated with NMDs, but the role they play in the development of these disorders is not yet well-understood. More than 25 syndromes resulting from abnormal neuronal migration have been described. Among them are syndromes with several different patterns of inheritance; genetic counseling thus differs greatly between syndromes.

Treatment: Treatment is symptomatic, and may include anti-seizure medication and special or supplemental education consisting of physical, occupational, and speech therapies.

Prognosis: The prognosis for children with NMDs varies depending on the specific disorder and the degree of brain abnormality and subsequent neurological losses.

Chapter 21

Cephalic Disorders

Cephalic disorders are congenital conditions that stem from damage to, or abnormal development of, the budding nervous system. Cephalic is a term that means head or head end of the body. Congenital means the disorder is present at, and usually before, birth. Although there are many congenital developmental disorders, this chapter briefly describes only cephalic conditions.

Cephalic disorders are not necessarily caused by a single factor but may be influenced by hereditary or genetic conditions or by environmental exposures during pregnancy such as medication taken by the mother, maternal infection, or exposure to radiation. Some cephalic disorders occur when the cranial sutures (the fibrous joints that connect the bones of the skull) join prematurely. Most cephalic disorders are caused by a disturbance that occurs very early in the development of the fetal nervous system.

The human nervous system develops from a small, specialized plate of cells on the surface of the embryo. Early in development, this plate of cells forms the neural tube, a narrow sheath that closes between the third and fourth weeks of pregnancy to form the brain and spinal cord of the embryo. Four main processes are responsible for the development of the nervous system: cell proliferation, the process in which nerve cells divide to form new generations of cells; cell migration, the process in which nerve cells move from their place of origin to the place where they will remain for life; cell differentiation, the process during

Excerpted from "Cephalic Disorders Fact Sheet," National Institute of Neurological Disorders and Stroke (NINDS), January 14, 2010.

which cells acquire individual characteristics; and cell death, a natural process in which cells die.

Damage to the developing nervous system is a major cause of chronic, disabling disorders, and sometimes death in infants, children, and even adults. The degree to which damage to the developing nervous system harms the mind and body varies enormously. Many disabilities are mild enough to allow those afflicted to eventually function independently in society. Others are not. Some infants, children, and adults die, others remain totally disabled, and an even larger population is partially disabled, functioning well below normal capacity throughout life.

Different Kinds of Cephalic Disorders

Anencephaly: A neural tube defect that occurs when the cephalic (head) end of the neural tube fails to close, usually between the 23rd and 26th days of pregnancy, resulting in the absence of a major portion of the brain, skull, and scalp. Infants with this disorder are born without a forebrain—the largest part of the brain consisting mainly of the cerebrum, which is responsible for thinking and coordination. The remaining brain tissue is often exposed—not covered by bone or skin.

Infants born with anencephaly are usually blind, deaf, unconscious, and unable to feel pain. Although some individuals with anencephaly may be born with a rudimentary brainstem, the lack of a functioning cerebrum permanently rules out the possibility of ever gaining consciousness. Reflex actions such as breathing and responses to sound or touch may occur. The disorder is one of the most common disorders of the fetal central nervous system. Approximately 1,000 to 2,000 American babies are born with anencephaly each year. The disorder affects females more often than males.

Recent studies have shown that the addition of folic acid to the diet of women of child-bearing age may significantly reduce the incidence of neural tube defects. Therefore it is recommended that all women of child-bearing age consume 0.4 milligrams (mg) of folic acid daily.

Colpocephaly: A disorder in which there is an abnormal enlargement of the occipital horns—the posterior or rear portion of the lateral ventricles (cavities or chambers) of the brain. This enlargement occurs when there is an underdevelopment or lack of thickening of the white matter in the posterior cerebrum. Colpocephaly is characterized by microcephaly (abnormally small head) and mental retardation. Other features may include motor abnormalities, muscle spasms, and seizures.

252

Although the cause is unknown, researchers believe that the disorder results from an intrauterine disturbance that occurs between the second and sixth months of pregnancy. Colpocephaly may be diagnosed late in pregnancy, although it is often misdiagnosed as hydrocephalus (excessive accumulation of cerebrospinal fluid in the brain). It may be more accurately diagnosed after birth when signs of mental retardation, microcephaly, and seizures are present.

There is no definitive treatment for colpocephaly. Anticonvulsant medications can be given to prevent seizures, and doctors try to prevent contractures (shrinkage or shortening of muscles). The prognosis for individuals with colpocephaly depends on the severity of the associated conditions and the degree of abnormal brain development. Some children benefit from special education.

Holoprosencephaly: A disorder characterized by the failure of the prosencephalon (the forebrain of the embryo) to develop. During normal development the forebrain is formed and the face begins to develop in the fifth and sixth weeks of pregnancy. Holoprosencephaly is caused by a failure of the embryo's forebrain to divide to form bilateral cerebral hemispheres (the left and right halves of the brain), causing defects in the development of the face and in brain structure and function.

There are three classifications of holoprosencephaly. Alobar holoprosencephaly, the most serious form in which the brain fails to separate, is usually associated with severe facial anomalies. Semilobar holoprosencephaly, in which the brain's hemispheres have a slight tendency to separate, is an intermediate form of the disease. Lobar holoprosencephaly, in which there is considerable evidence of separate brain hemispheres, is the least severe form. In some cases of lobar holoprosencephaly, the patient's brain may be nearly normal.

Although the causes of most cases of holoprosencephaly remain unknown, researchers know that approximately one-half of all cases have a chromosomal cause. There is no treatment for holoprosencephaly and the prognosis for individuals with the disorder is poor. Most of those who survive show no significant developmental gains. For children who survive, treatment is symptomatic. Although it is possible that improved management of diabetic pregnancies may help prevent holoprosencephaly, there is no means of primary prevention.

Hydranencephaly: A rare condition in which the cerebral hemispheres are absent and replaced by sacs filled with cerebrospinal fluid. Usually the cerebellum and brainstem are formed normally. An infant with hydranencephaly may appear normal at birth. However, after a few weeks the infant usually becomes irritable and has increased muscle tone (hypertonia). After several months of life, seizures and hydrocephalus may develop. Other symptoms may include visual impairment, lack of growth, deafness, blindness, spastic quadriparesis (paralysis), and intellectual deficits.

Hydranencephaly is an extreme form of porencephaly (a rare disorder, discussed later in this chapter, characterized by a cyst or cavity in the cerebral hemispheres) and may be caused by vascular insult (such as stroke) or injuries, infections, or traumatic disorders after the 12th week of pregnancy.

Diagnosis may be delayed for several months because the infant's early behavior appears to be relatively normal. There is no standard treatment for hydranencephaly. Treatment is symptomatic and supportive. Hydrocephalus may be treated with a shunt. The outlook for children with hydranencephaly is generally poor, and many children with this disorder die before age one. However, in rare cases, children with hydranencephaly may survive for several years or more.

Iniencephaly: A rare neural tube defect that combines extreme retroflexion (backward bending) of the head with severe defects of the spine. The affected infant tends to be short, with a disproportionately large head. Diagnosis can be made immediately after birth because the head is so severely retroflexed that the face looks upward. The skin of the face is connected directly to the skin of the chest and the scalp is directly connected to the skin of the back. Generally, the neck is absent.

Most individuals with iniencephaly have other associated anomalies such as anencephaly, cephalocele (a disorder in which part of the cranial contents protrudes from the skull), hydrocephalus, cyclopia, absence of the mandible (lower jaw bone), cleft lip and palate, cardiovascular disorders, diaphragmatic hernia, and gastrointestinal malformation. The disorder is more common among females.

The prognosis for those with iniencephaly is extremely poor. Newborns with iniencephaly seldom live more than a few hours. The distortion of the fetal body may also pose a danger to the mother's life.

Lissencephaly: A rare brain malformation characterized by microcephaly and the lack of normal convolutions (folds) in the brain. It is caused by defective neuronal migration, the process in which nerve cells move from their place of origin to their permanent location. Symptoms of the disorder may include unusual facial appearance, difficulty swallowing, failure to thrive, and severe psychomotor retardation. Anomalies of the hands, fingers, or toes, muscle spasms, and seizures may also occur. Lissencephaly may be diagnosed at or soon after birth.

Treatment for those with lissencephaly is symptomatic and depends on the severity and locations of the brain malformations. The prognosis for children with lissencephaly varies depending on the degree of brain malformation. Many individuals show no significant development beyond a 3- to 5-month-old level. Some may have near-normal development and intelligence. Many will die before the age of two. Respiratory problems are the most common causes of death.

Megalencephaly: Also called macrencephaly, this is a condition in which there is an abnormally large, heavy, and usually malfunctioning brain. By definition, the brain weight is greater than average for the age and gender of the infant or child. Head enlargement may be evident at birth or the head may become abnormally large in the early years of life.

Symptoms of megalencephaly may include delayed development, convulsive disorders, corticospinal (brain cortex and spinal cord) dysfunction, and seizures. Megalencephaly affects males more often than females.

The prognosis for individuals with megalencephaly largely depends on the underlying cause and the associated neurological disorders. Treatment is symptomatic. Megalencephaly may lead to a condition called macrocephaly.

Microcephaly: A neurological disorder in which the circumference of the head is smaller than average for the age and gender of the infant or child. Microcephaly may be congenital or it may develop in the first few years of life. The disorder may stem from a wide variety of conditions that cause abnormal growth of the brain, or from syndromes associated with chromosomal abnormalities.

Infants with microcephaly are born with either a normal or reduced head size. Subsequently the head fails to grow while the face continues to develop at a normal rate, producing a child with a small head, a large face, a receding forehead, and a loose, often wrinkled scalp. As the child grows older, the smallness of the skull becomes more obvious, although the entire body also is often underweight and dwarfed. Development of motor functions and speech may be delayed. In general, life expectancy for individuals with microcephaly is reduced and the prognosis for normal brain function is poor. The prognosis varies depending on the presence of associated abnormalities.

Porencephaly: An extremely rare disorder of the central nervous system involving a cyst or cavity in a cerebral hemisphere. The cysts or cavities are usually the remnants of destructive lesions, but are sometimes the result of abnormal development. The disorder can occur before or after birth. Porencephaly most likely has a number of different, often unknown causes, including absence of brain development and destruction of brain tissue. The presence of porencephalic cysts can sometimes be detected by transillumination of the skull in infancy.

Individuals with porencephaly may have poor or absent speech development, epilepsy, hydrocephalus, spastic contractures (shrinkage or shortening of muscles), and mental retardation. Treatment may include physical therapy, medication for seizure disorders, and a shunt for hydrocephalus. The prognosis for individuals with porencephaly varies according to the location and extent of the lesion. Some patients with this disorder may develop only minor neurological problems and have normal intelligence, while others may be severely disabled. Others may die before the second decade of life.

Schizencephaly: A rare developmental disorder characterized by abnormal slits, or clefts, in the cerebral hemispheres. Schizencephaly is a form of porencephaly. Individuals with clefts in both hemispheres, or bilateral clefts, are often developmentally delayed and have delayed speech and language skills and corticospinal dysfunction. Individuals with smaller, unilateral clefts (clefts in one hemisphere) may be weak on one side of the body and may have average or near-average intelligence. Patients with schizencephaly may also have varying degrees of microcephaly, mental retardation, hemiparesis (weakness or paralysis affecting one side of the body), or quadriparesis (weakness or paralysis affecting all four extremities), and may have reduced muscle tone (hypotonia). Most patients have seizures and some may have hydrocephalus.

Other Less Common Cephalic Disorders

Acephaly: Literally means absence of the head. It is a much rarer condition than anencephaly. The acephalic fetus is a parasitic twin attached to an otherwise intact fetus.

Exencephaly: A condition in which the brain is located outside of the skull. This condition is usually found in embryos as an early stage of anencephaly.

Macrocephaly: A condition in which the head circumference is larger than average for the age and gender of the infant or child. It is a descriptive rather than a diagnostic term and is a characteristic of a variety of disorders. Macrocephaly also may be inherited.

Micrencephaly: A disorder characterized by a small brain and may be caused by a disturbance in the proliferation of nerve cells. Micrencephaly may also be associated with maternal problems such as alcoholism, diabetes, or rubella (German measles). A genetic factor may play a role in causing some cases of micrencephaly.

Otocephaly: A lethal condition in which the primary feature is agnathia—a developmental anomaly characterized by total or virtual absence of the lower jaw. The condition is considered lethal because of a poorly functioning airway.

Craniostenoses: Deformities of the skull caused by the premature fusion or joining together of the cranial sutures. Cranial sutures are fibrous joints that join the bones of the skull together. The nature of these deformities depends on which sutures are affected.

Brachycephaly: This occurs when the coronal suture fuses prematurely, causing a shortened front-to-back diameter of the skull.

Oxycephaly: This is a term sometimes used to describe the premature closure of the coronal suture plus any other suture, or it may be used to describe the premature fusing of all sutures. Oxycephaly is the most severe of the craniostenoses.

Plagiocephaly: This results from the premature unilateral fusion (joining of one side) of the coronal or lambdoid sutures. It is a common finding at birth and may be the result of brain malformation, a restrictive intrauterine environment, or torticollis (a spasm or tightening of neck muscles).

Scaphocephaly: Applies to premature fusion of the sagittal suture. The sagittal suture joins together the two parietal bones of the skull. Scaphocephaly is the most common of the craniostenoses and is characterized by a long, narrow head.

Trigonocephaly: The premature fusion of the metopic suture (part of the frontal suture which joins the two halves of the frontal bone of the skull) in which a V-shaped abnormality occurs at the front of the skull. It is characterized by the triangular prominence of the forehead and closely set eyes.

Chapter 22

Cerebral Palsy

Doctors use the term cerebral palsy to refer to any one of a number of neurological disorders that appear in infancy or early childhood and permanently affect body movement and muscle coordination but aren't progressive, in other words, they don't get worse over time. The term cerebral refers to the two halves or hemispheres of the brain, in this case to the motor area of the brain's outer layer (called the cerebral cortex), the part of the brain that directs muscle movement; palsy refers to the loss or impairment of motor function.

Even though cerebral palsy affects muscle movement, it isn't caused by problems in the muscles or nerves. It is caused by abnormalities inside the brain that disrupt the brain's ability to control movement and posture.

In some cases of cerebral palsy, the cerebral motor cortex hasn't developed normally during fetal growth. In others, the damage is a result of injury to the brain either before, during, or after birth. In either case, the damage is not repairable and the disabilities that result are permanent.

Children with cerebral palsy exhibit a wide variety of symptoms, including:

- lack of muscle coordination when performing voluntary movements (ataxia);

- stiff or tight muscles and exaggerated reflexes (spasticity);

Excerpted from "Cerebral Palsy: Hope through Research," National Institute of Neurological Disorders and Stroke (NINDS), NIH Publication No. 06-159, updated December 18, 2009.

- walking with one foot or leg dragging;

- walking on the toes, a crouched gait, or a scissored gait;

- variations in muscle tone, either too stiff or too floppy;

- excessive drooling or difficulties swallowing or speaking;

- shaking (tremor) or random involuntary movements; and

- difficulty with precise motions, such as writing or buttoning a shirt.

The symptoms of cerebral palsy differ in type and severity from one person to the next, and may even change in an individual over time. Some people with cerebral palsy also have other medical disorders, including mental retardation, seizures, impaired vision or hearing, and abnormal physical sensations or perceptions.

Cerebral palsy doesn't always cause profound disabilities. While one child with severe cerebral palsy might be unable to walk and need extensive, lifelong care, another with mild cerebral palsy might be only slightly awkward and require no special assistance.

Cerebral palsy isn't a disease. It isn't contagious and it can't be passed from one generation to the next. There is no cure for cerebral palsy, but supportive treatments, medications, and surgery can help many individuals improve their motor skills and ability to communicate with the world.

The early signs of cerebral palsy usually appear before a child reaches three years of age. Parents are often the first to suspect that their baby's motor skills aren't developing normally. Parents who are concerned about their baby's development for any reason should contact their pediatrician. A doctor can determine the difference between a normal lag in development and a delay that could indicate cerebral palsy.

Causes: Research has given us a bigger and more accurate picture of the kinds of events that can happen during early fetal development, or just before, during, or after birth, that cause the particular types of brain damage that will result in congenital cerebral palsy. There are multiple reasons why cerebral palsy happens—as the result of genetic abnormalities, maternal infections or fevers, or fetal injury, for example. But, in all cases, the disorder is the result of four types of brain damage that cause its characteristic symptoms:

- Damage to the white matter of the brain (periventricular leukomalacia [PVL])

- Abnormal development of the brain (cerebral dysgenesis)

- Bleeding in the brain (intracranial hemorrhage)

- Brain damage caused by a lack of oxygen in the brain (hypoxic-ischemic encephalopathy or intrapartum asphyxia)

Risk factors: Just as there are particular types of brain damage that cause cerebral palsy, there are also certain medical conditions or events that can happen during pregnancy and delivery that will increase a baby's risk of being born with cerebral palsy. If a mother or her baby has any of these risk factors, it doesn't mean that cerebral palsy is inevitable, but it does increase the chance for the kinds of brain damage that cause it.

- Low birthweight and premature birth

- Multiple births

- Blood type incompatibility

- Exposure to toxic substances

- Mothers with thyroid abnormalities, mental retardation, or seizures

Different Forms of and Conditions Associated with Cerebral Palsy

The specific forms of cerebral palsy are determined by the extent, type, and location of a child's abnormalities. Doctors classify cerebral palsy according to the type of movement disorder involved—spastic (stiff muscles), athetoid (writhing movements), or ataxic (poor balance and coordination)—plus any additional symptoms. Doctors will often describe the type of cerebral palsy a child has based on which limbs are affected.

Spastic hemiplegia/hemiparesis: This type of cerebral palsy typically affects the arm and hand on one side of the body, but it can also include the leg. Children with spastic hemiplegia generally walk later and on tip-toe because of tight heel tendons. The arm and leg of the affected side are frequently shorter and thinner. Some children will develop an abnormal curvature of the spine (scoliosis). Depending on the location of the brain damage, a child with spastic hemiplegia may also have seizures. Speech will be delayed and, at best, may be competent, but intelligence is usually normal.

Spastic diplegia/diparesis: In this type of cerebral palsy, muscle stiffness is predominantly in the legs and less severely affects the arms and face, although the hands may be clumsy. Tendon reflexes are hyperactive. Toes point up. Tightness in certain leg muscles makes the legs move like the arms of a scissor. Children with this kind of cerebral palsy may require a walker or leg braces. Intelligence and language skills are usually normal.

Spastic quadriplegia/quadriparesis: This is the most severe form of cerebral palsy, often associated with moderate-to-severe mental retardation. It is caused by widespread damage to the brain or significant brain malformations. Children will often have severe stiffness in their limbs but a floppy neck. They are rarely able to walk. Speaking and being understood are difficult. Seizures can be frequent and hard to control.

Dyskinetic cerebral palsy (also includes athetoid, choreoathetoid, and dystonic cerebral palsies): This type of cerebral palsy is characterized by slow and uncontrollable writhing movements of the hands, feet, arms, or legs. In some children, hyperactivity in the muscles of the face and tongue makes them grimace or drool. They find it difficult to sit straight or walk. Children may also have problems coordinating the muscle movements required for speaking. Intelligence is rarely affected in these forms of cerebral palsy.

Ataxic cerebral palsy: This rare type of cerebral palsy affects balance and depth perception. Children will often have poor coordination and walk unsteadily with a wide-based gait, placing their feet unusually far apart. They have difficulty with quick or precise movements, such as writing or buttoning a shirt. They may also have intention tremor, in which a voluntary movement, such as reaching for a book, is accompanied by trembling that gets worse the closer their hand gets to the object.

Mixed types: It is common for children to have symptoms that don't correspond to any single type of cerebral palsy. Their symptoms are a mix of types. For example, a child with mixed cerebral palsy may have some muscles that are too tight and others that are too relaxed, creating a mix of stiffness and floppiness.

Other conditions associated with cerebral palsy: Many individuals with cerebral palsy have no additional medical disorders. However, because cerebral palsy involves the brain and the brain controls so many of the body's functions, cerebral palsy can also cause seizures, impair intellectual development, and affect vision, hearing, and behavior. Coping with these disabilities may be even more of a challenge than coping with the motor impairments of cerebral palsy. These additional medical conditions include mental retardation; seizure disorder; delayed growth and development; spinal deformities; impaired vision, hearing, or speech; drooling; incontinence; and abnormal sensations and perceptions.

Diagnosing Cerebral Palsy

Early signs of cerebral palsy may be present from birth. Most children with cerebral palsy are diagnosed during the first two years of life. But if a child's symptoms are mild, it can be difficult for a doctor to make a reliable diagnosis before the age of four or five.

Doctors diagnose cerebral palsy by evaluating a child's motor skills and taking a careful and thorough look at their medical history. In addition to checking for the most characteristic symptoms—slow development, abnormal muscle tone, and unusual posture—a doctor also has to rule out other disorders that could cause similar symptoms. Most important, a doctor has to determine that the child's condition is not getting worse. Although symptoms may change over time, cerebral palsy by definition is not progressive. Additional tests are often used to rule out other movement disorders that could cause the same symptoms as cerebral palsy. Neuroimaging techniques that allow doctors to look into the brain (such as a magnetic resonance imaging [MRI] scan) can detect abnormalities that indicate a potentially treatable movement disorder. If it is cerebral palsy, an MRI scan can also show a doctor the location and type of brain damage.

Other types of disorders can also be mistaken for cerebral palsy. For example, coagulation disorders (which prevent blood from clotting) can cause prenatal or perinatal strokes that damage the brain and cause symptoms characteristic of cerebral palsy. Because stroke is so often the cause of hemiplegic cerebral palsy, a doctor may find it necessary to perform diagnostic testing on children with this kind of cerebral palsy to rule out the presence of a coagulation disorder. If left undiagnosed, coagulation disorders can cause additional strokes and more extensive brain damage.

Managing Cerebral Palsy

Cerebral palsy can't be cured, but treatment will often improve a child's capabilities. Many children go on to enjoy near-normal adult lives if their disabilities are properly managed. In general, the earlier treatment begins, the better chance children have of overcoming developmental disabilities or learning new ways to accomplish the tasks that challenge them.

There is no standard therapy that works for every individual with cerebral palsy. Once the diagnosis is made, and the type of cerebral palsy is determined, a team of health care professionals will work with a child and his or her parents to identify specific impairments and needs, and then develop an appropriate plan to tackle the core disabilities that affect the child's quality of life.

A comprehensive management plan will pull in a combination of health professionals with expertise in physical therapy; occupational therapy; speech therapy; counseling and behavioral therapy; drugs to control seizures, relax muscle spasms, and alleviate pain; surgery to correct anatomical abnormalities or release tight muscles; braces and other orthotic devices; mechanical aids; and communication aids.

Doctors use tests and evaluation scales to determine a child's level of disability, and then make decisions about the types of treatments and the best timing and strategy for interventions. Early intervention programs typically provide all the required therapies within a single treatment center. Centers also focus on parents' needs, often offering support groups, babysitting services, and respite care.

Regardless of age or the types of therapy that are used, treatment doesn't end when an individual with cerebral palsy leaves the treatment center. Most of the work is done at home. Members of the treatment team often act as coaches, giving parents and children techniques and strategies to practice at home. Studies have shown that family support and personal determination are two of the most important factors in helping individuals with cerebral palsy reach their long-term goals.

Treatments for Cerebral Palsy

Physical therapy: Usually begun in the first few years of life or soon after the diagnosis is made, physical therapy is a cornerstone of cerebral palsy treatment. Physical therapy programs use specific sets of exercises and activities to work toward two important goals: preventing weakening or deterioration in the muscles that aren't being used (disuse atrophy), and keeping muscles from becoming fixed in a rigid, abnormal position (contracture).

Resistive exercise programs (also called strength training) and other types of exercise are often used to increase muscle performance, especially in children and adolescents with mild cerebral palsy. Daily bouts of exercise keep muscles that aren't normally used moving and active and less prone to wasting away. Exercise also reduces the risk of contracture, one of the most common and serious complications of cerebral palsy. Physical therapy alone or in combination with special braces (called orthotic devices) helps prevent contracture by stretching spastic muscles.

Occupational therapy: This kind of therapy focuses on optimizing upper body function, improving posture, and making the most of a child's mobility. An occupational therapist helps a child master the basic activities of daily living, such as eating, dressing, and using the bathroom alone. Fostering this kind of independence boosts self-reliance and self-esteem, and also helps reduce demands on parents and caregivers.

Recreational therapies: Recreational therapies, such as therapeutic horseback riding (also called hippotherapy), are sometimes used with mildly impaired children to improve gross motor skills. Parents of children who participate in recreational therapies usually notice an improvement in their child's speech, self-esteem, and emotional well-being.

Controversial physical therapies: Patterning, the Bobath technique, and conductive education are physical therapies which have not had documented evidence of value or effectiveness in producing consistent or significant improvements in study groups.

Speech and language therapy: About 20% of children with cerebral palsy are unable to produce intelligible speech. They also experience challenges in other areas of communication, such as hand gestures and facial expressions, and they have difficulty participating in the basic give and take of a normal conversation. These challenges will last throughout their lives.

Speech and language therapists (also known as speech therapists or speech-language pathologists) observe, diagnose, and treat the communication disorders associated with cerebral palsy. They can also help children with severe disabilities learn how to use special communication devices, such as a computer with a voice synthesizer, or a special board covered with symbols of everyday objects and activities to which a child can point to indicate his or her wishes.

Treatments for problems with eating and drooling are often necessary when children with cerebral palsy have difficulty eating and drinking because they have little control over the muscles that move their mouth, jaw, and tongue. They are also at risk for breathing food or fluid into the lungs. Some children develop gastroesophageal reflux disease (GERD, commonly called heartburn) in which a weak diaphragm can't keep stomach acids from spilling into the esophagus. The irritation of the acid can cause bleeding and pain.

Individuals with cerebral palsy are also at risk for malnutrition, recurrent lung infections, and progressive lung disease. The individuals most at risk for these problems are those with spastic quadriplegia.

Initially, children should be evaluated for their swallowing ability, which is usually done with a modified barium swallow study. Recommendations regarding diet modifications will be derived from the results of this study.

Drug Treatments

Oral medications such as diazepam, baclofen, dantrolene sodium, and tizanidine are usually used as the first line of treatment to relax stiff, contracted, or overactive muscles. These drugs are easy to use, except that dosages high enough to be effective often have side effects, among them drowsiness, upset stomach, high blood pressure, and possible liver damage with long-term use. Oral medications are most appropriate for children who need only mild reduction in muscle tone or who have widespread spasticity.

Doctors also sometimes use alcohol washes—injections of alcohol into muscles—to reduce spasticity. The benefits last from a few months to two years or more, but the adverse effects include a significant risk of pain or numbness, and the procedure requires a high degree of skill to target the nerve. The availability of new and more precise methods to deliver antispasmodic medications is moving treatment for spasticity toward chemo-denervation, in which injected drugs are used to target and relax muscles.

Botulinum toxin (BT-A), injected locally, has become a standard treatment for overactive muscles in children with spastic movement disorders such as cerebral palsy. BT-A relaxes contracted muscles by keeping nerve cells from over-activating muscle. Although BT-A is not approved by the Food and Drug Administration (FDA) for treating cerebral palsy, since the 1990s doctors have been using it off-label to relax spastic muscles. A number of studies have shown that it reduces spasticity and increases the range of motion of the muscles it targets. The relaxing effect of a BT-A injection lasts approximately three months. Because BT-A does not have FDA approval to treat spasticity in children, parents and caregivers should make sure that the doctor giving the injection is trained in the procedure and has experience using it in children.

Intrathecal baclofen therapy uses an implantable pump to deliver baclofen, a muscle relaxant, into the fluid surrounding the spinal cord. Studies have shown it reduces spasticity and pain and improves sleep. The pump is the size of a hockey puck and is implanted in the abdomen. It contains a refillable reservoir connected to an alarm that beeps when the reservoir is low. The pump is programmable with an electronic telemetry wand. The program can be adjusted if muscle tone is worse at certain times of the day or night. As a muscle-relaxing therapy, the baclofen pump is most appropriate for individuals with chronic, severe stiffness or uncontrolled muscle movement throughout the body. Doctors have successfully implanted the pump in children as young as three years of age.

Surgery

Orthopedic surgery is often recommended when spasticity and stiffness are severe enough to make walking and moving about difficult or painful. For many people with cerebral palsy, improving the appearance of how they walk—their gait—is also important. A more upright gait with smoother transitions and foot placements is the primary goal for many children and young adults.

In the operating room, surgeons can lengthen muscles and tendons that are proportionately too short. But first, they have to determine the specific muscles responsible for the gait abnormalities. In the past, doctors relied on clinical examination, observation of the gait, and the measurement of motion and spasticity to determine the muscles involved. Now, doctors have a diagnostic technique known as gait analysis.

Gait analysis uses cameras that record how an individual walks, force plates that detect when and where feet touch the ground, a special recording technique that detects muscle activity (known as electromyography), and a computer program that gathers and analyzes the data to identify the problem muscles. Using gait analysis, doctors can precisely locate which muscles would benefit from surgery and how much improvement in gait can be expected.

Most of the surgical procedures can be done on an outpatient basis or with a short inpatient stay. Children usually return to their normal lifestyle within a week. With shorter recovery times and new, less invasive surgical techniques, doctors can schedule surgeries at times that take advantage of a child's age and developmental abilities for the best possible result.

Selective dorsal rhizotomy (SDR): A surgical procedure recommended only for cases of severe spasticity when all of the more conservative treatments—physical therapy, oral medications, and intrathecal baclofen—have failed to reduce spasticity or chronic pain. In the procedure, a surgeon locates and selectively severs overactivated nerves at the base of the spinal column.

Spinal cord stimulation: Developed in the 1980s to treat spinal cord injury and other neurological conditions involving motor neurons. An implanted electrode selectively stimulates nerves at the base of the spinal cord to inhibit and decrease nerve activity. The effectiveness of spinal cord stimulation for the treatment of cerebral palsy has yet to be proven in clinical studies. It is considered a treatment alternative only when other conservative or surgical treatments have been unsuccessful at relaxing muscles or relieving pain.

Orthotic Devices

Orthotic devices—such as braces and splints—use external force to correct muscle abnormalities. The technology of orthotics has advanced over the past 30 years from metal rods that hooked up to bulky orthopedic shoes, to appliances that are individually molded from high-temperature plastics for a precise fit. Ankle-foot orthoses are frequently prescribed for children with spastic diplegia to prevent muscle contracture and to improve gait. Splints are also used to correct spasticity in the hand muscles.

Assistive Technology

Devices that help individuals move about more easily and communicate successfully at home, at school, or in the workplace can help a child or adult with cerebral palsy overcome physical and communication limitations. There are a number of devices that help individuals stand straight and walk, such as postural support or seating systems, open-front walkers, quadrupedal canes (lightweight metal canes with four feet), and gait poles. Electric wheelchairs let more severely impaired adults and children move about successfully.

The computer is probably the most dramatic example of a communication device that can make a big difference in the lives of people with cerebral palsy. Equipped with a computer and voice synthesizer, a child or adult with cerebral palsy can communicate successfully with others. For example, a child who is unable to speak or write but can make head movements may be able to control a computer using a special light pointer that attaches to a headband.

Alternative Therapies

Therapeutic (subthreshold) electrical stimulation, also called neuromuscular electrical stimulation (NES): Pulses electricity into the motor nerves to stimulate contraction in selective muscle groups. Many studies have demonstrated that NES appears to increase range of motion and muscular strength.

Hyperbaric oxygen therapy: Some children have cerebral palsy as the result of brain damage from oxygen deprivation. Proponents of hyperbaric oxygen therapy propose that the brain tissue surrounding the damaged area can be awakened by forcing high concentrations of oxygen into the body under greater than atmospheric pressure. A recent study compared a group of children who received no hyperbaric treatment to a group that received 40 treatments over eight weeks. On every measure of function (gross motor, cognitive, communication, and memory) at the end of two months of treatment and after a further three months of follow up, the two groups were identical in outcome. There was no added benefit from hyperbaric oxygen therapy.

Part Four

Brain Infections

Chapter 23

Acquired Immune Deficiency Syndrome (AIDS): Neurological Complications

AIDS (acquired immune deficiency syndrome) is a condition that occurs in the most advanced stages of human immunodeficiency virus (HIV) infection. It may take many years for AIDS to develop following the initial HIV infection. Although AIDS is primarily an immune system disorder, it also affects the nervous system and can lead to a wide range of severe neurological disorders.

How does AIDS affect the nervous system?

The virus does not appear to directly invade nerve cells but it jeopardizes their health and function. The resulting inflammation may damage the brain and spinal cord and cause symptoms such as confusion and forgetfulness, behavioral changes, severe headaches, progressive weakness, loss of sensation in the arms and legs, and stroke. Cognitive motor impairment or damage to the peripheral nerves is also common. Research has shown that the HIV infection can significantly alter the size of certain brain structures involved in learning and information processing.

In the United States, neurological complications are seen in more than 40% of adult patients with AIDS. They can occur at any age but tend to progress more rapidly in children. Nervous system complications in children may include developmental delays, loss of previously achieved milestones, brain lesions, nerve pain, smaller than normal

Excerpted from "Neurological Complications of AIDS Fact Sheet," National Institute of Neurological Disorders and Stroke (NINDS), February 12, 2010.

skull size, slow growth, eye problems, and recurring bacterial infections.

What are some of the neurological complications that are associated with AIDS?

AIDS-related disorders of the nervous system may be caused directly by the HIV virus, by certain cancers and opportunistic infections (illnesses caused by bacteria, fungi, and other viruses that would not otherwise affect people with healthy immune systems), or by toxic effects of the drugs used to treat symptoms. Other neuro-AIDS disorders of unknown origin may be influenced by but are not caused directly by the virus.

AIDS dementia complex (ADC), or HIV-associated encephalopathy, occurs primarily in persons with more advanced HIV infection. Symptoms include encephalitis (inflammation of the brain), behavioral changes, and a gradual decline in cognitive function, including trouble with concentration, memory, and attention. Persons with ADC also show progressive slowing of motor function and loss of dexterity and coordination. When left untreated, ADC can be fatal.

Central nervous system (CNS) lymphomas are cancerous tumors that either begin in the brain or result from a cancer that has spread from another site in the body. CNS lymphomas are almost always associated with the Epstein-Barr virus (a common human virus in the herpes family). Symptoms include headache, seizures, vision problems, dizziness, speech disturbance, paralysis, and mental deterioration. AIDS patients may develop one or more CNS lymphomas. Prognosis is poor due to advanced and increasing immunodeficiency.

Cryptococcal meningitis is seen in about 10% of untreated AIDS patients and in other persons whose immune systems have been severely suppressed by disease or drugs. It is caused by the fungus *Cryptococcus neoformans*, which is commonly found in dirt and bird droppings. The fungus first invades the lungs and spreads to the covering of the brain and spinal cord, causing inflammation. Symptoms include fatigue, fever, headache, nausea, memory loss, confusion, drowsiness, and vomiting. If left untreated, patients with cryptococcal meningitis may lapse into a coma and die.

Cytomegalovirus (CMV) infections can occur concurrently with other infections. Symptoms of CMV encephalitis include weakness in the arms and legs, problems with hearing and balance, altered mental states, dementia, peripheral neuropathy, coma, and retinal disease that may lead to blindness. CMV infection of the spinal cord and nerves can result in weakness in the lower limbs and some paralysis, severe lower back pain, and loss of bladder function. It can also cause pneumonia and gastrointestinal disease.

Herpes virus infections are often seen in AIDS patients. The herpes zoster virus, which causes chickenpox and shingles, can infect the brain and produce encephalitis and myelitis (inflammation of the spinal cord). It commonly produces shingles, which is an eruption of blisters and intense pain along an area of skin supplied by an infected nerve. In people exposed to herpes zoster, the virus can lay dormant in the nerve tissue for years until it is reactivated as shingles. This reactivation is common in persons with AIDS because of their weakened immune systems. Signs of shingles include painful blisters (like those seen in chickenpox), itching, tingling, and pain in the nerves.

AIDS patients may suffer from several different forms of neuropathy, or nerve pain, each strongly associated with a specific stage of active immunodeficiency disease. Peripheral neuropathy describes damage to the peripheral nerves, the vast communications network that transmits information from the brain and spinal cord to every other part of the body. Peripheral nerves also send sensory information back to the brain and spinal cord. HIV damages the nerve fibers that help conduct signals and can cause several different forms of neuropathy. Distal sensory polyneuropathy causes either a numbing feeling or a mild to painful burning or tingling sensation that normally begins in the legs and feet. These sensations may be particularly strong at night and may spread to the hands. Affected persons have a heightened sensitivity to pain, touch, or other stimuli. Onset usually occurs in the later stages of the HIV infection and may affect the majority of advanced-stage HIV patients.

Neurosyphilis, the result of an insufficiently treated syphilis infection, seems more frequent and more rapidly progressive in people with HIV infection. It may cause slow degeneration of the nerve cells and nerve fibers that carry sensory information to the brain. Symptoms, which may not appear for some decades after the initial infection and vary from patient to patient, include weakness, diminished reflexes, unsteady gait, progressive degeneration of the joints, loss of coordination, episodes of intense pain and disturbed sensation, personality changes, dementia, deafness, visual impairment, and impaired response to light. The disease is more frequent in men than in women. Onset is common during mid-life.

Progressive multifocal leukoencephalopathy (PML) primarily affects individuals with suppressed immune systems (including nearly 5% of people with AIDS). PML is caused by the JC virus, which travels to the brain, infects multiple sites, and destroys the cells that make myelin—the fatty protective covering for many of the body's nerve and brain cells. Symptoms include various types of mental deterioration, vision loss, speech disturbances, ataxia (inability to coordinate movements), paralysis, brain lesions, and ultimately, coma. Some patients may also have compromised memory and cognition, and seizures may occur. PML is relentlessly progressive and death usually occurs within six months of initial symptoms.

Psychological and neuropsychiatric disorders can occur in different phases of the HIV infection and AIDS and may take various and complex forms. Some illnesses, such as AIDS dementia complex, are caused directly by HIV infection of the brain, while other conditions may be triggered by the drugs used to combat the infection. Patients may experience anxiety disorder, depressive disorders, increased thoughts of suicide, paranoia, dementia, delirium, cognitive impairment, confusion, hallucinations, behavioral abnormalities, malaise, and acute mania.

Stroke brought on by cerebrovascular disease has been considered a somewhat rare complication of AIDS, although the association between AIDS and stroke may be much larger than previously thought. Researchers at the University of Maryland conducted the first population-based study to quantify an AIDS-associated stroke risk and found that AIDS increases the chances of suffering a stroke by as much as ten-fold. Researchers caution that additional studies are needed to confirm this association. Earlier studies have indicated that the HIV infection, other infections, or the body's immune system reaction to HIV may cause vascular abnormalities and make the blood vessels less responsive to changes in blood pressure, which could lead to rupture and hemorrhagic stroke.

Toxoplasma encephalitis, also called cerebral toxoplasmosis, occurs in about 10% of untreated AIDS patients. It is caused by the parasite *Toxoplasma gondii*, which is carried by cats, birds, and other animals and can be found in soil contaminated by cat feces and sometimes in raw or undercooked meat. Once the parasite invades the immune system, it remains there; however, the immune system in a healthy person can fight off the parasite, preventing disease. Symptoms include encephalitis, fever, severe headache that does not respond to treatment, weakness on one side of the body, seizures, lethargy, increased confusion, vision problems, dizziness, problems with speaking and walking, vomiting, and personality changes. Not all patients show signs of the infection.

Vacuolar myelopathy causes the protective myelin sheath to pull away from nerve cells of the spinal cord, forming small holes called vacuoles in nerve fibers. Symptoms include weak and stiff legs and unsteadiness when walking. Walking becomes more difficult as the disease progresses and many patients eventually require a wheelchair. Some patients also develop AIDS dementia. Vacuolar myelopathy may affect up to 30% of untreated adults with AIDS and its incidence may be even higher in HIV-infected children.

How are these disorders treated?

No single treatment can cure the neurological complications of AIDS. Some disorders require aggressive therapy while others are treated symptomatically.

Neuropathic pain is often difficult to control. Medicines range from analgesics sold over the counter to antiepileptic drugs, opiates, and some classes of antidepressants. Inflamed tissue can press on nerves, causing pain. Inflammatory and autoimmune conditions leading to neuropathy may be treated with corticosteroids, and procedures such as plasmapheresis (or plasma exchange) can clear the blood of harmful substances that cause inflammation.

Treatment options for AIDS- and HIV-related neuropsychiatric or psychotic disorders include antidepressants and anticonvulsants. Psychostimulants may also improve depressive symptoms and combat lethargy. Anti-dementia drugs may relieve confusion and slow mental decline, and benzodiazepines may be prescribed to treat anxiety. Psychotherapy may also help some patients.

Aggressive antiretroviral therapy is used to treat AIDS dementia complex, vacuolar myopathy, progressive multifocal leukoencephalopathy, and cytomegalovirus encephalitis. HAART, or highly active antiretroviral therapy, combines at least three drugs to reduce the amount of virus circulating in the blood and may also delay the start of some infections.

Other neuro-AIDS treatment options include physical therapy and rehabilitation, radiation therapy and chemotherapy to kill or shrink cancerous brain tumors that may be caused by the HIV virus, antifungal or antimalarial drugs to combat certain bacterial infections associated with the disorder, and penicillin to treat neurosyphilis.

Chapter 24

Brain Abscess

Definition: A brain abscess is a collection of immune cells, pus, and other material in the brain, usually from a bacterial or fungal infection.

Causes

Brain abscesses commonly occur when bacteria or fungi infect part of the brain. Swelling and irritation (inflammation) develops in response. Infected brain cells, white blood cells, live and dead bacteria, and fungi collect in an area of the brain. A membrane forms around this area and creates a mass.

While this immune response can protect the brain by isolating the infection, it can also do more harm than good. The brain swells. Because the skull cannot expand, the mass may put pressure on delicate brain tissue. Infected material can block the blood vessels of the brain.

The bacteria or fungi that cause a brain abscess commonly reach the brain through the blood. The source of the infection is often not found. However, the most common source is a lung infection. Bacteria or fungi may also travel from a nearby infected area (for example, an ear infection) or be introduced into the body during an injury (such as a gun or knife wound) or surgery.

In children with heart disease or a birth defect, such as those born with Tetralogy of Fallot, infections are more able to reach the brain from the intestines, teeth, or other body areas.

The following raise your risk of a brain abscess:

- A weakened immune system (such as in AIDS patients)
- Chronic disease, such as cancer or Osler-Weber-Rendu syndrome
- Drugs that suppress the immune system (corticosteroids or chemotherapy)
- Right-to-left heart shunts

Symptoms

Symptoms may develop slowly, over a period of two weeks, or they may develop suddenly. They may include the following:

- Aching of neck, shoulders, or back
- Changes in mental status:
  - Confusion
  - Decreasing responsiveness
  - Drowsiness
  - Eventual coma
  - Inattention
  - Irritability
  - Slow thought processes
- Decreased movement
- Decreased sensation
- Decreased speech (aphasia)
- Fever and chills
- Headache
- Language difficulties
- Loss of coordination
- Loss of muscle function
- Seizures
- Stiff neck, shoulders, or back
- Vision changes

- Vomiting

- Weakness

Exams and Tests

A brain and nervous system (neurological) exam will usually show increased intracranial pressure and problems with brain function.
Tests to diagnose a brain abscess may include:

- blood cultures,

- chest x-ray,

- complete blood count (CBC),

- cranial computed tomography (CT) scan,

- electroencephalogram (EEG),

- magnetic resonance imaging (MRI) of head, and

- testing for the presence of antibodies to organisms (including toxoplasma and *Tinea solium*).

A needle biopsy is usually performed to identify the cause of the infection.

Treatment

A brain abscess is a medical emergency. Pressure inside the skull may become high enough to be life threatening. You will need to stay in the hospital until the condition is stable. Some people may need life support.
Medication, not surgery, is recommended if you have:

- several abscesses (rare),

- a small abscess (less than two centimeters),

- an abscess deep in the brain,

- an abscess and meningitis,

- shunts in the brain for hydrocephalus (in some cases the shunt may need to be removed temporarily or replaced), or

- a disease that makes surgery dangerous.

You will get antibiotics. Antibiotics that work against a number of different bacteria (broad spectrum antibiotics) are most commonly used. You may be prescribed several different types of antibiotics to make sure treatment works.

Antifungal medications may also be prescribed if the infection is likely caused by a fungus.

Immediate treatment may be needed if an abscess is injuring brain tissue by pressing on it, or there is a large abscess with a large amount of swelling around that it is raising pressure in the brain.

Surgery is needed if :

- pressure in the brain continues or gets worse,

- the brain abscess does not get smaller after medication,

- the brain abscess contains gas (produced by some types of bacteria), or

- the brain abscess might break open (rupture).

Surgery consists of opening the skull, exposing the brain, and draining the abscess. Laboratory tests are often done to examine the fluid. This can help identify what is causing the infection, so that more appropriate antibiotics or antifungal drugs can be prescribed.

The surgical procedure used depends on the size and depth of the abscess. The entire abscess may be removed (excised) if it is near the surface and enclosed in a sac.

Needle aspiration guided by CT or MRI scan may be needed for a deep abscess. During this procedure, medications may be injected directly into the mass.

Certain diuretics and steroids may also be used to reduce swelling of the brain.

Outlook (prognosis): If untreated, a brain abscess is almost always deadly. With treatment, the death rate is about 10%–30%. The earlier treatment is received, the better. Some patients may have long-term neurological problems after surgery.

Possible complications:

- Epilepsy

- Meningitis that is severe and life threatening

- Permanent loss of vision, speech, movement

- Return (recurrence) of infection

When to contact a medical professional: Go to a hospital emergency room or call the local emergency number (such as 911) if you have symptoms of a brain abscess.

Prevention: You can reduce the risk of developing a brain abscess by treating any disorders that can cause them. Have a follow-up examination after infections are treated. Some people, including those with certain heart disorders, may receive antibiotics before dental or urological procedures to help reduce the risk.

Reference

Nath A. Brain abscess and parameningeal infections. In: Goldman L, Ausiello D, eds. *Cecil Medicine. 23rd ed.* Philadelphia, Pa: Saunders Elsevier; 2007: chap 438.

Chapter 25

Encephalitis

Chapter Contents

Section 25.1

Recognizing and Treating Encephalitis

"Encephalitis," November 2007, reprinted with permission from www. kidshealth.org. Copyright © 2007 The Nemours Foundation. This information was provided by KidsHealth, one of the largest resources online for medically reviewed health information written for parents, kids, and teens. For more articles like this one, visit www.KidsHealth.org, or www.TeensHealth.org.

Encephalitis is an inflammation (swelling) of the brain. Encephalitis is usually caused by a virus, but other things, including bacteria, may cause it as well. Although encephalitis sounds scary, most cases aren't serious.

What is encephalitis?

Encephalitis (pronounced: in-seh-fuh-lye-tus) is typically caused by three different groups of viruses. The herpes viruses is one group, and includes chickenpox, EBV (Epstein-Barr virus—the virus that causes mono), and herpes simplex (the virus that causes cold sores). The second group is made up of viruses and other germs that are transmitted by insects. Viruses like West Nile virus, which is transmitted through a mosquito bite, and the germs that cause Lyme disease and Rocky Mountain spotted fever, which are transmitted thorough tick bites, can also cause encephalitis. The third group is made up of viruses that cause childhood infections that used to be common. These include measles, mumps, and German measles. Because lots of countries immunize against these diseases, it's rarer today that a person will develop encephalitis as a result of an illness like measles or mumps.

Some cases of encephalitis are mild and symptoms only last for a short time. However, it is possible to develop a severe case of encephalitis that can be serious and possibly even life threatening. When a person has encephalitis, his or her brain becomes inflamed—inflammation means swelling and irritation.

Is it contagious?

Infection with many different viruses can lead to encephalitis. So how contagious the infection is depends on which virus caused it. Viruses like West Nile are only transmitted through the bite of infected insects; it's not possible to catch them from other people. But viruses like EBV are passed from person to person.

Even if a person catches a virus that can cause encephalitis, it does not mean that person will automatically develop the condition. In fact, very few of the people who are infected with these viruses actually develop encephalitis.

What are the signs and symptoms?

Encephalitis may cause fever, headache, poor appetite, loss of energy, or just a general sick feeling. In more severe cases, other symptoms might occur, including:

- high fever;

- severe headache;

- sensitivity to light (called photophobia, which means light hurts your eyes);

- nausea and vomiting;

- stiff neck;

- confusion;

- sleepiness, difficulty waking, or unconsciousness; and

- convulsions (seizures).

When encephalitis happens after a common illness like chickenpox, the signs and symptoms of that illness usually come before symptoms of inflammation in the brain. But encephalitis can also appear without warning. If you have symptoms of encephalitis, get in touch with your doctor right away.

How is it diagnosed and treated?

To diagnose encephalitis, the doctor may take blood samples and order a spinal tap (also called a lumbar puncture), a procedure that involves inserting a very thin needle into the lower back to remove some cerebrospinal fluid (CSF) that surrounds the brain and spinal cord. The samples will be sent to a laboratory to be checked for viruses or bacteria.

A special brain scan (a magnetic resonance image [MRI] or a computed tomography [CT] scan) also may be ordered to look for inflammation.

The doctor might also order an electroencephalogram (EEG), a test that records your brain waves and can reveal any abnormalities that are consistent with encephalitis.

Treatment for encephalitis depends on the virus or other germ that caused it. People with mild cases of encephalitis can recover at home as long as they're watched carefully by a parent or other adult in the household. Most cases of encephalitis just run their course and the person gets better without treatment.

Some viruses that cause encephalitis can be treated with medication. For example, acyclovir, an antiviral drug, can help treat encephalitis caused by the herpes simplex virus. In addition, steroid medications can be used to reduce swelling in the brain (these aren't the same as the dangerous performance-enhancing steroids that some athletes use). Because antibiotics are not effective against viruses, they're not used to treat viral encephalitis.

Severe cases of encephalitis require a hospital stay so the patient can be carefully monitored and medical treatment is close at hand if needed. For people who have had severe encephalitis that has affected some of the brain's functions, doctors may recommend physical therapy or speech therapy to help with recovery.

How long does it last?

The worst symptoms of encephalitis generally last up to one week, but full recovery may take weeks or longer. Because encephalitis affects the brain, people with severe cases can sometimes develop problems like seizures, difficulties with muscle coordination, and learning disabilities.

Can I prevent encephalitis?

The best way to prevent encephalitis is to avoid getting infected with the viruses or other germs that can cause it. Regular hand washing will help limit the spread of some of these germs. Staying as healthy as possible by eating a balanced diet and getting plenty of rest can help keep your immune system in shape. Immunizations are also an important way to protect people from diseases like chickenpox and measles.

In areas where viruses are transmitted by insect bites, protect yourself by wearing long sleeves and pants and applying an insect repellent. Also, try to avoid unnecessary outdoor activities at dawn and dusk when mosquitoes are most likely to bite.

Section 25.2

Rabies Virus Causes Encephalomyelitis

Excerpted from "Human Rabies Prevention—United States, 2008," *Morbidity and Mortality Weekly Report (MMWR)*, May 23, 2008, Centers for Disease Control and Prevention (CDC). The full document is available at http://www.cdc.gov/mmwr/preview/mmwrhtml/rr5703a1.htm.

Rabies is a zoonotic disease caused by ribonucleic acid (RNA) viruses in the Family *Rhabdoviridae*, Genus *Lyssavirus*. The virus is typically present in the saliva of clinically ill mammals and is transmitted through a bite. After entering the central nervous system of the next host, the virus causes an acute, progressive encephalomyelitis that is almost always fatal. The incubation period in humans is usually several weeks to months, but ranges from days to years.

As a result of improved canine vaccination programs and stray animal control, a marked decrease in domestic animal rabies cases in the United States occurred after World War II. In 2006, a total of 79 cases of rabies were reported in domestic dogs, none of which was attributed to enzootic dog-to-dog transmission, and three cases were reported in humans. The infectious sources of the 79 cases in dogs were wildlife reservoirs or dogs that were translocated from localities where canine rabies virus variants still circulate. None of the 2006 human rabies cases was acquired from indigenous domestic animals.

Unlike the situation in developing countries, wild animals are the most important potential source of infection for both humans and domestic animals in the United States. Most reported cases of rabies occur among carnivores, primarily raccoons, skunks, foxes, and various species of bats. Rabies among insectivorous bats occurs throughout the continental United States. Hawaii remains consistently rabies-free. For the past several decades, the majority of naturally acquired, indigenous human rabies cases in the United States have resulted from variants of rabies viruses associated with insectivorous bats. The lone human case reported in the United States during 2005 and two of the three human rabies cases in 2006 were attributed to bat exposures. During 2004, two of the eight human rabies cases resulted from bat exposures.

Approximately 16,000–39,000 persons come in contact with potentially rabid animals and receive rabies postexposure prophylaxis each year. To appropriately manage potential human exposures to rabies, the risk for infection must be accurately assessed. Administration of rabies postexposure prophylaxis is a medical urgency, not a medical emergency, but decisions must not be delayed. Prophylaxis is occasionally complicated by adverse reactions, but these reactions are rarely severe.

For these recommendations, data on the safety and efficacy of active and passive rabies vaccination were derived from both human and animal studies. Because controlled human trials cannot be performed, studies describing extensive field experience and immunogenicity studies from certain areas of the world were reviewed. These studies indicated that postexposure prophylaxis combining wound treatment, local infiltration of rabies immune globulin (RIG), and vaccination is uniformly effective when appropriately administered. However, rabies has occasionally developed among humans when key elements of the rabies postexposure prophylaxis regimens were omitted or incorrectly administered. Timely and appropriate human pre-exposure and postexposure prophylaxis will prevent human rabies; however, the number of persons receiving prophylaxis can be reduced if other basic public health and veterinary programs are working to prevent and control rabies. Practical and accurate health education about rabies, domestic animal vaccination and responsible pet care, modern stray animal control, and prompt diagnosis can minimize unnecessary animal exposures, alleviate inherent natural risks after exposure, and prevent many circumstances that result in the need for rabies prophylaxis.

Section 25.3

Arboviral Encephalitides

Text in this section is excerpted from "Information on Arboviral Encephalitides," Centers for Disease Control and Prevention (CDC) November 7,
2005. Reviewed in January, 2010 by Dr. David A. Cooke, MD, FACP, Diplomate, American Board of Internal Medicine. Table 25.1 is excerpted from
"Confirmed and Probable California Serogroup Viral (mainly La Crosse)
Encephalitis Cases, Human, United States, 1964–2008, By State (as of
4/7/2009)," National Center for Infectious Diseases, Centers for Disease
Control and Prevention (CDC), April 7, 2009.

Arthropod-borne viruses, also called arboviruses, are viruses that
are maintained in nature through biological transmission between sus-
ceptible vertebrate hosts by blood-feeding arthropods (mosquitoes, psy-
chodids, ceratopogonids, and ticks). Vertebrate infection occurs when
the infected arthropod takes a blood meal. The term arbovirus has no
taxonomic significance. Arboviruses that cause human encephalitis are
members of three virus families: the *Togaviridae* (genus Alphavirus),
Flaviviridae, and *Bunyaviridae*.

All arboviral encephalitides are zoonotic, being maintained in complex life cycles involving a nonhuman primary vertebrate host and a
primary arthropod vector. These cycles usually remain undetected
until humans encroach on a natural focus, or the virus escapes this
focus via a secondary vector or vertebrate host as the result of some
ecologic change. Humans and domestic animals can develop clinical
illness but usually are dead-end hosts because they do not produce
significant viremia, and do not contribute to the transmission cycle.
Many arboviruses that cause encephalitis have a variety of different
vertebrate hosts and some are transmitted by more than one vector.
Maintenance of the viruses in nature may be facilitated by vertical
transmission (for example, the virus is transmitted from the female
through the eggs to the offspring).

Arboviral encephalitides have a global distribution, but there are
four main virus agents of encephalitis in the United States: eastern
equine encephalitis (EEE), western equine encephalitis (WEE), St.
Louis encephalitis (SLE) and La Crosse (LAC) encephalitis, all of
which are transmitted by mosquitoes. Another virus, Powassan, is

a minor cause of encephalitis in the northern United States, and is transmitted by ticks. A new Powassan-like virus has recently been isolated from deer ticks. Most cases of arboviral encephalitis occur from June through September, when arthropods are most active. In milder (warmer) parts of the country, where arthropods are active late into the year, cases can occur into the winter months.

The majority of human infections are asymptomatic or may result in a nonspecific flu-like syndrome. Onset may be insidious or sudden with fever, headache, myalgias, malaise, and occasionally prostration. Infection may, however, lead to encephalitis, with a fatal outcome or permanent neurologic sequelae. Fortunately, only a small proportion of infected persons progress to frank encephalitis.

Because the arboviral encephalitides are viral diseases, antibiotics are not effective for treatment and no effective antiviral drugs have yet been discovered. Treatment is supportive, attempting to deal with problems such as swelling of the brain, loss of the automatic breathing activity of the brain and other treatable complications like bacterial pneumonia.

There are no commercially available human vaccines for these U.S. diseases. There is a Japanese encephalitis vaccine available in the U.S. A tick-borne encephalitis vaccine is available in Europe. An equine vaccine is available for EEE, WEE and Venezuelan equine encephalitis (VEE). Arboviral encephalitis can be prevented in two major ways: personal protective measures and public health measures to reduce the population of infected mosquitoes. Personal measures include reducing time outdoors particularly in early evening hours, wearing long pants and long sleeved shirts and applying mosquito repellent to exposed skin areas. Public health measures often require spraying of insecticides to kill juvenile (larvae) and adult mosquitoes.

La Crosse encephalitis: Discovered in La Crosse, Wisconsin in 1963, the virus has since then been identified in several Midwestern and Mid-Atlantic states. During an average year, about 75 cases of LAC encephalitis are reported to the Centers for Disease Control and Prevention (CDC). Most cases of LAC encephalitis occur in children under 16 years of age.

LAC encephalitis initially presents as a nonspecific summertime illness with fever, headache, nausea, vomiting, and lethargy. Severe disease occurs most commonly in children under the age of 16 and is characterized by seizures, coma, paralysis, and a variety of neurological sequelae after recovery. Death from LAC encephalitis occurs in less than 1% of clinical cases.

Eastern equine encephalitis (EEE): Caused by a virus transmitted to humans and equines by the bite of an infected mosquito. EEE virus is an alphavirus that was first identified in the 1930s and currently occurs in focal locations along the eastern seaboard, the Gulf Coast and some inland Midwestern locations of the United States. While small outbreaks of human disease have occurred in the United States, equine epizootics can be a common occurrence during the summer and fall.

It takes from 4–10 days after the bite of an infected mosquito for an individual to develop symptoms of EEE. These symptoms begin with a sudden onset of fever, general muscle pains, and a headache of increasing severity. Many individuals will progress to more severe symptoms such as seizures and coma. Approximately one-third of all people with clinical encephalitis caused by EEE will die from the disease and of those who recover, many will suffer permanent brain damage with many of those requiring permanent institutional care.

Western equine encephalitis (WEE): The alphavirus WEE was first isolated in California in 1930 from the brain of a horse with encephalitis, and remains an important cause of encephalitis in horses and humans in North America, mainly in western parts of the USA and Canada. Human WEE cases are usually first seen in June or July. Most WEE infections are asymptomatic or present as mild, nonspecific illness. Patients with clinically apparent illness usually have a sudden onset with fever, headache, nausea, vomiting, anorexia and malaise, followed by altered mental status, weakness and signs of meningeal irritation. Children, especially those under one year old, are affected more severely than adults and may be left with permanent sequelae, which is seen in 5% to 30% of young patients. The mortality rate is about 3%.

St. Louis encephalitis: In the United States, the leading cause of epidemic flavivirus encephalitis is St. Louis encephalitis (SLE) virus. SLE is the most common mosquito-transmitted human pathogen in the U.S. While periodic SLE epidemics have occurred only in the Midwest and Southeast, SLE virus is distributed throughout the lower 48 states. Since 1964, there have been 4,437 confirmed cases of SLE with an average of 193 cases per year (range of 4–1,967). However, less than 1% of SLE viral infections are clinically apparent and the vast majority of infections remain undiagnosed. Illness ranges in severity from a simple febrile headache to meningoencephalitis, with an overall case-fatality ratio of 5%–15%. The disease is generally milder

Table 25.1. Confirmed and Probable California Serogroup Viral (mainly La Crosse) Neuro-Invasive Disease Cases, Human, United States, 2000–2008, by State (as of 4/7/2009) *(continued on next page)*

State	2000	2001	2002	2003	2004	2005	2006	2007	2008	Total
Alabama		1				1				2
Alaska										0
Arizona										0
Arkansas										5
California										0
Colorado	1									1
Connecticut		1								1
Delaware										0
Dist. of Columbia										0
Florida				2		1				3
Georgia	2		1		5	1		1	2	12
Hawaii										0
Idaho										0
Illinois	3	5	8	11	8			1		36
Indiana	2	5	4		2		3			16
Iowa	4	2	3		2		1	1		13
Kansas										0
Kentucky	2		2	3					1	8
Louisiana			1	3	3	1	2		1	11
Maine										0

Table 25.1. (continued) Confirmed and Probable California Serogroup Viral (mainly La Crosse) Neuro-Invasive Disease Cases, Human, United States, 2000–2008, by State (as of 4/7/2009)

State	2000	2001	2002	2003	2004	2005	2006	2007	2008	Total
Maryland		1								1
Massachusetts										0
Michigan			11				2			13
Minnesota	8	12	13	3	2	2	1	1	1	43
Mississippi		8	1	1		1			1	12
Missouri										0
Montana										0
Nebraska										0
Nevada										0
New Hampshire										0
New Jersey										0
New Mexico										0
New York								2	5	7
North Carolina	6	10	17	17	13	31	17	9	8	128
North Dakota										0
Ohio	18	19	25	20	26	14	11	9	9	151
Oklahoma										0
Oregon										0
Pennsylvania	1									1
Rhode Island										0

Table 25.1. (continued) Confirmed and Probable California Serogroup Viral (mainly La Crosse) Neuro-Invasive Disease Cases, Human, United States, 2000–2008, by State (as of 4/7/2009)

State	2000	2001	2002	2003	2004	2005	2006	2007	2008	Total
South Carolina							1			1
South Dakota										0
Tennessee	19	17	15	19	13	2	7	13	6	111
Texas			2							2
Utah										0
Vermont										0
Virginia		2	2	4	2	2			2	14
Washington										0
West Virginia	40	44	40	23	30	15	16	11	14	233
Wisconsin	6	7	22	9	4	3	2	2	4	59
Wyoming										0
Totals:	112	134	167	113	112	73	64	50	55	880

in children than in adults, but in those children who do have disease, there is a high rate of encephalitis. The elderly are at highest risk for severe disease and death.

Powassan encephalitis (POW): A flavivirus and currently the only well documented tick-borne transmitted arbovirus occurring in the United States and Canada. Recently a Powassan-like virus was isolated from the deer tick, Ixodes scapularis. Its relationship to POW and its ability to cause human disease has not been fully elucidated. POW's range in the United States is primarily in the upper tier states. Patients who recover may have residual neurological problems.

Venezuelan equine encephalitis: Like EEE and WEE viruses, Venezuelan equine encephalitis (VEE) is an alphavirus and causes encephalitis in horses and humans and is an important veterinary and public health problem in Central and South America.

Other arboviral encephalitides: Many other arboviral encephalitides occur throughout the world. Most of these diseases are problems only for those individuals traveling to countries where the viruses are endemic. These include Japanese encephalitis, tick-borne encephalitis; West Nile encephalitis, and Murray Valley encephalitis.

Section 25.4

Acute Disseminated Encephalomyelitis

"Acute Disseminated Encephalomyelitis Information Page," National Institute of Neurological Disorders and Stroke (NINDS), August 16, 2007.

Acute disseminated encephalomyelitis (ADEM) is characterized by a brief but intense attack of inflammation in the brain and spinal cord that damages myelin—the protective covering of nerve fibers. It often follows viral infection, or less often, vaccination for measles, mumps, or rubella. The symptoms of ADEM come on quickly, beginning with encephalitis-like symptoms such as fever, fatigue, headache, nausea and vomiting, and in severe cases, seizures and coma. It may also damage white matter (brain tissue that takes its name from the white color of myelin), leading to neurological symptoms such as visual loss (due to inflammation of the optic nerve) in one or both eyes, weakness even to the point of paralysis, and difficulty coordinating voluntary muscle movements (such as those used in walking). ADEM is sometimes misdiagnosed as a severe first attack of multiple sclerosis (MS), since some of the symptoms of the two disorders, particularly those caused by white matter injury, may be similar. However, ADEM usually has symptoms of encephalitis (such as fever or coma), as well as symptoms of myelin damage (visual loss, paralysis), as opposed to MS, which doesn't have encephalitis symptoms. In addition, ADEM usually consists of a single episode or attack, while MS features many attacks over the course of time. Doctors will often use imaging techniques, such as MRI (magnetic resonance imaging), to search for old and new lesions (areas of damage) on the brain. Old inactive brain lesions on MRI suggest that the condition may be MS rather than ADEM, since MS often causes brain lesions before symptoms become obvious. In rare situations, brain biopsy may show findings that allow differentiation between ADEM and severe, acute forms of MS. Children are more likely than adults to have ADEM.

Treatment: For ADEM, treatment is targeted at suppressing inflammation in the brain using anti-inflammatory drugs. Most individuals respond to intravenous corticosteroids such as methylprednisolone.

When corticosteroids fail to work, plasmapheresis or intravenous immunoglobulin therapy has been shown to produce improvement. Additional treatment is symptomatic and supportive.

Prognosis: Corticosteroid therapy can shorten the duration of neurological symptoms and halt further progression of the disease in the short term, but the long term prognosis for individuals with ADEM varies. For most, recovery begins within days, and half will recover completely. Others may have mild to moderate lifelong impairment. Severe cases of ADEM can be fatal. Some individuals who initially diagnosed as having ADEM will later be reclassified as MS, but there is currently no method to determine whom those individuals will be.

Chapter 26

Meningitis

Meningitis is an inflammation of the membranes that cover the brain and spinal cord. People sometimes refer to it as spinal meningitis. Meningitis is usually caused by a viral or bacterial infection. Knowing whether meningitis is caused by a virus or bacterium is important because the severity of illness and the treatment differ depending on the cause. Viral meningitis is generally less severe and clears up without specific treatment. But, bacterial meningitis can be quite severe and may result in brain damage, hearing loss, or learning disabilities. For bacterial meningitis, it is also important to know which type of bacteria is causing the meningitis because antibiotics can prevent some types from spreading and infecting other people. Before the 1990s, *Haemophilus influenzae* type b (Hib) was the leading cause of bacterial meningitis. Hib vaccine is now given to all children as part of their routine immunizations. This vaccine has reduced the number of cases of Hib infection and the number of related meningitis cases. Today, *Streptococcus pneumoniae* and *Neisseria meningitidis* are the leading causes of bacterial meningitis.

High fever, headache, and stiff neck are common symptoms of meningitis in anyone over the age of two years. These symptoms can develop over several hours, or they may take 1–2 days. Other symptoms may include nausea, vomiting, discomfort looking into bright lights, confusion, and sleepiness. In newborns and small infants, the classic

This chapter begins with excerpts from "Meningitis Questions and Answers," Centers for Disease Control and Prevention (CDC), June 24, 2009; and concludes with excerpts from "Meningitis: Prevention," CDC, updated August 6, 2009.

symptoms of fever, headache, and neck stiffness may be absent or difficult to detect. Infants with meningitis may appear slow or inactive, have vomiting, be irritable, or be feeding poorly. As the disease progresses, patients of any age may have seizures.

Bacterial meningitis: Early diagnosis and treatment are very important. If symptoms occur, the patient should see a doctor immediately. The diagnosis is usually made by growing bacteria from a sample of spinal fluid. The spinal fluid is obtained by performing a spinal tap, in which a needle is inserted into an area in the lower back where fluid in the spinal canal can be collected. Identification of the type of bacteria responsible is important for selection of correct antibiotics.

Bacterial meningitis can be treated with a number of effective antibiotics. It is important, however, that treatment be started early in the course of the disease. Appropriate antibiotic treatment of most common types of bacterial meningitis should reduce the risk of dying from meningitis to below 15%, although the risk is higher among the elderly.

Some forms of bacterial meningitis are contagious. The bacteria can mainly be spread from person to person through the exchange of respiratory and throat secretions. This can occur through coughing, kissing, and sneezing. Fortunately, none of the bacteria that cause meningitis are as contagious as things like the common cold or the flu. Also, the bacteria are not spread by casual contact or by simply breathing the air where a person with meningitis has been. There are vaccines against Hib, against some serogroups of *N. meningitidis* and many types of *Streptococcus pneumoniae*. The vaccines are safe and highly effective.

Viral meningitis: Meningitis caused by viral infections is sometimes called aseptic meningitis. Viral (aseptic) meningitis is serious but rarely fatal in people with normal immune systems. Usually, the symptoms last from 7–10 days and the patient recovers completely. Bacterial meningitis, on the other hand, can be very serious and result in disability or death if not treated promptly. Often, the symptoms of viral meningitis and bacterial meningitis are the same. For this reason, if you think you or your child has meningitis, see your doctor as soon as possible.

Different viral infections can lead to viral meningitis. But most cases in the United States, particularly during the summer and fall months, are caused by enteroviruses (which include enteroviruses, coxsackieviruses, and echoviruses). Most people who are infected with enteroviruses either have no symptoms or only get a cold, rash, or mouth sores with low-grade fever. And, only a small number of people with enterovirus infections go on to develop meningitis. Symptoms can appear quickly or they can also take several days to appear, usually after a cold or runny nose, diarrhea, vomiting, or other signs of infection show up.

The exact cause of viral meningitis can sometimes be found through tests that show which virus has infected a patient; however, identifying the exact virus causing meningitis may be difficult. Because the symptoms of viral meningitis are similar to those of bacterial meningitis, which is usually more severe and can be fatal, it is important for people suspected of having meningitis to seek medical care and have their spinal fluid tested.

There is no specific treatment for viral meningitis. Most patients completely recover on their own within two weeks. Antibiotics do not help viral infections, so they are not useful in the treatment of viral meningitis. Doctors often will recommend bed rest, plenty of fluids, and medicine to relieve fever and headache.

Different viruses that cause viral meningitis are spread in different ways. Enteroviruses, the most common cause of viral meningitis, are most often spread through direct contact with an infected person's stool. The virus is spread through this route mainly among small children who are not yet toilet trained. It can also be spread this way to adults changing the diapers of an infected infant. Enteroviruses and other viruses (such as mumps and varicella-zoster virus) can also be spread through direct or indirect contact with respiratory secretions (saliva, sputum, or nasal mucus) of an infected person. The viruses can also stay on surfaces for days and can be transferred from objects. Viruses also can spread directly when infected people cough or sneeze and send droplets containing the virus into the air we breathe.

The time from when a person is infected until they develop symptoms (incubation period) is usually between 3–7 days for enteroviruses. An infected person is usually contagious from the time they develop symptoms until the symptoms go away. Young children and people with low immune systems may spread the infection even after symptoms have resolved.

Prevention

Keeping up to date with recommended immunizations is the best defense. Good hygiene is also an important way to prevent most infections. Avoid sharing drinking glasses, water bottles, eating utensils, tissues, and lip-gloss or lipsticks. Wash hands often with soap. If you are pregnant, you can reduce your risk of listeriosis (an infection caused by listeria bacteria) by cooking meats thoroughly and by avoiding cheeses made from unpasteurized milk.

Bacterial meningitis prevention: Routine immunizations can be very effective in preventing meningitis. There are vaccines against *Haemophilus influenzae* serotype b (Hib), measles, meningococcus, mumps, pneumococcus, and polio that can protect against meningitis caused by these organisms. There are vaccines for the three main causes of bacterial meningitis: *Streptococcus pneumoniae, Haemophilus influenzae* serotype b (Hib), and *Neisseria meningitidis*:

Viral meningitis prevention: Preventing the spread of viruses can be difficult, especially since sometimes people are infected with a virus (like enterovirus), but they do not appear sick. In such cases, people can still spread the virus to others. Following good hygiene practices, being vaccinated, and avoiding mosquito bites can help lower your chances of becoming infected with viruses or of passing one on to someone else.

Fungal meningitis prevention: There is little evidence that specific activities can lead to developing fungal meningitis, although avoiding exposure to environments likely to contain fungal elements is prudent. People who are immunosuppressed should try to avoid bird droppings, digging, and dusty activities, particularly if they live in a geographic region where *Histoplasma, Coccidioides*, or *Blastomyces* exists.

Chapter 27

Neurocysticercosis

Cysticercosis is an infection caused by the pork tapeworm, *Taenia solium*. Infection occurs when the tapeworm larvae enter the body and form cysticerci (cysts). When cysticerci are found in the brain, the condition is called neurocysticercosis.

The tapeworm that causes cysticercosis is found worldwide. Infection is found most often in rural, developing countries with poor hygiene where pigs are allowed to roam freely and eat human feces. This allows the tapeworm infection to be completed and the cycle to continue. Infection can occur, though rarely, if you have never traveled outside of the United States. Taeniasis and cysticercosis are very rare in Muslim countries where eating pork is forbidden.

Cysticercosis is spread by accidentally swallowing pork tapeworm eggs. Tapeworm eggs are passed in the bowel movement of a person who is infected. These tapeworm eggs are spread through food, water, or surfaces contaminated with feces. This can happen by drinking contaminated water or food, or by putting contaminated fingers to your mouth. A person who has a tapeworm infection can reinfect themselves (autoinfection). Once inside the stomach, the tapeworm egg hatches, penetrates the intestine, travels through the bloodstream and may develop into cysticerci in the muscles, brain, or eyes.

Symptoms will depend on the location and number of cysticerci in your body.

Excerpted from "Cysticercosis," Centers for Disease Control and Prevention (CDC), March 31, 2008.

Cysticerci in the muscles: Generally do not cause symptoms. However, you may be able to feel lumps under your skin.

Cysticerci in the eyes: Although rare, cysticerci may float in the eye and cause blurry or disturbed vision. Infection in the eyes may cause swelling or detachment of the retina.

Neurocysticercosis (cysticerci in the brain, spinal cord): Symptoms of neurocysticercosis depend upon where and how many cysticerci (often called lesions) are found in the brain. Seizures and headaches are the most common symptoms. However, confusion, lack of attention to people and surroundings, difficulty with balance, or swelling of the brain (called hydrocephalus) may also occur. Death can occur suddenly with heavy infections.

How long will I be infected before symptoms begin?

Symptoms can occur months to years after infection, usually when the cysts are in the process of dying. When this happens, the brain can swell. The pressure caused by swelling is what causes most of the symptoms of neurocysticercosis. Most people with cysticerci in muscles will not have symptoms of infection.

Diagnosis: Can be difficult and may require several testing methods. Your health care provider will ask you about where you have traveled and your eating habits. Diagnosis of neurocysticercosis is usually made by magnetic resonance imaging (MRI) or computed tomography (CT) brain scans. Blood tests are available to help diagnose an infection, but may not always be accurate. If surgery is necessary, confirmation of the diagnosis can be made by the laboratory.

Treatment: Infections are generally treated with anti-parasitic drugs in combination with anti-inflammatory drugs. Surgery is sometimes necessary to treat cases in the eyes, cases that are not responsive to drug treatment, or to reduce brain edema (swelling). Not all cases of cysticercosis are treated. The decision of whether or not to treat neurocysticercosis is based upon the number of lesions found in the brain and the symptoms you have. When only one lesion is found, often treatment is not given. It there is more than one lesion, specific anti-parasitic treatment is generally recommended. Also, if the brain lesion is considered calcified (this means that a hard shell has formed around the tapeworm larvae), the cysticerci is considered dead and specific anti-parasitic treatment is not beneficial. As the cysticerci die, the lesion will shrink. The swelling will go down, and often symptoms (such as seizures) will go away.

Can infection spread from person to person?

No. Cysticercosis is not spread from person to person. However, a person infected with the intestinal tapeworm stage of the infection (*T. solium*) will shed tapeworm eggs in their bowel movements. Tapeworm eggs that are accidentally swallowed by another person can cause infection. Family members may also be tested. Because the tapeworm infection can be difficult to diagnose, your health care provider may ask you to submit several stool specimens over several days to examine your stools for evidence of a tapeworm.

How can I prevent cysticercosis and other disease causing germs?

- Avoid eating raw or undercooked pork and other meats.

- Do not eat meat of pigs that are likely to be infected with the tapeworm.

- Wash hands with soap and water after using the toilet and before handling food, especially when traveling in developing countries.

- Wash and peel all raw vegetables and fruits before eating. Avoid food that may be contaminated with feces.

- Drink only bottled or boiled (one minute) water or carbonated (bubbly) drinks in cans or bottles. Do not drink fountain drinks or any drinks with ice cubes. Another way to make water safe is by filtering it through an "absolute 1-micron or less" filter and dissolving iodine tablets in the filtered water. Absolute 1-micron filters can be found in camping and outdoor supply stores.

Part Five

Acquired and Traumatic Brain Injuries

Chapter 28

Head Injury:
Identification and First Aid

Definition: A head injury is any trauma that leads to injury of the scalp, skull, or brain. The injuries can range from a minor bump on the skull to serious brain injury.

Head injury is classified as either closed or open (penetrating):

- A closed head injury means you received a hard blow to the head from striking an object, but the object did not break the skull.

- An open, or penetrating, head injury means you were hit with an object that broke the skull and entered the brain. This usually happens when you move at high speed, such as going through the windshield during a car accident. It can also happen from a gunshot to the head.

There are several types of brain injuries, including:

- concussion, the most common type of traumatic brain injury, in which the brain is shaken;

- contusion, which is a bruise on the brain;

- subarachnoid hemorrhage; and

- subdural hematoma.

"Head Injury," © 2009 A.D.A.M., Inc. Reprinted with permission.

Considerations: Every year, millions of people have a head injury. Most of these injuries are minor because the skull provides the brain with considerable protection. The symptoms of minor head injuries usually go away on their own. More than half a million head injuries a year, however, are severe enough to require hospitalization.

Learning to recognize a serious head injury, and implementing basic first aid, can make the difference in saving someone's life. In patients who have suffered a severe head injury, there are often other organ systems injured. For example, a head injury is sometimes accompanied by a spinal injury.

Causes: Common causes of head injury include traffic accidents, falls, physical assault, and accidents at home, work, outdoors, or while playing sports. Some head injuries result in prolonged or nonreversible brain damage. This can occur as a result of bleeding inside the brain or forces that damage the brain directly. These more serious head injuries may cause coma; chronic headaches; loss of or change in sensation, hearing, vision, taste, or smell; paralysis; seizures; or speech and language problems.

Symptoms: The symptoms of a head injury can occur immediately or develop slowly over several hours or days. Even if the skull is not fractured, the brain can bang against the inside of the skull and be bruised. The head may look fine, but complications could result from bleeding or swelling inside the skull.

When encountering a person who just had a head injury, try to find out what happened. If he or she cannot tell you, look for clues and ask witnesses. In any serious head trauma, always assume the spinal cord is also injured.

The following symptoms suggest a more serious head injury—other than a concussion or contusion—and require emergency medical treatment:

- Changes in, or unequal size of, pupils

- Convulsions

- Distorted features of the face

- Fluid draining from nose, mouth, or ears (may be clear or bloody)

- Fracture in the skull or face, bruising of the face, swelling at the site of the injury, or scalp wound

- Impaired hearing, smell, taste, or vision

- Inability to move one or more limbs

- Irritability (especially in children), personality changes, or unusual behavior

- Loss of consciousness, confusion, or drowsiness

- Low breathing rate or drop in blood pressure

- Restlessness, clumsiness, or lack of coordination

- Severe headache

- Slurred speech or blurred vision

- Stiff neck or vomiting

- Symptoms improve, and then suddenly get worse (change in consciousness)

First Aid: Get medical help immediately if the person:

- becomes unusually drowsy;

- behaves abnormally;

- develops a severe headache or stiff neck;

- loses consciousness, even briefly;

- vomits more than once.

For a moderate to severe head injury, take the following steps:

1. Call 911.

2. Check the person's airway, breathing, and circulation. If necessary, begin rescue breathing and cardiopulmonary resuscitation (CPR).

3. If the person's breathing and heart rate are normal but the person is unconscious, treat as if there is a spinal injury. Stabilize the head and neck by placing your hands on both sides of the person's head, keeping the head in line with the spine and preventing movement. Wait for medical help.

4. Stop any bleeding by firmly pressing a clean cloth on the wound. If the injury is serious, be careful not to move the person's head. If blood soaks through the cloth, do not remove it. Place another cloth over the first one.

5. If you suspect a skull fracture, do not apply direct pressure to the bleeding site, and do not remove any debris from the wound. Cover the wound with sterile gauze dressing.

6. If the person is vomiting, roll the head, neck, and body as one unit to prevent choking. This still protects the spine, which you must always assume is injured in the case of a head injury. (Children often vomit once after a head injury. This may not be a problem, but call a doctor for further guidance.)

7. Apply ice packs to swollen areas.

For a mild head injury, no specific treatment may be needed. However, closely watch the person for any concerning symptoms over the next 24 hours. The symptoms of a serious head injury can be delayed. While the person is sleeping, wake him or her every 2–3 hours and ask simple questions to check alertness, such as "What is your name?"

If a child begins to play or run immediately after getting a bump on the head, serious injury is unlikely. However, as with anyone with a head injury, closely watch the child for 24 hours after the incident.

Over-the-counter pain medicine, such as acetaminophen, may be used for a mild headache. Do not take aspirin, ibuprofen, or other anti-inflammatory medications because they can increase the risk of bleeding.

*   Do not wash a head wound that is deep or bleeding a lot.
*   Do not remove any object sticking out of a wound.
*   Do not move the person unless absolutely necessary.
*   Do not shake the person if he or she seems dazed.
*   Do not remove a helmet if you suspect a serious head injury.
*   Do not pick up a fallen child with any sign of head injury.
*   Do not drink alcohol within 48 hours of a serious head injury.

When to contact a medical professional: Call 911 if:

*   there is severe head or facial bleeding;
*   the person is confused, drowsy, lethargic, or unconscious;
*   the person stops breathing; or
*   you suspect a serious head or neck injury, or the person develops any signs or symptoms of a serious head injury.

Prevention

- Always use safety equipment during activities that could result in head injury. These include seat belts, bicycle or motorcycle helmets, and hard hats.

- Obey traffic signals when riding a bicycle. Be predictable so that other drivers will be able to determine your course.

- Be visible. Do not ride a bicycle at night unless you wear bright, reflective clothing and have proper headlamps and flashers.

- Use age-appropriate car seats or boosters for babies and young children.

- Make sure that children have a safe area in which to play.

- Supervise children of any age.

- Do not drink and drive, and do not allow yourself to be driven by someone whom you know or suspect has been drinking alcohol or is otherwise impaired.

References

Heegaard WG, Biros MH. Head. In: Marx J. *Rosen's Emergency Medicine: Concepts and Clinical Practice*. 6th ed. St. Louis, Mo: Mosby; 2006:chap. 38.

Atabaki SM. Pediatric head injury. *Pediatr Rev*. 2007;28(6):215–224.

Chapter 29

Preventing Brain Injuries

A concussion is a brain injury. Concussions are caused by a bump, blow, or jolt to the head. They can range from mild to severe and can disrupt the way the brain normally works. Most people will only experience symptoms from a concussion for a short period of time. But sometimes concussion can lead to long-lasting problems. The best way to protect yourself and your family from concussions is to prevent them from happening.

There are many ways to reduce the chances that you or your family members will have a concussion or more serious brain injury:

Wear a seat belt every time you drive or ride in a motor vehicle.

Buckle your child in the car using a child safety seat, booster seat, or seat belt (according to the child's height, weight, and age). Children should start using a booster seat when they outgrow their child safety seats (usually when they weigh about 40 pounds). They should continue to ride in a booster seat until the lap and shoulder belts in the car fit properly and in accordance with state laws.

Never drive while under the influence of alcohol or drugs.

Wear a helmet and make sure your children wear helmets that are fitted and maintained properly when doing the following:

Excerpted from "Heads Up: Preventing Concussion," Centers for Disease Control and Prevention (CDC), 2007.

- Riding a bike, motorcycle, snowmobile, scooter, or all-terrain vehicle

- Playing a contact sport, such as football, ice hockey, lacrosse, or boxing

- Using in-line skates or riding a skateboard

- Batting and running bases in baseball or softball

- Riding a horse

- Skiing, sledding, or snowboarding

Use the right protective equipment (should be fitted and maintained properly in order to provide the expected protection) during athletic games and practices:

- Follow the safety rules and the rules of the sport.

- Practice good sportsmanship.

- Do not return to play with a known or suspected concussion until you have been evaluated and given permission by an appropriate health care professional.

Make living areas safer for seniors:

- Remove tripping hazards such as throw rugs and clutter in walkways.

- Place nonslip mats in the bathtub and on shower floors.

- Install grab bars next to the toilet and in the tub or shower.

- Install handrails on both sides of stairways.

- Improve lighting throughout the home.

- Maintain a regular exercise program to improve lower body strength and balance.

Make living areas safer for children:

- Install window guards to keep young children from falling out of open windows.

- Use safety gates at the top and bottom of stairs when young children are around.

- Keep stairs clear of clutter.

- Secure rugs and using rubber mats in bathtubs.

- Do not allow children to play on fire escapes or on other unsafe platforms.

Playgrounds:

- Make sure the surface on your child's playground is made of shock-absorbing material, such as hardwood mulch or sand, and is maintained to an appropriate depth.

Chapter 30

Concussion (Mild Traumatic Brain Injury)

Chapter Contents

Section 30.1

Facts about Concussion and Brain Injury

Excerpted from "Heads Up: Facts for Physicians about Mild
Traumatic Brain Injury (MTBI)," Centers for Disease Control
and Prevention (CDC), 2007.

The term mild traumatic brain injury (MTBI) is used interchange-
ably with the term concussion. An MTBI or concussion is defined as
a complex pathophysiologic process affecting the brain, induced by
traumatic biomechanical forces secondary to direct or indirect forces
to the head. MTBI is caused by a blow or jolt to the head that disrupts
the function of the brain. This disturbance of brain function is typically associated with normal structural neuroimaging findings. MTBI
results in a constellation of physical, cognitive, emotional and sleep-
related symptoms and may or may not involve a loss of consciousness.
Duration of symptoms is highly variable and may last from several
minutes to days, weeks, months, or even longer in some cases.

Magnitude of MTBI

- An estimated 75%–90% of the 1.4 million traumatic brain injury
  (TBI)-related deaths, hospitalizations, and emergency department
  visits that occur each year are concussions or other forms of
  MTBI.

- Approximately 1.6–3.8 million sports and recreation-related
  traumatic brain injuries occur in the United States each year.
  Most of these are MTBI that are not treated in a hospital or
  emergency department.

- Blasts are an important cause of MTBI among military personal
  in war zones.

- Direct medical costs and indirect costs such as lost productivity
  from MTBI totaled an estimated $12 billion in the U.S. in 2000.

- Individuals with a history of concussion are at an increased risk
  of sustaining a subsequent concussion.

- Duration of symptoms is highly variable and may last from several minutes to days, weeks, months, or even longer in some cases. Research shows that recovery time may be longer for children and adolescents.

- Symptoms or deficits that continue beyond three months may be a sign of post-concussion syndrome.

- With proper diagnosis and management, most patients with MTBI recover fully.

Neuropathophysiology of MTBI: Unlike more severe TBI, the disturbance of brain function from MTBI is related more to dysfunction of brain metabolism rather than to structural injury or damage. Clinical signs and symptoms of MTBI such as poor memory, speed of processing, fatigue, and dizziness result from this underlying neurometabolic cascade.

Physical signs and symptoms:

- Headache
- Nausea
- Vomiting
- Balance problems
- Dizziness
- Visual problems
- Fatigue
- Sensitivity to light
- Sensitivity to noise
- Numbness/tingling
- Dazed or stunned

Cognitive signs and symptoms:

- Feeling mentally foggy
- Feeling slowed down
- Difficulty concentrating
- Difficulty remembering

- Forgetful of recent information or conversations
- Confused about recent events
- Answers questions slowly
- Repeats questions

Emotional signs and symptoms:

- Irritability
- Sadness
- More emotional
- Nervousness

Sleep problems:

- Drowsiness
- Sleeping less than usual
- Sleeping more than usual
- Trouble falling asleep

Diagnosis: MTBI can be challenging to diagnose as symptoms of MTBI are common to those of other medical conditions (such as post-traumatic stress disorder [PTSD], depression, and headache syndromes), and the onset or recognition of symptoms may occur days or weeks after the initial injury. A systematic assessment of the injury and its manifestations is essential to proper management and reduced morbidity.

Section 30.2

Children's Concussion Recovery: No Sports, No Schoolwork, No Text Messages

Text in this section is from "Concussion Experts: For Kids—No Sports, No Schoolwork, No Text Messages," June 8, 2009; and "Post-Concussion Home/School Instructions," © Children's National Medical Center (www. childrensnational.org). Reprinted with permission.

Concussion Experts: For Kids—No Sports, No Schoolwork, No Text Messages

When it comes to concussions, children and teens require different treatment, according to international experts who recently published consensus recommendations. *The British Journal of Sports Medicine's* new guidelines state children and teens must be strictly monitored and activities restricted until fully healed. These restrictions include no return to the field of play, no return to school, and no cognitive activity.

The new consensus is from the International Conference on Concussion in Sports. Children's pediatric concussion expert and neuropsychologist Gerard Gioia, PhD, participated in the panel, and played a key role in delineating the differences between children, adolescents and teens, and adult athletes. "These consensus recommendations mark the first time that international experts have focused on specialized treatment for kids," said Dr. Gioia, chief of Neuropsychology at Children's National. "This conference of experts has led the way in developing protocols for adult athletes, and now international protocols take into consideration that the developing brain of the child and adolescent requires special consideration. The guidelines also point to the important role parents, coaches, and teachers play in assessing and treating young athletes."

For children and adolescents, the guidance strongly reiterates several key points for coaches, parents, and physicians:

- Injury to the developing brain, especially repeat concussions, may increase the risk of long-term effects in children, so no return-to-play until completely symptom free.

- No child or adolescent athlete should ever return to play on the same day of an injury—regardless of level of athletic performance.

- Children and adolescents may need a longer period of full rest and then gradual return to normal activities than adults.

- For children, cognitive rest is a key to recovery. While restrictions on physical activity restrictions are also important, cognitive rest must be carefully adhered to, including limits on cognitive stressors such as academic activities and at-home and social activities including text messaging, video games, and television watching.

The group's recommendations for children and adolescents were based on the fact that though 80% to 90% of adult concussions resolve in seven to ten days, for children and adolescents, the recovery time is often longer. In all cases, the decision to return-to-play should be made based on the individual's progress, not a standard time period. Careful post-injury evaluation of the injured student-athlete is essential.

Post-Concussion Home and School Instructions*

You have been diagnosed with a concussion (also known as a mild traumatic brain injury). The following instructions are provided to assist your recovery. Following these instructions can also prevent further injury.

Returning to Daily Activities

Following a concussion, rest is the key. The injured person:

- should not participate in any high risk activities (for example: sports, physical education [PE], riding a bike) or other physical activities that increase his/her normal heart rate;

- limit activities that require a lot of lengthy mental activity or concentration (such as homework, schoolwork, job-related activities, extended video game playing), as this can make the symptoms worse;

- get good sleep (no late nights or sleep overs) and take naps if tired or drowsy;

- will need help from parents, teachers, coaches, and athletic trainers to help manage their activity level, it is hard to change from the normal routine; and

- should be informed that during recovery, it is normal to feel frustrated and sad when you do not feel right and you can't be as active as usual.

It is okay to use acetaminophen (Tylenol) for headaches; use ice pack on head and neck as needed for comfort; eat a light diet; go to sleep; or rest (no strenuous activity or sports).

There is no need to check eyes with a flashlight, wake up every hour, test reflexes, or stay in bed.

Do not drink alcohol, drive while symptomatic, exercise or lift weights, or take ibuprofen (Advil, Motrin), aspirin, naproxen, or other non-steroidal anti-inflammatory medications until told by a physician.

Returning to School

- Inform the teacher(s), school nurse, school psychologist or counselor, and administrator(s) about your child/adolescent's injury and symptoms. Share a copy of these instructions with them.

- Students who experience symptoms of concussion often need extra help to perform school-related activities and may not perform at their best on classroom or standardized tests. Rest breaks during the school day can also be helpful. As symptoms decrease during recovery, the extra help or supports can be removed slowly.

School personnel should watch for:

- increased problems paying attention or concentration;

- increased problems remembering or learning new information;

- longer time needed to complete tasks or assignments;

- greater irritability, less able to cope with stress; or

- increase in symptoms (for example: headache, tiredness) when doing schoolwork.

Returning to Sports and Recreation

- Your son or daughter should never return to sports participation or active recreation with any symptoms unless directed by a qualified health professional.

- No return to physical education class.

- No physical activity at recess.

- No return to sports practices or games.

- Be sure that the physical education teacher and all coaches are aware of the injury and symptoms.

- When appropriate, have the student check in with the athletic trainer on the first day he or she returns.

- It is normal for the child or adolescent to feel frustrated, sad, and even angry because they cannot return to sports or recreation right away. With any injury, a full recovery will lower the chances of getting hurt again. It is better to miss one or two games than the whole season.

Serious Signs to Watch For

Please watch carefully for any of the following serious signs and symptoms. The best guideline is to note symptoms that worsen, and behaviors that are a change in your son or daughter. If you observe any of the following signs, call your doctor or go to your emergency department immediately.

- Headaches that worsen

- Seizures

- Neck pain

- Look very drowsy, can't be awakened

- Repeated vomiting

- Slurred speech

- Can't recognize people or places

- Increasing confusion

- Weakness or numbness in arms or legs

- Unusual behavior change

- Significant irritability

- Change in state of consciousness

*Adapted from ACE Care Plan "Heads Up: Brain Injury in Your Practice" (2007); National Athletic Trainers' Association Position Statement: Management of Sport-Related Concussion (2004).

Chapter 31

Traumatic Brain Injury (TBI)

Chapter Contents

Section 31.1

Facts about TBI

This section begins with an excerpt from "Traumatic Brain Injury Overview," Centers for Disease Control and Prevention (CDC), April 1, 2008; and continues with excerpts from "Traumatic Brain Injury: Hope through Research," National Institute of Neurological Disorders and Stroke (NINDS), NIH Publication No. 02–2478, updated February 9, 2010. Figures 31.1, 31.2, 31.3, and 31.4 are excerpted from "Traumatic Brain Injury Model Systems National Database Update, 2009," a publication of the Traumatic Brain Injury Model Systems National Data and Statistical Center, Englewood, CO, © 2009. Reprinted with permission.

Overview of Traumatic Brain Injury

Traumatic brain injuries (TBI) contribute to a substantial number of deaths and cases of permanent disability annually. The Centers for Disease Control and Prevention (CDC) estimates that at least 5.3 million Americans, about 2% of the United States' (U.S.) population, currently have a long-term or lifelong need for help to perform activities of daily living as a result of a TBI.

The severity of a TBI may range from mild (a brief change in mental status or consciousness) to severe (an extended period of unconsciousness or amnesia) after the injury. Approximately 75% of TBIs that occur each year are concussions or other forms of mild TBI.

Recent data shows that, on average, approximately 1.4 million people sustain a TBI each year in the United States. Of those 50,000 die, 235,000 are hospitalized; and 1.1 million are treated and released from an emergency department.

Among children ages 0–14 years, TBI results in an estimated 2,685 deaths, 37,000 hospitalizations, and 435,000 emergency department visits.

The number of people with TBI who are not seen in an emergency department or who receive no care is unknown.

Groups at risk:

- Males are about twice as likely as females to sustain a TBI.

- The two age groups at highest risk for TBI are 0–4 year olds and 15–19 year olds.

- Adults age 75 years or older have the highest rates of TBI-related hospitalization and death.

- Certain military duties (for example, paratrooper) increase the risk of sustaining a TBI.

- African Americans have the highest death rate from TBI.

- TBI hospitalization rates are highest among African Americans and American Indians/Alaska Natives (AI/AN).

Traumatic Brain Injury: What You Need to Know

TBI, a form of acquired brain injury, occurs when a sudden trauma causes damage to the brain. The damage can be focal (confined to one area of the brain), or diffuse (involving more than one area of the brain). TBI can result from a closed head injury or a penetrating head injury. A closed injury occurs when the head suddenly and violently hits an object but the object does not break through the skull. A penetrating injury occurs when an object pierces the skull and enters brain tissue.

Symptoms of a TBI can be mild, moderate, or severe, depending on the extent of the damage to the brain. Some symptoms are evident immediately, while others do not surface until several days or weeks after the injury. A person with a mild TBI may remain conscious or may experience a loss of consciousness for a few seconds or minutes.

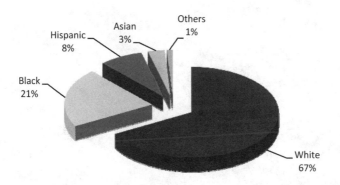

Figure 31.1. *Race or Ethnicity of Individuals with TBI (n=8777) (Source: Traumatic Brain Injury Model Systems National Data and Statistical Center, Englewood, CO, © 2009. Reprinted with permission.)*

The person may also feel dazed or not like himself for several days or weeks after the initial injury. Other symptoms of mild TBI include headache, confusion, lightheadedness, dizziness, blurred vision or tired eyes, ringing in the ears, bad taste in the mouth, fatigue or lethargy, a change in sleep patterns, behavioral or mood changes, and trouble with memory, concentration, attention, or thinking.

A person with a moderate or severe TBI may show these same symptoms, but may also have a headache that gets worse or does not go away, repeated vomiting or nausea, convulsions or seizures, inability to awaken from sleep, dilation of one or both pupils of the eyes, slurred speech, weakness or numbness in the extremities, loss of coordination, or increased confusion, restlessness, or agitation. Small children with moderate to severe TBI may show some of these signs as well as signs specific to young children, such as persistent crying, inability to be consoled, or refusal to nurse or eat. Anyone with signs of moderate or severe TBI should receive medical attention as soon as possible.

Half of all TBIs are due to transportation accidents involving automobiles, motorcycles, bicycles, and pedestrians. These accidents are the major cause of TBI in people under age 75. For those 75 and older, falls cause the majority of TBIs. Approximately 20% of TBIs are due to violence, such as firearm assaults and child abuse, and about 3% are due to sports injuries. Fully half of TBI incidents involve alcohol use.

The cause of the TBI plays a role in determining the patient's outcome. For example, approximately 91% of firearm TBIs (two-thirds of which may be suicidal in intent) result in death, while only 11% of TBIs from falls result in death.

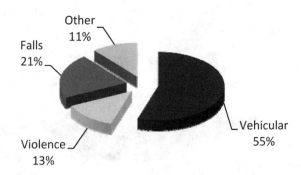

Figure 31.2. *Causes of Injury (n=8749) (Source: Traumatic Brain Injury Model Systems National Data and Statistical Center, Englewood, CO, © 2009. Reprinted with permission.)*

Medical care of TBI: Medical care usually begins when paramedics or emergency medical technicians arrive on the scene of an accident or when a TBI patient arrives at the emergency department of a hospital. Because little can be done to reverse the initial brain damage caused by trauma, medical personnel try to stabilize the patient and focus on preventing further injury. As soon as medical personnel have stabilized the head-injured patient, they assess the patient's condition by measuring vital signs and reflexes and by performing a neurological examination.

Immediate post-injury complications: Sometimes, health complications occur in the period immediately following a TBI. These complications are not types of TBI, but are distinct medical problems that arise as a result of the injury. Although complications are rare, the risk increases with the severity of the trauma. Complications of TBI include immediate seizures, hydrocephalus or post-traumatic ventricular enlargement, cerebral spinal fluid (CSF) leaks, infections, vascular injuries, cranial nerve injuries, pain, bed sores, multiple organ system failure in unconscious patients, and polytrauma (trauma to other parts of the body in addition to the brain).

General trauma: Most TBI patients have injuries to other parts of the body in addition to the head and brain. Physicians call this polytrauma. These injuries require immediate and specialized care and can complicate treatment of and recovery from the TBI. Other medical complications that may accompany a TBI include pulmonary (lung) dysfunction; cardiovascular (heart) dysfunction from blunt chest trauma; gastrointestinal dysfunction; fluid and hormonal imbalances; and other isolated complications, such as fractures, nerve injuries, deep vein thrombosis, excessive blood clotting, and infections.

Disabilities from a TBI: Disabilities resulting from a TBI depend upon the severity of the injury, the location of the injury, and the age and general health of the patient. Some common disabilities include problems with cognition (thinking, memory, and reasoning), sensory processing (sight, hearing, touch, taste, and smell), communication (expression and understanding), and behavior or mental health (depression, anxiety, personality changes, aggression, acting out, and social inappropriateness).

Within days to weeks of the head injury approximately 40% of TBI patients develop a host of troubling symptoms collectively called postconcussion syndrome (PCS). A patient need not have suffered a concussion or loss of consciousness to develop the syndrome and many patients with mild TBI suffer from PCS. Symptoms include headache, dizziness, vertigo (a sensation of spinning around or of objects spinning around the patient), memory problems, trouble concentrating, sleeping problems, restlessness, irritability, apathy, depression, and anxiety. These symptoms may last for a few weeks after the head injury. The syndrome is more prevalent in patients who had psychiatric symptoms, such as depression or anxiety, before the injury.

Cognition is a term used to describe the processes of thinking, reasoning, problem solving, information processing, and memory. Most patients with severe TBI, if they recover consciousness, suffer from cognitive disabilities, including the loss of many higher level mental skills. The most common cognitive impairment among severely head-injured patients is memory loss, characterized by some loss of specific memories and the partial inability to form or store new ones.

Many patients with mild to moderate head injuries who experience cognitive deficits become easily confused or distracted and have problems with concentration and attention. They also have problems with higher level, so-called executive functions, such as planning, organizing, abstract reasoning, problem solving, and making judgments, which may make it difficult to resume pre-injury work-related activities. Recovery from cognitive deficits is greatest within the first six months after the injury and more gradual after that.

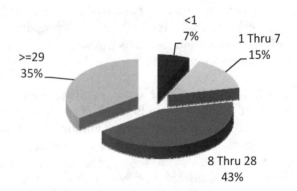

Figure 31.3. *Severity of TBI Based on Days of Post-Traumatic Amnesia (mean = 24.9 days; n = 6536) (Source: Traumatic Brain Injury Model Systems National Data and Statistical Center, Englewood, CO, © 2009. Reprinted with permission.)*

Many TBI patients have sensory problems, especially problems with vision. Patients may not be able to register what they are seeing or may be slow to recognize objects. Also, TBI patients often have difficulty with hand-eye coordination.

Language and communication problems are common disabilities in TBI patients. Some may experience aphasia, defined as difficulty with understanding and producing spoken and written language; others may have difficulty with the more subtle aspects of communication, such as body language and emotional, non-verbal signals.

In non-fluent aphasia, also called Broca aphasia or motor aphasia, TBI patients often have trouble recalling words and speaking in complete sentences. They may speak in broken phrases and pause frequently. Most patients are aware of these deficits and may become extremely frustrated. Patients with fluent aphasia, also called Wernicke aphasia or sensory aphasia, display little meaning in their speech, even though they speak in complete sentences and use correct grammar. Patients with global aphasia have extensive damage to the portions of the brain responsible for language and often suffer severe communication disabilities.

TBI patients may have problems with spoken language if the part of the brain that controls speech muscles is damaged. In this disorder, called dysarthria, the patient can think of the appropriate language, but cannot easily speak the words because they are unable to use the muscles needed to form the words and produce the sounds. These language deficits can lead to miscommunication, confusion, and frustration for the patient as well as those interacting with him or her.

Most TBI patients have emotional or behavioral problems that fit under the broad category of psychiatric health. Family members of TBI patients often find that personality changes and behavioral problems are the most difficult disabilities to handle. Psychiatric problems that may surface include depression, apathy, anxiety, irritability, anger, paranoia, confusion, frustration, agitation, insomnia or other sleep problems, and mood swings. Problem behaviors may include aggression and violence, impulsivity, disinhibition, acting out, noncompliance, social inappropriateness, emotional outbursts, childish behavior, impaired self-control, impaired self awareness, inability to take responsibility or accept criticism, egocentrism, inappropriate sexual activity, and alcohol or drug abuse or addiction.

Long-term problems associated with a TBI: In addition to immediate post-injury complications, other long-term problems can develop after a TBI. These include Parkinson disease and other motor

335

problems, Alzheimer disease, dementia pugilistica, and post-traumatic dementia.

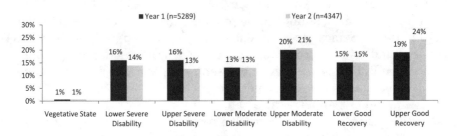

Figure 31.4. *Glasgow Outcome Scale-Extended (Source: Traumatic Brain Injury Model Systems National Data and Statistical Center, Englewood, CO, © 2009. Reprinted with permission.)*

Section 31.2

Impact of a Recent TBI on Family Members

"Understanding TBI–Part 4: The impact of a recent TBI on family members and what they can do to help with recovery," Copyright © 2009 Model Systems Knowledge Translation System (MSKTC). This publication was produced by the TBI Model Systems in collaboration with the Model Systems Knowledge Translation Center (http://msktc.washington.edu) with funding from the National Institute on Disability and Rehabilitation Research in the U.S. Department of Education, Grant no. H133A060070.

How does brain injury affect family members?

For most family members, life is not the same after TBI. We want you to know that you are not alone in what you are feeling. While everyone's situation is a bit different, there are some common problems that many family members experience such as less time for you, financial difficulties, role changes of family members, problems with communication, and lack of support from other family members and friends. These are just some of the problems that family members may face after injury. Sometimes these problems can seem too much and you may become overwhelmed, not seeing any way out. Family members have commonly reported feeling sad, anxious, angry, guilty, and frustrated.

Ways to reduce stress: Since the injury, you have likely been under a great deal of stress. A little stress is part of life, but stress that goes on for a long time can have a negative effect on the mind and body. Stress is related to medical problems such as heart disease, cancer, and stroke.

- Stress can make you do things less well because it affects your ability to concentrate, to be organized, and to think clearly.

- Stress also has a negative effect on your relationships with other people because it makes you irritable, less patient, and more likely to lash out at others.

- Stress can lead to depression and/or anxiety.

If you are under constant stress, you are not going to be as helpful to your injured family member or anyone else. If you do not take the time to rest and care for yourself, you will get fewer things done, which will lead to more stress. If you won't do this for yourself, do it for your injured family member. They will be better off if you are healthy and rested. Here are some suggestions for ways to reduce stress and stay healthy. These things have worked for many people, but not all of them may work for you. The important thing is that you begin thinking about ways to improve your life.

Learn to relax: Taking a few moments to relax can help you be more ready for the things you need to do. Learning to relax is not easy, especially in your current situation. There are relaxation techniques that can help you such as breathing deeply and focusing on your breathing, stating a word or phrase that has positive meaning (such as peace), or visual imagery. In order to train your body and mind to relax, you need to practice often. Don't give up if it doesn't work right away. If you keep practicing these techniques, you will feel more relaxed in the long run, and you will find that you're able to function better in all areas of your life.

Learn which coping strategies work for you: No matter what was going on in your life before, the injury has caused changes. You may never have experienced anything similar to the injury, and some of your usual coping strategies may not work in your current situation.

The best thing that you can do for yourself is to be open to trying new ways of coping and find out what works for you.

Some coping strategies that others have found helpful:

- Take time for yourself.

- Keep a regular schedule for yourself.

- Get regular exercise such as taking a 20–30 minute walk each day.

- Participate in support groups.

- Maintain a sense of humor.

- Be more assertive about getting the support you need.

- Change roles and responsibilities within the family.

Learn how to reward yourself: Everyone needs something to look forward to. You'll probably say, "I have no time; it's impossible." Just remember that you will be more ready to do the things you have to do if you take some time to do some things that you want to do. Even if you have very limited time, you can find some small way to reward yourself. Promise yourself a cup of your favorite coffee or an opportunity to watch a good television (TV) show or read something you enjoy.

Problem Solving for Caregivers

Sometimes you may feel overwhelmed by problems. There may be so many problems that you're not sure which one to tackle first. You can only solve one problem at a time, so pick one. Use the following problem-solving steps to find a good solution. Try to choose a smaller problem to solve first. This will give you practice and make you more confident about solving bigger problems. If you deal with problems in this way, they may seem easier to handle.

Steps in Problem Solving

1. Identify the problem: What is the problem? Define it as clearly and specifically as possible. Remember that you can only solve one problem at a time.

2. Brainstorm solutions: What can be done? Think of as many things as you can. Don't worry about whether they sound silly or realistic. This is the time to think about all possibilities, even the ones that you don't think will happen. Be creative.

338

3. Evaluate the alternatives: Now you will start thinking about the consequences of the ideas you came up with in Step 2. For each idea, make a list of positives on one side of the page and a list of negatives on the other side.

4. Choose a solution: Pick the solution with the best consequences based on your list of positives and negatives. Keep in mind that having more positives than negatives is not always the best rule. Sometimes you will have one negative that outweighs many positives.

5. Try the solution: Try out the idea you have chosen. Give it more than one chance to work. If it doesn't work right away, try to figure out why. Was there some consequence you didn't think of? Is there another problem in the way that could be easily solved?

6. If your first solution doesn't work, try another one: Don't give up. Everything doesn't always work out the first time. You can learn from your mistakes; they may help you to choose a better solution next time.

Ways Family Members Can Help the Injured Person

The treatment team can provide you with guidance in how to help the person while not giving them too much or too little assistance. Attending therapy when possible and working with the therapists and nurses are the best ways to learn to help the person before discharge from the hospital.

The following recommendations are intended to help families and caregivers care for their loved one once they have returned home. Not all of the following recommendation may apply to your situation.

Provide structure and normalcy to daily life:

- Establish and maintain a daily routine—this helps the person feel more secure in their environment.

- Place objects the person needs within easy reach.

- Have the person rest frequently. Don't let the person get fatigued.

- Be natural with the person and help them to maintain their former status in the family. Communication is important to the person's recovery. Although they may not be able to speak, they should continue to be involved in as normal a social world as possible.

- Include the person in family activities and conversations.

- Keep a calendar of activities visible on the wall. Cross off days as they pass.

- Maintain a photo album with labeled pictures of family members, friends, and familiar places.

Provide support in a respectful way:

- Try not to overwhelm the person with false optimism by saying statements like "You will be alright," or "You will be back to work in no time."

- Point out every gain the person has made since the onset of the injury. Avoid comparing speech, language or physical abilities prior to the injury with how they are now. Look ahead and help the person to do the same.

- Treat the person as an adult by not talking down to them.

- Respect the person's likes and dislikes regarding food, dress, entertainment, music, and so forth.

- Avoid making the person feel guilty for mistakes and accidents such as spilling something.

- If the person has memory problems, explain an activity as simply as possible before you begin. Then as you do the activity, review with the person each step in more detail.

Avoid over-stimulation: Agitation can be heightened by too much activity and stimulation.

- Restrict the number of visitors (one or two at a time).

- Not more than one person should speak at a time.

- Use short sentences and simple words.

- Present only one thought or command at a time and provide extra response time.

- Use a calm, soft voice when speaking with the person.

- Keep stimulation to one sense (hearing, visual, or touch) at a time.

- Avoid crowded places such as shopping malls and stadiums.

Safety tips: The person who has confusion or impaired judgment may be unable to remember where dangers lie or to judge what is dangerous (stairs, stoves, medications). Fatigue and inability to make the body do what one wants can lead to injury. Therefore, it is very important that a brain injured person live in an environment that has been made as safe as possible. The following are some safety guidelines to use in the home:

- Keep clutter out of the hallway and off stairs or anywhere the person is likely to walk. Remove small rugs that could cause tripping or falls.

- Remove breakables and dangerous objects (matches, knives, and guns).

- Keep medications in a locked cabinet or drawer.

- Get the doctor's consent before giving the person over-the-counter medication.

- Limit access to potentially dangerous areas (bathrooms, basement) by locking doors if the person tends to wander. Have the person wear an identification bracelet in case he or she wanders outside.

- Keep the person's bed low. If they fall out of the bed, you may want to place the mattress on the floor or install side rails.

- Make sure rooms are well lit, especially in the evening. Night lights can help prevent falls.

- Have someone stay with the person who is severely confused or agitated.

- Keep exit doors locked. Consider some type of exit alarm, such as a bell attached to the door.

- Consider a mat alarm under a bedside rug to alert others if the person gets up during the night.

Things that can be more dangerous after a TBI and should be resumed only after consulting a health care professional include contact sports, horseback riding, swimming, hunting or access to firearms, power tools or sharp objects, riding recreational vehicles, and cooking without supervision.

Individuals with brain injury should receive permission from a health care professional prior to using alcohol or other substances at any point after their injury. Also, no driving until approved by your doctor.

Section 31.3

Difficulties with Cognition, Emotions, or Fatigue after TBI

This section includes: "Cognitive Problems after Traumatic Brain Injury," "Emotional Problems after Traumatic Brain Injury," and "Fatigue and Traumatic Brain Injury," Copyright © 2009 Model Systems Knowledge Translation System (MSKTC). These publications were produced by the TBI Model Systems in collaboration with the Model Systems Knowledge Translation Center (http://msktc.washington.edu) with funding from the National Institute on Disability and Rehabilitation Research in the U.S. Department of Education, Grant no. H133A060070.

Cognition

Cognition is the act of knowing or thinking. It includes the ability to choose, understand, remember, and use information. Cognition includes the following:

- Attention and concentration

- Processing and understanding information

- Memory

- Communication

- Planning, organizing, and assembling

- Reasoning, problem-solving, decision-making, and judgment

- Controlling impulses and desires and being patient

How does TBI affect cognition and what can be done about it?

After a TBI it is common for people to have problems with attention, concentration, speech and language, learning and memory, reasoning, planning, and problem-solving.

Attention and concentration: A person with TBI may be unable to focus, pay attention, or attend to more than one thing at a time.

This may result in restlessness and being easily distracted; having difficulty finishing a project or working on more than one task at a time; or problems carrying on long conversations or sitting still for long periods of time. Since attention skills are considered a "building block" of higher level skills (such as memory and reasoning), people with attention or concentration problems often show signs of other cognitive problems as well.

What can be done to improve attention and concentration?

- Decrease the distractions. For example, work in a quiet room.

- Focus on one task at a time.

- Begin practicing attention skills on simple, yet practical activities (such as reading a paragraph or adding numbers) in a quiet room. Gradually make the tasks harder (read a short story or balance a checkbook) or work in a more noisy environment.

- Take breaks when you get tired.

Problems with processing and understanding information: After brain injury, a person's ability to process and understand information often slows down, resulting in the following problems:

- Taking longer to grasp what others are saying.

- Taking more time to understand and follow directions.

- Having trouble following television shows, movies, and so forth.

- Taking longer to read and understand written information including books, newspapers, or magazines.

- Being slower to react. This is especially important for driving, which may become unsafe if the person cannot react fast enough to stop signs, traffic lights or other warning signs. Individuals with TBI should not drive until their visual skills and reaction time have been tested by a specialist.

- Being slower to carry out physical tasks, including routine activities like getting dressed or cooking.

What can be done to improve the ability to process and understand information?

- Place your full attention on what you are trying to understand. Decrease distractions.

- Allow more time to think about the information before moving on.

- Re-read information as needed. Take notes and summarize in your own words.

- If needed, ask people to repeat themselves, to say something in a different way, or to speak slower. Repeat what you just heard to make sure you understood it correctly.

Language and communication problems: Communication problems can cause persons with TBI to have difficulty understanding and expressing information in some of the following ways:

- Difficulty thinking of the right word

- Trouble starting or following conversations or understanding what others say

- Rambling or getting off topic easily

- Difficulty with more complex language skills, such as expressing thoughts in an organized manner

- Trouble communicating thoughts and feelings using facial expressions, tone of voice and body language (non-verbal communication)

- Having problems reading others' emotions and not responding appropriately to another person's feelings or to the social situation

- Misunderstanding jokes or sarcasm

What can be done to improve language and communication?

Work with a speech therapist to identify areas that need work. Communication problems can keep improving for a long time after the injury. Tips for family members wanting to help include the following:

- Use kind words and a gentle tone of voice. Be careful not to "talk down" to the person.

- When talking with the injured person, ask every so often if he or she understands what you are saying, or ask the person a question to determine if he or she understood what you said.

- Do not speak too fast or say too much at once.

- Develop a signal (like raising a finger) that will let the injured person know when he or she has gotten off topic. Practice this ahead of time. If signals don't work, try saying "We were talking about..."

- Limit conversations to one person at a time.

Problems learning and remembering new information: Persons with TBI may have trouble learning and remembering new information and events. They may have difficulty remembering events that happened several weeks or months before the injury (although this often comes back over time). Persons with TBI are usually able to remember events that happened long ago. They may have problems remembering entire events or conversations. Therefore, the mind tries to "fill in the gaps" of missing information and recalls things that did not actually happen. Sometimes bits and pieces from several situations are remembered as one event. These false memories are not lies.

What can be done to improve memory problems?

- Put together a structured routine of daily tasks and activities.

- Be organized and have a set location for keeping things.

- Learn to use memory aids such as memory notebooks, calendars, daily schedules, daily task lists, computer reminder programs and cue cards.

- Devote time and attention to review and practice new information often.

- Be well rested and try to reduce anxiety as much as possible.

- Speak with your doctor about how medications may affect your memory.

Planning and organization problems: Persons with TBI may have difficulty planning their day and scheduling appointments. They may have trouble with tasks that require multiple steps done in a particular order, such as laundry or cooking.

What can be done to improve planning and organization?

- Make a list of things that need to be done and when. List them in order of what should be done first.

- Break down activities into smaller steps.

- When figuring out what steps you need to do first to complete an activity, think of the end goal and work backwards.

Problems with reasoning, problem solving, and judgment: Individuals with TBI may have difficulty recognizing when there is a problem, which is the first step in problem-solving. They may have trouble analyzing information or changing the way they are thinking (being flexible). When solving problems, they may have difficulty deciding the best solution, or get stuck on one solution and not consider other, better options. They may make quick decisions without thinking about the consequences, or not use the best judgment.

What can be done to improve reasoning and problem-solving?

- A speech therapist or psychologist experienced in cognitive rehabilitation can teach an organized approach for daily problem-solving.

- Work through a step-by-step problem-solving strategy in writing: define the problem; brainstorm possible solutions; list the pros and cons of each solution; pick a solution to try; evaluate the success of the solution; and try another solution if the first one doesn't work.

Inappropriate, embarrassing, or impulsive behavior: Individuals with brain injuries may lack self-control and self-awareness, and as a result they may behave inappropriately or impulsively (without thinking it through) in social situations. They may deny they have cognitive problems, even if these are obvious to others. They may say hurtful or insensitive things, act out of place, or behave in inconsiderate ways. They may lack awareness of social boundaries and others' feelings, such as being too personal with people they don't know well or not realizing when they have made someone uncomfortable.

Impulsive and socially inappropriate behavior results from decreased reasoning abilities and lack of control. The injured person may not reason that "If I say or do this, something bad is going to happen." Self-awareness requires complex thinking skills that are often weakened after brain injury.

Things family members can do:

- Think ahead about situations that might bring about poor judgment.

346

- Give realistic, supportive feedback as you observe inappropriate behavior.

- Provide clear expectations for desirable behavior before events.

- Plan and rehearse social interactions so they will be predictable and consistent.

- Establish verbal and non-verbal cues to signal the person to "stop and think." For example, you could hold up your hand to signal "stop," shake your head "no," or say a special word you have both agreed on. Practice this ahead of time.

- If undesired behavior occurs, stop whatever activity you are doing. For example, if you are at the mall, return home immediately.

Cognitive outcome, recovery, and rehabilitation: Cognition is usually evaluated by a neuro-psychologist. Since there are many factors that can affect how someone will improve cognitively, it is very difficult to predict how much someone will recover. With practice, cognitive problems usually improve to some degree.

Cognitive rehabilitation is therapy to improve cognitive skills and has two main approaches, remediation and compensation. Remediation focuses on improving skills that have been lost or impaired. Compensation helps you learn to use different ways to achieve a goal.

Discuss your concerns with your physician or treatment provider: You should discuss any questions or concerns you have with a physiatrist (rehabilitation specialist) or the rehabilitation team. It is important to mention new problems as they develop. New problems could be the result of medication or require further evaluation.

Emotional Problems after Traumatic Brain Injury

Brain injury and emotions: A brain injury can change the way people feel or express emotions. An individual with TBI can have several types of emotional problems.

Difficulty controlling emotions or mood swings: Some people may experience emotions very quickly and intensely but with very little lasting effect. For example, they may get angry easily but get over it quickly. Or they may seem to be on an emotional roller coaster in which they are happy one moment, sad the next and then angry. This is called emotional lability.

347

What causes this problem?

Mood swings and emotional lability are often caused by damage to the part of the brain that controls emotions and behavior. Often there is no specific event that triggers a sudden emotional response. This may be confusing for family members who may think they accidentally did something that upset the injured person. In some cases the brain injury can cause sudden episodes of crying or laughing. These emotional expressions or outbursts may not have any relationship to the way the persons feels (in other words, they may cry without feeling sad or laugh without feeling happy). In some cases the emotional expression may not match the situation (such as laughing at a sad story). Usually the person cannot control these expressions of emotion.

What can be done about it?

Fortunately, this situation often improves in the first few months after injury, and people often return to a more normal emotional balance and expression. If you are having problems controlling your emotions, it is important to talk to a physician or psychologist to find out the cause and get help with treatment. Counseling for the family can be reassuring and allow them to cope better on a daily basis. Several medications may help improve or stabilize mood. You should consult a physician familiar with the emotional problems caused by brain injury.

What family members and others can do:

- Remain calm if an emotional outburst occurs, and avoid reacting emotionally yourself.

- Take the person to a quiet area to help him or her calm down and regain control.

- Acknowledge feelings and give the person a chance to talk about feelings.

- Provide feedback gently and supportively after the person gains control.

- Gently redirect attention to a different topic or activity.

Anxiety: Anxiety is a feeling of fear or nervousness that is out of proportion to the situation. People with brain injury may feel anxious without exactly knowing why. Or they may worry and become anxious about making too many mistakes, or failing at a task, or if they feel they are being criticized. Many situations can be harder to handle after brain injury and cause anxiety, such as being in crowds, being rushed, or adjusting to sudden changes in plan.

Some people may have sudden onset of anxiety that can be overwhelming (panic attacks). Anxiety may be related to a very stressful situation—sometimes the situation that caused the injury—that gets replayed in the person's mind over and over and interferes with sleep (post-traumatic stress disorder). Since each form of anxiety calls for a different treatment, anxiety should always be diagnosed by a mental health professional or physician.

What causes anxiety after TBI?

Difficulty reasoning and concentrating can make it hard for the person with TBI to solve problems. This can make the person feel overwhelmed, especially if he or she is being asked to make decisions. Anxiety often happens when there are too many demands on the injured person, such as returning to employment too soon after injury. Time pressure can also heighten anxiety. Situations that require a lot of attention and information processing can make people with TBI anxious. Examples of such situations might be crowded environments, heavy traffic, or noisy children.

What can be done about anxiety?

- Try to reduce the environmental demands and unnecessary stresses that may be causing anxiety.

- Provide reassurance to help calm the person and allow them to reduce their feelings of anxiety when they occur.

- Add structured activities into the daily routine, such as exercising, volunteering, church activities, or self-help groups.

- Anxiety can be helped by certain medications, by psychotherapy (counseling) from a mental health professional who is familiar with TBI, or a combination of medications and counseling.

Depression: Feeling sad is a normal response to the losses and changes a person faces after TBI. Feelings of sadness, frustration, and loss are common after brain injury. These feelings often appear during the later stages of recovery, after the individual has become more aware of the long-term situation. If these feelings become overwhelming or interfere with recovery, the person may be suffering from depression.

Symptoms of depression include feeling sad or worthless, changes in sleep or appetite, difficulty concentrating, withdrawing from others, loss of interest or pleasure in life, lethargy (feeling tired and sluggish), or thoughts of death or suicide. Because signs of depression are also symptoms of a brain injury itself, having these symptoms doesn't necessarily mean the injured person is depressed. The problems are more likely to mean depression if they show up a few months after the injury rather than soon after it.

What causes depression?

Depression can arise as the person struggles to adjust to temporary or lasting disability and loss or to changes in one's roles in the family and society caused by the brain injury. Depression may also occur if the injury has affected areas of the brain that control emotions. Both biochemical and physical changes in the brain can cause depression.

What can be done about depression?

- Anti-depressant medications, psychotherapy (counseling) from a mental health professional who is familiar with TBI, or a combination of the two, can help most people who have depression.

- Aerobic exercise and structured activities during each day can sometimes help reduce depression.

- Depression is not a sign of weakness, and it is not anyone's fault. Depression is an illness. A person cannot get over depression by simply wishing it away, using more willpower, or toughening up.

- It is best to get treatment early to prevent needless suffering. Don't wait.

Temper outbursts and irritability: Family members of individuals with TBI often describe the injured person as having a short fuse, flying off the handle easily, being irritable or having a quick temper. Studies show that up to 71% of people with TBI are frequently irritable. The injured person may yell, use bad language, throw objects, slam fists into things, slam doors, or threaten or hurt family members or others.

Temper outbursts after TBI are likely caused by several factors, including: injury to the parts of the brain that control emotional expression; frustration and dissatisfaction with the changes in life brought on by the injury, such as loss of one's job and independence; feeling isolated, depressed, or misunderstood; difficulty concentrating, remembering, expressing oneself, or following conversations, all of which can lead to frustration; tiring easily; or pain.

What can be done about temper problems?

Reducing stress and decreasing irritating situations can remove some of the triggers for temper outbursts and irritability. People with brain injury can learn some basic anger management skills such as self-calming strategies, relaxation, and better communication methods. A psychologist or other mental health professional familiar with TBI can help. Certain medications can be prescribed to help control temper outbursts.

Family members can help by changing the way they react to the temper outbursts:

- Understand that being irritable and getting angry easily is due to the brain injury. Try not to take it personally.

- Do not try to argue with the injured person during an outburst. Instead, let him or her cool down for a few minutes first.

- Do not try to calm the person down by giving in to his or her demands.

- Set some rules for communication. Let the injured person know that it is not acceptable to yell at, threaten, or hurt others. Refuse to talk to the injured person when he or she is yelling or throwing a temper tantrum.

- After the outburst is over, talk about what might have led to the outburst. Encourage the injured person to discuss the problem in a calm way. Suggest other outlets, such as leaving the room and taking a walk (after letting others know when he or she will return) when the person feels anger coming on.

Questions to ask your physician or treatment provider to better understand your problem: If you or your family members are experiencing anxiety, feelings of sadness or depression, irritability or mood swings, consider asking your doctor:

- Would psychological counseling be helpful?

- Would an evaluation by a psychiatrist be helpful?

- Are there medications that can help?

351

More about medications: If you or your family member tries a medication for one of these problems, it is very important to work closely with the physician or other health care provider who prescribes them. Always make a follow-up appointment to let him or her know how the medication is working, and report any unusual reactions between appointments. Remember:

- There can be a delay until the beneficial effects of medications are felt.

- Doses might need to be adjusted by your doctor for maximum benefit.

- You may need to try one or more different medications to find the one that works best for you.

- Except in an emergency, you should not stop taking a prescribed medication without consulting your doctor.

Peer and other support: Remember, too, that not all help comes from professionals. You may benefit from the following:

- A brain injury support group—some are specialized for the person with TBI, others are for family members, and others are open to everyone affected by brain injury.

- Peer mentoring, in which a person who has coped with brain injury for a long time gives support and suggestions to someone who is struggling with similar problems.

- Check with your local Brain Injury Association chapter to find out more about these resources. Visit http://www.biausa.org online to find brain injury resources near you.

- Talk to a friend, family member, member of the clergy, or someone else who is a good listener.

Fatigue

What is fatigue?

Fatigue is a feeling of exhaustion, tiredness, weariness, or lack of energy. After TBI, you may have more than one kind of fatigue:

1. Physical fatigue: "I'm tired and I need to rest. I'm dragging today."

2. Psychological fatigue: "I just can't get motivated to do anything. Being depressed wears me out; I just don't feel like doing anything."

3. Mental fatigue: "After a while, I just can't concentrate anymore. It's hard to stay focused. My mind goes blank."

Why is fatigue important?

When you are fatigued, you are less able to think clearly or do physical activities. If you are overwhelmed by fatigue, you have less energy to care for yourself or do things you enjoy. Fatigue can have a negative effect on your mood, physical functioning, attention, concentration, memory, and communication. It can interfere with your ability to work or enjoy leisure activities. It can make activities such as driving dangerous.

Fatigue is one of the most common problems people have after a traumatic brain injury. As many as 70% of survivors of TBI complain of mental fatigue.

What causes fatigue?

Fatigue is normal for anyone after hard work or a long day. In persons with TBI, fatigue often occurs more quickly and frequently than it does in the general population. The cause of fatigue after TBI is not clear but may be due to the extra effort and attention it takes to do even simple activities such as walking or talking clearly. Brain function may be less efficient than before the injury.

Physical fatigue can come from muscle weakness. The body needs to work harder to do things that were easy before the TBI. Physical fatigue gets worse in the evening and is better after a good night's sleep. Often this kind of fatigue will lessen as the individual gets stronger, more active, and back to his or her old life.

Psychological fatigue is associated with depression, anxiety, and other psychological conditions. This type of fatigue gets worse with stress. Sleep may not help at all, and the fatigue is often at its worst when you wake up in the morning.

Mental fatigue comes from the extra effort it takes to think after your brain is injured. Many common tasks take much more concentration than they did before. Working harder to think and stay focused can make you mentally tired.

Certain conditions are known to cause or increase fatigue including: depression, sleep problems such as sleep apnea, seasonal allergies, hypothyroidism or other endocrine gland disorders, respiratory or cardiac problems, headaches, lack of physical exercise, vitamin deficiency or poor nutrition, stress, low red blood cell counts (anemia), and medications commonly used after TBI such as muscle relaxers and pain medication.

What can be done to decrease fatigue?

Pay attention to what triggers your fatigue, and learn to identify the early signs of fatigue, such as becoming more irritable or distracted. Stop an activity before getting tired.

Get more sleep and rest: If you have insomnia, tell your doctor. There may be a medical condition causing this, or there may be useful treatments.

Set a regular schedule of going to bed and awakening the same time every day—your body and mind will be more efficient. Include some regular rest breaks or naps. Be careful to limit naps to 30 minutes and avoid evening naps.

Alcohol and marijuana will generally make fatigue worse.

Caffeine (coffee, cola products) should be avoided after lunch if sleeping is a problem.

Resume activities gradually, over weeks or even months.

Start with familiar tasks at home or work that you can complete without fatigue. Gradually increase the complexity of each task, taking breaks as needed.

Improve your time management:
- Plan and follow a daily schedule. Using a calendar or planner can help manage mental fatigue.
- Prioritize activities. Finish what is most important first.
- Do things that require the most physical or mental effort earlier in the day, when you are fresher.
- Avoid over-scheduling.
- If visitors make you tired, limit time with them.

Exercise daily: Research has shown that people with TBI who exercise have better mental function and alertness. Over time, exercise and being more active helps lessen physical and mental fatigue and builds stamina. It also may decrease depression and improve sleep.

Talk to your doctor:

- Discuss medical or physical problems that may be causing fatigue.

- Have your doctor review all your current medications.

- Tell your doctor if you think you might be depressed so treatment can be started.

- Ask your doctor if there are any blood tests that could help to find out what is causing your fatigue.

Section 31.4

TBI Often Causes Sleep Problems

"Sleep and Traumatic Brain Injury," Copyright © 2009 Model Systems Knowledge Translation System (MSKTC). This publication was produced by the TBI Model Systems in collaboration with the Model Systems Knowledge Translation Center (http://msktc.washington.edu) with funding from the National Institute on Disability and Rehabilitation Research in the U.S. Department of Education, Grant no. H133A060070.

Many people who have brain injuries suffer from sleep disturbances. Not sleeping well can increase or worsen depression, anxiety, fatigue, irritability, and one's sense of well-being. It can also lead to poor work performance and traffic or workplace accidents. A review of sleep disorder studies and surveys suggest that sleep disorders are three times more common in TBI patients than in the general population and that nearly 60% of people with TBI experience long-term difficulties with sleep. Women were more likely to be affected than men. Sleep problems are more likely to develop as the person ages.

Sleep disturbances have been found in people with all severities of brain injuries from mild to severe. Sleep is a complex process that involves many parts of the brain. For this reason, and depending on the location and extent of injury, many different kinds of sleep disturbances can occur after brain injury.

Common sleep disorders:

- Insomnia: Difficulty with falling asleep or staying asleep, or sleep that does not make you feel rested. Insomnia can worsen other problems resulting from brain injury, including behavioral and cognitive (thinking) difficulties. Insomnia makes it harder to learn new things. Insomnia is typically worse directly after injury and often improves as time passes.

- Excessive daytime sleepiness: Extreme drowsiness.

- Delayed sleep phase syndrome: Mixed-up sleep patterns.

- Narcolepsy: Falling asleep suddenly and uncontrollably during the day.

Common sleep syndromes:

- Restless leg syndrome (RLS): Urge to move the legs because they feel uncomfortable, especially at night or when lying down.

- Bruxism: Grinding or clenching teeth.

- Sleep apnea: Brief pauses in breathing during sleep, resulting in reduced oxygen flow to the brain and causing loud snoring and frequent awakening.

- Periodic limb movement disorder (PLMD): Involuntary movement of legs and arms during sleep.

- Sleepwalking: Walking or performing other activities while sleeping and not being aware of it.

What causes sleep problems?

Physical and chemical changes: The internal clock in the brain controls when people sleep and wake every day. If injured, the brain may not be able to tell the body to fall asleep or wake up. There are chemicals in our body that help us to sleep. An injury can change the way that these chemicals affect the body. If brain mechanisms for starting and stopping sleep are injured, a condition called post-traumatic hypersomnia may result in which a person sleeps many hours more than normal.

Changes in breathing control: Sometimes the brain's ability to control breathing during sleep becomes altered after a TBI, resulting in periods of apnea (when breathing actually stops for long enough for blood oxygen levels to drop). This is called sleep apnea. Other factors may affect the chance of having sleep apnea such as family history or being overweight.

Medications: Medications taken after a brain injury may cause problems going to sleep or staying asleep, or can make people sleepy during the day and unable to participate in activities.

- Prescription drugs for treating asthma and depression may cause insomnia. Also, stimulants that are meant to treat daytime sleepiness can cause insomnia if taken too close to bedtime. These problems can often be avoided by adjusting the timing of the medication or by substituting a different drug, of course, in consultation with your physician. Many other medications can cause sedation (sleepiness), as well.

- Most over-the-counter sleep aid medications contain an antihistamine (commonly diphenhydramine) and are not recommended for people with TBI because they may cause disturbances in memory and new learning. Retention of urine, dry mouth, nighttime falls, and constipation are also possible side effects of this class of medications.

Daytime sleeping (napping) and physical inactivity: Napping during the day is likely to disturb sleep at night. Inactivity or lack of exercise can also worsen sleep.

Pain: Many people who have suffered brain injuries also experience pain in other parts of the body. This discomfort may disturb sleep. Medications taken to relieve pain may also affect sleep.

Depression: Depression is much more common in persons with traumatic brain injury than in the general population. Sleep problems such as difficulty falling asleep and early morning waking are common symptoms of depression.

Alcohol: While alcohol may help bring on sleep, drinking alcohol before bedtime is likely to interfere with normal sleep rather than improve it.

Caffeine and nicotine: Nicotine from tobacco may cause sleep disturbances and is often overlooked. Caffeine can disturb sleep when consumed in the afternoon or evening.

What can be done to improve sleep?

Changes in behavior and environment are the first line to treating sleep difficulties.

Daytime Suggestions

- Set an alarm to try to wake up at the same time every day.

- Include meaningful activities in your daily schedule.

- Get off the couch and limit television (TV) watching.

- Exercise every day. People with TBI who exercise regularly report fewer sleep problems.

- Try to get outdoors for some sunlight during the daytime. If you live in an area with less sun in the wintertime, consider trying light box therapy.

- Don't nap more than 20 minutes during the day.

Nighttime Suggestions

- Try to go to bed at the same time every night and set your alarm for the next day.

- Follow a bedtime routine. For example, put out your clothes for morning, brush your teeth, and then read or listen to relaxing music for ten minutes before turning out the light.

- Avoid caffeine, nicotine, alcohol, and sugar for five hours before bedtime.

- Avoid eating prior to sleep to allow time to digest, but also do not go to bed hungry, as this can also wake you from sleep.

- Do not exercise within two hours of bedtime, but stretching or meditation may help with sleep.

- Do not eat, read, or watch TV while in bed.

- Keep stress out of the bedroom. For example, do not work or pay bills there.

- Create a restful atmosphere in the bedroom, protected from distractions, noise, extreme temperatures, and light.

- If you don't fall asleep in 30 minutes, get out of bed and do something relaxing or boring until you feel sleepy.

Talk to your doctor: If your sleep problems persist, talk to your doctor to explore safe and effective solutions. Evaluation of sleep problems should include a thorough history of such problems, medication review, an assessment of your bedtime routines, and a comprehensive medical evaluation. Before recommending any action, your physician will explore with you a variety of possible causes for your sleep problems, including pain or depression. If necessary, he or she may recommend a polysomnographic evaluation (also known as a sleep lab). Based on your symptoms, medical history, and specific needs, your doctor will be able to make a personalized treatment plan to help you achieve restful sleep.

Treatment Options

Non-pharmacological therapies:

* If mood or emotional issues such as anxiety or depression are causing sleep difficulties, psychotherapy (counseling) may be an appropriate treatment.

* Sleep restriction may improve sleeping patterns by restricting the number of hours spent in bed to the actual number of hours slept.

* For those with anxiety, relaxation therapy can help create a restful environment both in your bedroom and in your body and mind.

* Use of special bright lights (phototherapy) has been shown in studies to help promote sleep. When exposed to these lights at strategic times in the day, you may be able to sleep more at night. However, consult with your doctor first, as these bright lights can cause eyestrain and headaches.

Medications: Ask your doctor about medications that can help you sleep through the night or keep you awake during the day. Special care is necessary when choosing a medication in order to avoid daytime sedation or worsening of cognitive and behavior problems.

Natural remedies: Some consumers have found herbal teas, melatonin, and valerian useful for sleep problems, and these are sold in health food and drug stores with no prescription needed. However, these remedies have multiple drug interactions, and you should tell your doctor if you are using them.

Section 31.5

TBI Can Affect Ability to Drive

"Driving after Traumatic Brain Injury," Copyright © 2009 Model Systems Knowledge Translation System (MSKTC). This publication was produced by the TBI Model Systems in collaboration with the Model Systems Knowledge Translation Center (http://msktc.washington.edu) with funding from the National Institute on Disability and Rehabilitation Research in the U.S. Department of Education, Grant no. H133A060070.

Driving is an important part of a person's independent lifestyle and integration into the community. Because we take our driving skills for granted, it is easy to forget that driving is the most dangerous thing we do in our everyday lives. A brain injury can affect the skills needed to drive safely. If and when an injured person may safely return to driving should be addressed early in recovery. The injured person, family members, and health professionals should all be included in this important decision. If anyone has concerns that that driving may put the injured person or others in danger, health professionals may recommend pre-driving testing.

A brain injury can disrupt and slow down skills that are essential for good driving, such as:

- ability to maintain a constant position in a lane;

- having accurate vision;

- maintaining concentration over long periods of time;

- memory functioning, such as recalling directions;

- figuring out solutions to problems;

- hand-eye coordination;

- reaction time; and

- safety awareness and judgment.

Studies indicate that even mild thinking difficulties, which may not be recognized by the injured person, may add to increased risks while driving.

Warning signs of unsafe driving:

- Driving too fast or slow

- Not observing signs or signals

- Judging distance inaccurately when stopping or turning

- Slow to make decisions

- Becoming easily frustrated or confused

- Having accidents or near misses

- Drifting across lane markings into other lanes

- Getting lost easily, even in familiar areas

How often do individuals with TBI return to driving?

Between 40–60% of people with moderate to severe brain injuries return to driving after their injury. To lessen the risk of crashes, people with TBI may place limitations on their driving habits. They may drive less frequently than they did before the injury or drive only at certain times (such as during daylight), on familiar routes, or when there is less traffic. Having experienced a seizure after the TBI may be a barrier to driving. States often require that a person be free of seizures for a period of time, such as six months, before resuming driving. People who want to return to driving need to check with the laws in their state.

Driving evaluations and training: A driving evaluation is a crucial step in determining a person's ability to drive following recovery from a TBI. Research studies indicate that most TBI survivors are not thoroughly evaluated for driving skills before they begin driving after the injury, and this may put TBI survivors at risk for a crash.

While there is no standardized assessment test or process, a typical driving evaluation has two parts:

- Preliminary evaluation: A review of cognitive (thinking) abilities, including reaction time, judgment, reasoning, and visual spatial skills. Recommendations regarding the need for adaptive equipment and additional skills training are based on the results of the evaluation.

- On-the-road evaluation: A test of the mechanical operation of a vehicle, either using a driving simulator or driving a vehicle on the roadway in the presence of the evaluator. This evaluation is used to assess safe driving skills in various traffic environments, as well as basic driving skills while a client uses the appropriate adaptive driving equipment.

Current research indicates that many individuals with TBI can become competent, safe drivers when given the proper training. Training serves to improve specific driving skills. Sometimes this involves practicing driving under the supervision of a driving evaluator. In some cases, a training program might focus on specific skills such as rapid understanding of visual information. Evaluations and training are often provided by professionals certified through the Association for Driver Rehabilitation (ADED). A list of certified professionals may be found on the ADED website, http://www.driver-ed.org.

Vehicle modifications: If an individual with TBI has physical disabilities but has well-preserved cognitive functions, the individual may be able to resume driving with adaptive equipment or other modifications to the vehicle. Recommendations for adaptive equipment and modifications could include hand-controlled gas and brake systems, spinner knobs for steering, left foot accelerator, or lifts for entering and exiting the vehicle.

Legal and insurance considerations: A person who wishes to resume driving must have a valid driver's license. In some states, there must be a formal evaluation performed by a licensing bureau before resuming driving after a brain injury. Insurance may also be required. The person should check local regulations relating to licenses and insurance.

Other transportation options: Accessible and reliable transportation is the most critical part of community integration following a TBI. If a person is not able to drive, there may be other options for transportation. Family members can provide transportation, and public transportation such as buses can be used. Some communities provide public transportation specifically for disabled riders.

Should you be driving?

1. Discuss your ability to drive with your doctor and/or health professionals and family members.

2. Get a professional evaluation to determine your driving ability.

3. Based on your evaluation you may be allowed to drive, need training or vehicle modification before returning to driving, or will need to use other transportation options.

Section 31.6

Employment after TBI

This section is excerpted from "Frequently Asked Questions about Trau-
matic Brain Injury (TBI) and Employment," and "Tips for Communicating
with People with Traumatic Brain Injury (TBI) and Post-Traumatic Stress
Disorder (PTSD)," U. S. Department of Labor: America's Heroes at Work,
2008. Figure 31.5 is excerpted from "Traumatic Brain Injury Model Systems
National Database Update, 2009," a publication of the Traumatic Brain
Injury Model Systems National Data and Statistical Center, Englewood,
CO, © 2009. Reprinted with permission.

Are traumatic brain injuries (TBI) disabilities under the Americans with Disabilities Act (ADA)?

The ADA has a general definition of disability that each person
must meet. Therefore, some people with TBI will meet the criteria for
having a disability under the ADA and some will not. A person has a
disability if he or she has a physical or mental impairment that substantially limits one or more major life activities, a record of such an
impairment, or is regarded as having such an impairment. Information
about how to determine whether a person has a disability under the
ADA is available at www.eeoc.gov/policy/docs/902cm.html.

Are employees (or applicants) with TBI required to disclose their disability to their employers?

No. Employees need only disclose their disability if or when they
need an accommodation to perform the essential functions of the job.
Applicants never have to disclose a disability on a job application, or in
the job interview, unless they need an accommodation to assist them
in the application or interview process.

Can an employer ask an employee with TBI to submit to a medical examination?

Yes, if the need for the medical examination is job-related, consistent with business necessity, and conducted after an offer has been
made. People with brain injuries (or any disability) do not have to

submit to a medical exam or answer any medical questions until after they have been conditionally offered a job.

Why does employment play such an important role in the recovery of individuals with TBI?

Employment enables many people with disabilities, including those with TBI, to fully participate in society. For example, employment provides income that is key to individual and family economic health and general well-being, and builds skills for the future. It also provides greater social interaction and connections that can reduce isolation and build social capital. Finally, employment provides a valued social role in our society and helps create a sense of personal efficacy and social integration that contributes to greater life satisfaction. According to the National Council on Disability, people who regain employment following the onset of an injury or a disability report higher life satisfaction and better adjustment than do people who are not employed. For these reasons, gainful employment can be one important component in the recovery and rehabilitation of individuals with TBI.

What challenges might people with TBI encounter in the workplace?

Although recovery from mild brain injuries (concussions) is generally uncomplicated and complete, some individuals continue to experience

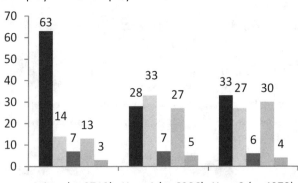

Figure 31.5. *Occupational Status (Source: Traumatic Brain Injury Model Systems National Data and Statistical Center, Englewood, CO, © 2009. Reprinted with permission.)*

cognitive or mood difficulties. Most workplace difficulties associated with TBI are related to attention span, short-term memory, and organization. For some, headaches and mental fatigue may persist.

What sorts of jobs are well-suited for people with TBI?

Because the effects of TBI vary widely, there are no occupations that any particular person with TBI is disqualified from pursuing. However, certain characteristics provide the greatest potential for workplace achievement and success including regular daily schedules, routine tasks, low levels of distracting noise and light, regular breaks, and access to memory aids (such as voice recorders and task checklists).

How can employers help people with TBI do their jobs more effectively?

Though the time period needed for workplace accommodations can often be short, a variety of promising practices can help people with TBI succeed in the workplace. These include the following:

- Schedule-reminders (telephone, pagers, alarm clocks)
- Scheduled rest breaks to prevent stimulus overload and fatigue
- Work task checklists and clipboards
- Tape recorders as memory aids
- Stop watches for time management
- Job coaches who make frequent, scheduled site visits
- Supportive phone calls after work
- Role playing exercises related to the job
- Periodic evaluation forms completed by supervisors or job coaches
- Job-site accommodations including adaptive technology
- Job sharing with another employee
- Mentoring by a co-worker or retired worker
- Setting reasonable expectations for task completion
- Limiting multi-tasking

- Scheduling more difficult or challenging tasks at the beginning of the work shift to account for fatigue

- Recognizing accomplishments through positive reinforcement

Note: Those with mild TBI generally do not need all of these adjustments or accommodations.

Tips for Communicating with People with Traumatic Brain Injury (TBI)

Not everyone has experience communicating with people with disabilities. However, it should not be intimidating. Appropriate etiquette when interacting with people with disabilities is based primarily on respect and courtesy.

General tips for communicating with people with disabilities:

- When introduced to a person with a disability, it is appropriate to offer to shake hands. People with limited hand use or who wear an artificial limb can usually shake hands. (Shaking hands with the left hand is an acceptable greeting.)

- If you offer assistance to the person, wait until the offer is accepted. Then listen to or ask for instructions.

- Treat adults as adults. Address people who have disabilities by their first names only when extending the same familiarity to all others.

- Don't be afraid to ask questions when you're unsure of what to do.

Tips for communicating with people with TBI:

- Some people with TBI may have trouble concentrating or organizing their thoughts. If you are in a public area with many distractions, consider moving to a quiet or private location, and try focusing on short-term goals.

- Be prepared to repeat what you say, orally or in writing. Some people with TBI may have short-term memory deficits.

- If you are not sure whether the person understands you, offer assistance completing forms or understanding written instructions and provide extra time for decision-making. Wait for the individual to accept the offer of assistance; do not over-assist or be patronizing.

• Be patient, flexible, and supportive. Take time to understand the individual, make sure the individual understands you, and avoid interrupting the person.

Section 31.7

Outcomes of TBI

This section includes excerpts from "Trial Compares Methods for Brain Injury Rehab," *VA Research Currents*, January 2009, U.S. Department of Veterans Affairs; and excerpts from "Victimization of Persons with Traumatic Brain Injury or Other Disabilities," Centers for Disease Control and Prevention (CDC), February 1, 2007.

Trial Compares Methods for Brain Injury Rehabilitation

Researchers from the Defense and Veterans Brain Injury Center (DVBIC) have published the results of one of the first studies of its kind: a randomized clinical trial comparing different treatment approaches for those with traumatic brain injury (TBI). The study appeared in the December 2008 issue of the *Archives of Physical Medicine and Rehabilitation*. It compared two rehabilitation approaches: cognitive didactic versus functional-experiential.

While the findings suggest pluses to both methods, the cognitive approach resulted in better short-term gains in mental function and was more effective in helping younger patients return to work or school. The functional method led to higher rates of independent living among older patients. Both methods had been validated in prior research but had never been tested head-to-head.

Long-term gains from both approaches: "Our results show long-term functional improvements in both groups," said lead author Rodney Vanderploeg, PhD, a research psychologist at the Tampa VA Medical Center and University of South Florida. At one year after treatment, he said, about six in ten study participants overall were employed and living independently. "This is remarkable," wrote Vanderploeg and colleagues, "given that none were capable of work or independent living at baseline" and 90% had brain injuries that were considered severe.

The study included 360 veterans or active duty troops, mostly men, with moderate to severe TBI. Enrollment for the study ran from 1996 to May 2003, shortly after the onset of the war in Iraq. As such, most of the participants sustained their injuries not in combat but in vehicle crashes, falls, or other incidents.

Younger patients fare better with cognitive method: Over a month or two, each group received about two hours per day of therapy specific to their study arm. For example, the cognitive group worked on paper-and-pencil or computerized tests that became progressively more difficult, with the explicit goal of sharpening their mental skills. The functional group, on the other hand, received extra help going through the physical motions of everyday activities such as dining and grooming.

Each group also received additional physical, occupational, and speech therapy in which the therapists used either a cognitive or functional approach. In the cognitive group, therapists offered more verbal instruction and encouraged learning through trial and error. They asked questions such as "How do you think you did?" or "What do you need to do now?" to promote thinking and self awareness. In the functional group, therapists did less verbal teaching and emphasized "learning by doing." They offered more hands-on, step-by-step support to help patients successfully complete tasks. The aim was to ingrain the physical movements and thereby promote implicit learning.

Results

The researchers tested participants' cognitive abilities and everyday functioning before and after treatment and one year later. Among the findings:

Overall function was similar between the two groups after one year: For example, in the cognitive study arm, 65 out of 167 participants (38%) were working or in school. In the functional group, the rate was 68 out of 164 (35.4%). The difference was not statistically significant. (Follow-up data were not available on all 360 study participants.)

Immediate post-treatment cognitive function was better in the cognitive group: This was measured with tests in areas such as comprehension, expression, social interaction, problem solving and memory. Cognitive-arm participants also reported fewer memory problems after one year.

Younger patients (those age 30 or under) in the cognitive arm had a higher rate of return to work or school than their age peers in the functional arm. On the other hand, older patients and those with more years of education in the functional arm were more likely to be living independently at one year than similar participants in the cognitive group.

The study authors offered a tentative analysis of why younger and older patients may have benefited differently from the two approaches: "…These findings suggest that the cognitive treatment not only better enhances cognitive recovery but also lays a stronger foundation for the development of work-related cognitive skills. This effect appears to be most prominent in younger patients, who may benefit more from the higher level of structure and teaching provided in the cognitive approach to treatment. The functional approach generally provided less structure and did not offer problem-solving strategies and approaches. Older or more educated persons, who may already have internalized structure and independence, seemed to benefit more from the direct living skills emphasized in the functional interventions."

Victimization of Persons with Traumatic Brain Injury or Other Disabilities

Victimization is harm caused on purpose. It is not an accident and can happen anywhere. While anyone can be victimized, people with disabilities are at greater risk for victimization than people without disabilities. This information provides a general overview of victimization and the risks to people with traumatic brain injury (TBI) and other disabilities.

Victimization includes:

- physical violence with or without a weapon;

- sexual violence of any kind including rape;

- emotional abuse, including verbal attacks or being humiliated; and

- neglect of personal needs for daily life, including medical care or equipment.

369

In the United States, people with disabilities are four to ten times more likely to be victimized than people without them. Children with disabilities are more than twice as likely to be victimized as children without them.

The two most common places for victimization are in hospitals and at home. Victims usually know the person who harms them. They can be health care workers, intimate partners, or family members. More men than women cause harm to people with disabilities.

Why are people with a TBI at risk for victimization?

A TBI may cause problems that can increase risk. Known problems include difficulty understanding risky situations or avoiding risky persons; difficulty controlling one's temper which causes others to get angry; and behavioral problems, such as drinking too much.

What can be done to help a friend or family member who is being victimized?

* Don't be afraid to voice your concern for their safety.

* Acknowledge that they are in a very difficult and scary situation.

* Be supportive.

* Don't be judgmental.

* Encourage them to talk to people who can provide help and guidance.

* Help them plan safety steps so that they will know what to do and how to reduce their risk of harm when they are being victimized.

* Remember that you cannot rescue them.

Getting Help

National Domestic Violence Hotline
Toll-Free: 800-799-SAFE
Toll-Free TTY: 800-787-3224

This hotline is available 24 hours a day, seven days a week. Confidential services include crisis intervention, safety planning, and referrals to local service providers. Assistance is available in English and Spanish, and in other languages.

Chapter 32

Abusive Head Trauma (Shaken Baby Syndrome)

Abusive head trauma, inflicted traumatic brain injury, or AHT (also called shaken baby, shaken impact syndrome or SBS) is a form of inflicted head trauma. AHT can be caused by direct blows to the head, dropping or throwing a child, or shaking a child. Head trauma is the leading cause of death in child abuse cases in the United States.

How These Injuries Happen

Unlike other forms of inflicted head trauma, abusive head trauma results from injuries caused by someone vigorously shaking a child. Because the anatomy of infants puts them at particular risk for injury from this kind of action, the vast majority of victims are infants younger than one year old. The average age of victims is between three and eight months, although these injuries are occasionally seen in children up to four years old.

The perpetrators in these cases are most often parents or caregivers. Common triggers are frustration or stress when the child is crying. Unfortunately, the shaking may have the desired effect: although at first the baby cries more, he or she may stop crying as the brain is damaged.

Approximately 60% of identified victims of shaking injury are male, and children of families who live at or below the poverty level are at an increased risk for these injuries as well as any type of child abuse. It is estimated that the perpetrators in 65% to 90% of cases are males—usually either the baby's father or the mother's boyfriend, often someone in his early twenties.

When someone forcefully shakes a baby, the child's head rotates about the neck uncontrollably because infants' neck muscles aren't well developed and provide little support for their heads. This violent movement pitches the infant's brain back and forth within the skull, sometimes rupturing blood vessels and nerves throughout the brain and tearing the brain tissue. The brain may strike the inside of the skull, causing bruising and bleeding to the brain.

The damage can be even greater when a shaking episode ends with an impact (hitting a wall or a crib mattress, for example), because the forces of acceleration and deceleration associated with an impact are so strong. After the shaking, swelling in the brain can cause enormous pressure within the skull, compressing blood vessels and increasing overall injury to its delicate structure.

Normal interaction with a child, like bouncing the baby on a knee, will not cause these injuries, although it's important to never shake a baby under any circumstances because gentle shaking can rapidly escalate.

What Are the Effects?

AHT often causes irreversible damage. In the worst cases, children die due to their injuries.

Children who survive may have:

- partial or total blindness,

- hearing loss,

- seizures,

- developmental delays,

- impaired intellect,

- speech and learning difficulties,

- problems with memory and attention,

- severe mental retardation,

- cerebral palsy.

Even in milder cases, in which babies looks normal immediately after the shaking, they may eventually develop one or more of these problems. Sometimes the first sign of a problem isn't noticed until the child enters the school system and exhibits behavioral problems or learning difficulties. But by that time, it's more difficult to link these problems to a shaking incident from several years before.

Signs and Symptoms

In any abusive head trauma case, the duration and force of the shaking, the number of episodes, and whether impact is involved all affect the severity of the infant's injuries. In the most violent cases, children may arrive at the emergency room unconscious, suffering seizures, or in shock. But in many cases, infants may never be brought to medical attention if they don't exhibit such severe symptoms.

In less severe cases, a child who has been shaken may experience:

- lethargy,
- irritability,
- vomiting,
- poor sucking or swallowing,
- decreased appetite,
- lack of smiling or vocalizing,
- rigidity,
- seizures,
- difficulty breathing,
- altered consciousness,
- unequal pupil size,
- an inability to lift the head,
- an inability to focus the eyes or track movement.

Diagnosis

Many cases of AHT are brought in for medical care as silent injuries. In other words, parents or caregivers don't often provide a history that the child has had abusive head trauma or a shaking injury, so doctors don't know to look for subtle or physical signs. This can sometimes result in children having injuries that aren't identified in the medical system.

And again, in many cases, babies who don't have severe symptoms may never be brought to a doctor. Many of the less severe symptoms such as vomiting or irritability may resolve and can have many nonabusive causes.

Unfortunately, unless a doctor has reason to suspect child abuse, mild cases (in which the infant seems lethargic, fussy, or perhaps isn't feeding well) are often misdiagnosed as a viral illness or colic. Without a diagnosis of child abuse and any resulting intervention with the parents or caregivers, these children may be shaken again, worsening any brain injury or damage.

If shaken baby syndrome is suspected, doctors may look for:

- hemorrhages in the retinas of the eyes;

- skull fractures;

- swelling of the brain;

- subdural hematomas (blood collections pressing on the surface of the brain);

- rib and long bone (bones in the arms and legs) fractures;

- bruises around the head, neck, or chest.

The Child's Development and Education

What makes AHT so devastating is that it often involves a total brain injury. For example, a child whose vision is severely impaired won't be able to learn through observation, which decreases the child's overall ability to learn.

The development of language, vision, balance, and motor coordination, all of which occur to varying degrees after birth, are particularly likely to be affected in any child who has AHT. Such impairment can require rigorous physical and occupational therapy to help the child acquire skills that would have developed on their own had the brain injury not occurred. As they get older, kids who were shaken as babies may require special education and continued therapy to help with language development and daily living skills, such as dressing themselves.

Before age three, a child can receive speech or physical therapy through the Department of Public Health early intervention services. Federal law requires that each state provide these services for children who have developmental disabilities as a result of being abused. Some schools are also increasingly providing information and developmental assessments for kids under the age of three. Parents can turn to a variety of rehabilitation and other therapists for early intervention services for children after abusive head trauma. Developmental assessments can assist in improving education outcomes as well as the overall well-being of the child. After a child who's been diagnosed with abusive head trauma turns three, it's the school district's responsibility to provide additional special educational services.

Preventing AHT

Abusive head trauma is 100% preventable. A key aspect of prevention is increasing awareness of the potential dangers of shaking. Finding ways to alleviate the parent or caregiver's stress at the critical moments when a baby is crying can significantly reduce the risk to the child. Some hospital-based programs have helped new parents identify and prevent shaking injuries and understand how to respond when infants cry.

The National Center on Shaken Baby Syndrome offers a prevention program, the Period of Purple Crying, which seeks to help parents and other caregivers understand crying in normal infants. By defining and describing the sometimes inconsolable infant crying that can sometimes cause stress, anger, and frustration in parents and caregivers, the program hopes to educate and empower people to prevent AHT.

One method that may help is author Dr. Harvey Karp's *Five S's*:

1. Shushing (using white noise or rhythmic sounds that mimic the constant whir of noise in the womb, with things like vacuum cleaners, hair dryers, clothes dryers, a running tub, or a white noise compact disk [CD]).

2. Side or stomach positioning (placing the baby on the left side— to help digestion—or on the belly while holding him or her, then putting the sleeping baby in the crib or bassinet on his or her back).

3. Sucking (letting the baby breastfeed or bottle-feed, or giving the baby a pacifier or finger to suck on).

4. Swaddling (wrapping the baby up snugly in a blanket to help him or her feel more secure).

5. Swinging gently (rocking in a chair, using an infant swing, or taking a car ride to help duplicate the constant motion the baby felt in the womb).

If a baby in your care won't stop crying, you can also try the following:

- Make sure the baby's basic needs are met (for example, he or she isn't hungry and doesn't need to be changed).

- Check for signs of illness, like fever or swollen gums.

- Rock or walk with the baby.

- Sing or talk to the baby.

- Offer the baby a pacifier or a noisy toy.

- Take the baby for a ride in a stroller or strapped into a child safety seat in the car.

- Hold the baby close against your body and breathe calmly and slowly.

- Call a friend or relative for support or to take care of the baby while you take a break.

- If nothing else works, put the baby on his or her back in the crib, close the door, and check on the baby in ten minutes.

- Call your doctor if nothing seems to be helping your infant, in case there is a medical reason for the fussiness.

To prevent potential AHT, parents and caregivers of infants need to learn how to respond to their own stress. It's important to talk to anyone caring for your baby about the dangers of shaking and how it can be prevented.

Chapter 33

Brain Aneurysm

A cerebral aneurysm (also known as an intracranial or intracerebral aneurysm) is a weak or thin spot on a blood vessel in the brain that balloons out and fills with blood. The bulging aneurysm can put pressure on a nerve or surrounding brain tissue. It may also leak or rupture, spilling blood into the surrounding tissue (called a hemorrhage). Some cerebral aneurysms, particularly those that are very small, do not bleed or cause other problems. Cerebral aneurysms can occur anywhere in the brain, but most are located along a loop of arteries that run between the underside of the brain and the base of the skull.

Cerebral aneurysms can be congenital, resulting from an inborn abnormality in an artery wall. Cerebral aneurysms are also more common in people with certain genetic diseases, such as connective tissue disorders and polycystic kidney disease, and certain circulatory disorders, such as arteriovenous malformations (snarled tangles of arteries and veins in the brain that disrupt blood flow). Other causes include trauma or injury to the head, high blood pressure, infection, tumors, atherosclerosis and other diseases of the vascular system, cigarette smoking, and drug abuse. Aneurysms that result from an infection in the arterial wall are called mycotic aneurysms. Cancer-related aneurysms are often associated with primary or metastatic tumors of the head and neck. Drug abuse, particularly the habitual

Excerpted from "Cerebral Aneurysm Fact Sheet," National Institute of Neurological Disorders and Stroke (NINDS), NIH Publication No. 08–5505, updated February 3, 2010.

use of cocaine, can inflame blood vessels and lead to the development of brain aneurysms.

There are three types of cerebral aneurysm. A saccular aneurysm (known as a berry aneurysm) is a rounded or pouch-like sac of blood that is attached by a neck or stem to an artery or a branch of a blood vessel. This most common form of cerebral aneurysm is typically found on arteries at the base of the brain. A lateral aneurysm appears as a bulge on one wall of the blood vessel, while a fusiform aneurysm is formed by the widening along all walls of the vessel.

Aneurysms are also classified by size. Small aneurysms are less than 11 millimeters in diameter (about the size of a large pencil eraser), larger aneurysms are 11–25 millimeters (about the width of a dime), and giant aneurysms are greater than 25 millimeters in diameter (more than the width of a quarter).

Brain aneurysms can occur in anyone, at any age. They are more common in adults than in children and slightly more common in women than in men. People with certain inherited disorders are also at higher risk. All cerebral aneurysms have the potential to rupture and cause bleeding within the brain. The incidence of reported ruptured aneurysm is about 27,000 individuals per year in the United States, most commonly in people between ages 30 and 60 years.

Aneurysms may burst and bleed into the brain, causing serious complications, including hemorrhagic stroke, permanent nerve damage, or death. Once it has burst, the aneurysm may burst again and bleed into the brain, and additional aneurysms may also occur. More commonly, rupture may cause a subarachnoid hemorrhage—bleeding into the space between the skull bone and the brain. A delayed, serious complication of subarachnoid hemorrhage is hydrocephalus, in which the excessive buildup of cerebrospinal fluid in the skull dilates fluid pathways (ventricles) that can swell and press on the brain tissue. Another delayed postrupture complication is vasospasm, in which other blood vessels in the brain contract and limit blood flow to vital areas of the brain can cause stroke or tissue damage.

Symptoms: Most cerebral aneurysms do not show symptoms until they either become very large or burst. Small, unchanging aneurysms generally will not produce symptoms, whereas a larger aneurysm that is steadily growing may press on tissues and nerves. Symptoms may include pain above and behind the eye; numbness, weakness, or paralysis on one side of the face; dilated pupils; and vision changes. When an aneurysm hemorrhages, an individual may experience a sudden and extremely severe headache, double vision, nausea, vomiting, stiff neck, or loss of consciousness. Individuals usually describe the headache as "the worst headache of my life" and it is generally different in severity and intensity from other headaches people may experience. "Sentinel" or warning headaches may result from an aneurysm that leaks for days to weeks prior to rupture. Only a minority of individuals have a sentinel headache prior to aneurysm rupture.

Diagnosis: Most cerebral aneurysms go unnoticed until they rupture or are detected by brain imaging that may have been obtained for another condition.

Treatment: Not all cerebral aneurysms burst. Some people with very small aneurysms may be monitored to detect any growth or onset of symptoms and to ensure aggressive treatment of coexisting medical problems and risk factors. Each case is unique, and considerations for treating an unruptured aneurysm include the type, size, and location of the aneurysm; risk of rupture; the individual's age, health, and personal and family medical history; and risk of treatment.

Two surgical options are available for treating cerebral aneurysms, both of which carry some risk to the individual (such as possible damage to other blood vessels, the potential for aneurysm recurrence and rebleeding, and the risk of post-operative stroke). Microvascular clipping involves cutting off the flow of blood to the aneurysm. A related procedure is an occlusion, in which the surgeon clamps off (occludes) the entire artery that leads to the aneurysm. This procedure is often performed when the aneurysm has damaged the artery. Endovascular embolization is an alternative to surgery. This procedure may need to be performed more than once during the person's lifetime.

Other treatment for cerebral aneurysm is symptomatic and may include anticonvulsants to prevent seizures and analgesics to treat headache. Vasospasm can be treated with calcium channel-blocking drugs and sedatives may be ordered if the person is restless. A shunt may be surgically inserted into a ventricle several months following rupture if the buildup of cerebrospinal fluid is causing harmful pressure on surrounding tissue. Individuals who have suffered a subarachnoid hemorrhage often need rehabilitative, speech, and occupational therapy to regain lost function and learn to cope with any permanent disability.

Prevention: There are no known ways to prevent a cerebral aneurysm from forming. People with a diagnosed brain aneurysm should carefully control high blood pressure, stop smoking, and avoid cocaine use or other stimulant drugs. They should also consult with a doctor about the benefits and risks of taking aspirin or other drugs that thin the blood. Women should check with their doctors about the use of oral contraceptives.

An unruptured aneurysm may go unnoticed throughout a person's lifetime. A burst aneurysm, however, may be fatal or could lead to hemorrhagic stroke, vasospasm (the leading cause of disability or death following a burst aneurysm), hydrocephalus, coma, or short-term and/or permanent brain damage.

Prognosis: Largely dependent on the age and general health of the individual whose aneurysm has burst including: other preexisting neurological conditions, location of the aneurysm, extent of bleeding (and rebleeding), and time between rupture and medical attention. It is estimated that about 40% of individuals whose aneurysm has ruptured do not survive the first 24 hours; up to another 25% die from complications within six months. People who experience subarachnoid hemorrhage may have permanent neurological damage. Other individuals may recover with little or no neurological deficit. Delayed complications from a burst aneurysm may include hydrocephalus and vasospasm. Early diagnosis and treatment are important.

Individuals who receive treatment for an unruptured aneurysm generally require less rehabilitative therapy and recover more quickly than persons whose aneurysm has burst. Recovery from treatment or rupture may take weeks to months.

Chapter 34

Cavernous Angioma

Chapter Contents

Section 34.1

What We Know and Don't Know about Cavernous Angioma

This section includes "About Cavernous Angioma," and "Questions to Ask Your Doctor," © 2009 Angioma Alliance. Reprinted with permission. Visit www.angiomaalliance.org for additional information.

About Cavernous Angioma

Cavernous angiomas are vascular lesions comprised of clusters of abnormally dilated blood vessels. These lesions can be found in the brain, spinal cord, and rarely, in other areas of the body including the skin and retina. Multiple names refer to this condition:

- cavernous angioma

- cavernous hemangioma

- cerebral cavernous malformation (CCM)

- cavernoma

Cavernous angiomas are typically described as having a raspberry-like appearance due to their composition of multiple bubble-like structures called caverns. Each cavern is filled with blood and lined by a specialized cell layer called the endothelium. Endothelial cells are the basic building blocks that work in conjunction with other cell types to form blood vessels. In the case of cavernous angioma, the bubble-like caverns are grossly dilated vessels that leak due to defects in the endothelial cells and due to the loss of other structural components that are required for normal vessel walls. Patients may present with a single or multiple cavernous angioma lesions. Lesion size is variable ranging from microscopic to a few inches in diameter and the lesions may cause a wide variety of symptoms including seizures, stroke symptoms, hemorrhages, and headaches.

Incidence: Cavernous angiomas are estimated to occur in approximately one out of every 100–200 people, that is 0.5–1% of the general population. While presentation of cavernous angioma is not uncommon in children, individuals often shown the first sign of symptoms in their 20s or 30s. Cavernous angiomas can continue to form later in life; therefore incidence rates and number of angiomas per person are higher among adults. Generally, more than 30% of those with cavernous angioma eventually will develop symptoms.

Familial cavernous angioma: For at least 20% of those with the illness, cavernous angioma is hereditary. This form of the illness is often associated with multiple cavernous angiomas. While familial cavernous angioma can happen in any family, it occurs at a higher rate among Mexican-American families. This prevalence in Mexican-American families is due to a specific genetic mutation which has been passed through more than 17 generations within this cultural group. Each child of someone with the familial form has a 50% chance of inheriting the illness. Recent research has shown that there are three genes that cause the familial form of cavernous angioma; inheritance of a causative mutation in any one of three genes can lead to the illness.

Sporadic cavernous angioma: In addition to the familial form, cavernous angioma may arise sporadically. Under this condition, there is no associated inherited genetic mutation. The sporadic form typically presents as a solitary cavernous angioma that may be present at birth or may develop later in life. Because sporadic lesions do not arise following the same genetic inheritance as with familial cases, related family members will not have a predisposition for the condition. Additionally, children of those with sporadic cavernous angioma may have no greater chance of developing the disorder than anyone else in the general public (one out of 100–200 individuals).

Associated venous angioma: Up to 40% of solitary cavernous angiomas may develop in the vicinity of another vascular anomaly called a venous angioma. The venous angioma, also known as venous malformation or venous developmental anomaly, usually does not create problems unless it is associated with a cavernous angioma. It may make surgery more difficult; the goal is not to disturb the venous angioma while removing the cavernous angioma.

Other vascular malformations: The cavernous angioma is part of a spectrum of lesions known as angiographically occult vascular malformations related to the fact that they are not visible on an angiogram. Cavernous angiomas cannot be seen on angiogram because they are low-flow anomalies in which blood flows through the lesion slowly. This is one quality that makes cavernous angiomas different from arteriovenous malformations which are high blood flow lesions that are readily visible on angiogram.

Symptoms: Cavernous angioma symptoms are highly variable among individuals; in some cases no symptoms may be present. However, when symptoms do manifest they often depend on the location of the angioma and on the strength of the angioma walls and their propensity for bleeding. Cavernous angiomas can cause seizures. A person who suffers from seizures is said to have epilepsy. There are many types of seizure including mild absence seizures and dramatic tonic-clonic seizures. Seizures tend to worsen with age and frequency. Most cases of epilepsy can be well controlled with medications. The type of seizure a person experiences depends, in part, on the location of the cavernous angioma. If a person has seizures and more than one cavernous angioma, it may be difficult to pinpoint which cavernous angioma is the cause of the seizures.

In addition to seizures, cavernous angiomas can cause neurological deficits such as weaknesses in arms or legs, vision problems, balance problems, or memory and attention problems. As with seizure, the type of deficit is associated with which part of the brain or spinal cord the cavernous angioma is located. Symptoms may come and go as the cavernous angioma changes in size with bleeding and reabsorption of blood.

Cavernous angiomas can bleed in a number of different ways:

- Angiomas can bleed slowly within the walls of the angioma and remain quite small. A small hemorrhage may not require surgery, and may be reabsorbed by the body. However, continued small hemorrhages in the same cavernous angioma often cause deterioration in function.

- Angiomas can bleed more profusely within the walls of the angioma. This can cause them to increase in size and to put pressure on the surrounding brain tissue.

- Finally, angiomas may bleed through a weak spot in the angioma wall into the surrounding brain tissue. This is called an overt hemorrhage.

The risk of hemorrhage is dependent on the number of angiomas. The higher the number, the greater the chance of one or more hemorrhages occurring sometime over a lifetime. On average, cavernous angiomas that have bled in the past are those that are the most likely to bleed again, particularly in the first two years after their initial bleed. It is also important to note that a hemorrhage in a cavernous angioma in the brain stem can be life threatening, as the brainstem is responsible for regulating critical life processes including breathing and heart-beat.

Finally, those with cavernous angioma may experience headache. This seems to be true particularly when a lesion has undergone recent bleed activity.

Cavernous Angioma Statistics

• One in 100–200 people have at least one cavernous angioma.

• At least 30% of those with a cavernous angioma eventually will develop symptoms.

• At least 20% of those with cavernous angioma have the familial form of the illness.

• Up to 40% of solitary cavernous angiomas may have an associated venous angioma.

• Age at first diagnosis: Under 20 (25–30%); age 20–40 (60%); over 40 (10–15%)

• Primary symptom: Seizure (30%); neurological deficit (25%); hemorrhage (15%); headache (5%)

• Odds of your child having cavernous angioma:

    • If you have sporadic cavernous angioma, your child is at no greater risk for developing a cavernous angioma than anyone in the general public; that is a one in 200 chance (0.5%).

    • If you have familial cavernous angioma, your child may have a one in two chance (50%) of inheriting the causative mutation and developing cavernous angioma.

Diagnosis and Treatment

Cavernous angiomas are diagnosed most often when they become symptomatic. Although cavernous angiomas have been known since the 1930s, they have not been reliably diagnosed until the advent of the MRI (magnetic resonance imaging) in the 1980s. Previously, the illness may have been misdiagnosed as multiple sclerosis or as a seizure disorder with no known cause. Cavernous angiomas are not visible on angiogram and were only inconsistently visible on computed axial tomography (CAT) scans. An MRI scan, with and without contrast and with gradient echo sequences, read by an experienced physician remains the best means of diagnosing this illness. The MRI scan may need to be repeated to assess change in the size of a cavernous angioma, recent bleeding, or the appearance of new lesions.

Most cavernous angiomas are observed for change in appearance, recent hemorrhage, or clinical symptoms. Medications are available to treat seizures and headaches caused by cavernous angiomas. Surgery is advocated for cavernous angiomas with recent hemorrhage, those which are expanding in size, and in some cases, those which are causing seizures. Radiosurgery, by gamma knife, linear accelerator, or new shaped beam techniques, is a controversial treatment that has been used on cavernous angiomas too dangerous to reach through traditional surgery. For familial cases of cavernous angioma, genetic testing is another option for diagnosis.

Surgery: Cerebral cavernous angiomas are surgically removed (resected) using a craniotomy, or opening the skull. This is usually performed under general anesthesia, except in cases where mapping of the brain while awake is needed. Cavernous angiomas in the spine are removed using laminectomy or unroofing of the vertebrae.

Surgery for cavernous angioma has been made safer using the operating microscope (microsurgery) and image guided surgical navigation (also known as computer-assisted or frameless stereotaxy) to reach the cavernous angioma with as little disruption to normal brain or spinal cord as possible. Risks of any surgery, including cavernous angioma, include stroke, paralysis, coma, or death, although these complications are rare with modern surgery performed by expert neurosurgeons. Surgery on cavernous angioma in the brain stem and spinal cord is more risky, but these cavernous angiomas are more dangerous if left alone. While recovery is different for everyone, many patients leave the hospital within a few days and resume normal life within a few weeks of surgery. However, people with neurological deficits may require a prolonged period of rehabilitation.

What We Don't Know about Cavernous Angioma

While researchers continue to make discoveries about cavernous angioma every day, many important research questions remain. Genetic researchers and a growing number of other researchers are working to determine the cause of the illness and the mechanisms by which the defective blood vessels are formed. We don't know most of the factors that lead to angioma bleeding and re-bleeding. Efforts to uncover what causes a particular cavernous angioma to bleed will help us to be able to reduce the risk of bleeding. We don't know how to remove a cavernous angioma without brain surgery. Less intrusive removal methods may allow for treatment of more angiomas before they become problematic.

Questions to Ask Your Doctor

When you are first diagnosed, it is likely you will feel overwhelmed by the sudden and many choices you must make. Which doctor? Which hospital? Surgery? What next? Sometimes it is hard to think clearly and get the answers you need to make informed decisions. Angioma Alliance's Surgery Support Committee has put together a list of questions you should ask your physician. You will probably want extra time to consider the information you receive, so make sure you or someone you trust takes thorough notes for your review later.

General Questions

1. What size is the cerebral cavernous malformation (cavernous angioma, CCM)?

2. How many CCM do I have?

3. What is the exact location of the CCM?

4. What functions does this area of the brain perform?

5. Do there appear to be any venous or other malformations in the vicinity of the CCM?

6. Does it appear to have bled previously?

7. In your opinion, what are the conditions under which you recommend surgery to remove a CCM?

8. Are there any other treatments you consider?

9. What tests do you recommend? (MRI, functional MRI, magnetic resonance angiography [MRA], angiogram, and so forth)

10. If I had another bleed, what deficits would you expect?

11. What symptoms would warrant a call to you or a trip to the emergency room (ER)?

12. Should I have my children (or anyone else in my family) tested?

13. Is there a genetic test to diagnose CCM?

14. Should I be concerned about possible cavernous malformations in other areas of my body? Should my spine be scanned?

15. Is this a rare disorder?

16. How did I get/develop a CCM?

17. Are there any vitamins or supplements I should take to improve my situation?

18. Can I exercise?

19. Can I participate in sports? What about contact sports such as football or snowboarding that might include a blow to the head?

20. Can I fly in an airplane?

21. What restrictions in activities do you recommend?

22. Are you concerned about my blood pressure?

23. What medications, prescriptions and over the counter, do you recommend I avoid? Are there any vitamins or supplements to avoid?

24. Is travel to higher elevations safe?

25. Can I drink alcohol or caffeinated beverages?

Management

1. How often will I have follow up tests (and which ones)?

2. How often will I follow up with you?

3. What will you be looking for while monitoring me? (What changes are you looking for?)

4. Is there anything I can do to minimize the risk of a bleed (or re-bleed)?

5. What is the risk of re-bleed?

6. Is this risk cumulative?

7. How would I know if I had another bleed? (for example, what symptoms would you expect to see?)

8. What would cause you to recommend surgery?

Surgery Resection Recommendation

1. How long would you estimate the surgery to take?

2. How long would you estimate for recovery from surgery?

3. How long will I be in the hospital?

4. When do you expect I will be able to return to work and/or daily responsibilities?

5. What, if any, additional deficits would be possible as a result of the surgery?

6. Would you anticipate any of the deficits to be permanent?

7. Can my CCM come back after surgery?

Surgeon's Background

1. How many of these have you seen?

2. Do you have a cerebrovascular specialization?

3. How many CCM have you removed surgically?

4. (If you have a brainstem CCM) How many of these were brainstem CCM?

Section 34.2

Raising Children with or at Risk for Cavernous Angioma

Note: We use the term cavernous malformation as a synonym for cavernous angioma, cavernous hemangioma, and cavernoma. Venous malformations (venous angioma, DVA) and arteriovenous malformations (AVM) are different types of vascular malformations and information for these conditions is not included here.

My infant can't tell me when she has a headache. What are the symptoms of a cavernous malformation hemorrhage in an infant?

It is difficult to determine when an infant is having trouble with cavernous malformations versus when they are having a normal childhood illness. Those who have experienced raising an infant with this illness can identify with the anxiety this engenders. In general, there are several ways to distinguish whether a behavior warrants a trip to the pediatrician versus a trip to the emergency room (ER) or the neurosurgeon.

If your baby starts to demonstrate unusual irritability and a new onset sleep problem without fever, this may be a first sign. The baby may be having a normal reaction to teething, may have a virus, an earache, or any number of other childhood illnesses. However, pressure from a cavernous malformation bleed is greater when a baby is sleeping because gravity is not helping to move blood away from the head, making frequent awakenings common. Babies also become irritable while a cavernous malformation is bleeding much as an adult would. Although not a reason to panic, a trip to the pediatrician would be a good choice to help identify the source of the baby's symptoms.

There are more serious signs of hemorrhage that warrant a call to the neurosurgeon and perhaps a trip to the ER. Signs to watch include:

1. Your baby loses a function that she could once perform such as rolling over, holding up her head, crawling, or babbling.

2. Changes in your baby's eyes: Keeping tabs on your baby's eyes is important—look for a pupil that is suddenly larger in one eye than the other (unequal pupils), eyes jumping left to right or up and down when the baby is trying to look straight ahead (nystagmus), or both eyes no longer looking in the same direction (strabismus).

3. A first tonic-clonic seizure not related to fever.

4. Feeling your baby's soft spot (fontanel) and becoming familiar with how raised it is can help you monitor him or her. If the fontanel becomes raised above where it usually is, this may be a sign of increased pressure in the brain.

5. If your baby experiences projectile vomiting, particularly along with any of the other signs, it is important to call the neurosurgeon. Projectile vomiting is vomiting with some force behind it. For example, if your baby is in his or her rear-facing car seat and vomits, it's probably not projectile vomiting if he or she is only soiled the front of her clothes. If he or she is soiled anything beyond the car seat you would want to suspect projectile vomiting. Also, if your baby vomits in his or her bed and does not have other symptoms of illness, this would warrant a call to the doctor.

6. If your baby holds his or her head to one side or the other and appears to be unable to straighten his or her neck, this is called torticollis and may indicate a hemorrhage in the area of the brain called the posterior fossa.

7. Finally, if your child loses consciousness, you will want to call the neurosurgeon and emergency services.

What are the symptoms of a cavernous malformation hemorrhage in a child over two years?

Please read the symptoms for children already listed, because many of these continue to apply to older children. Additionally, preschool age and older children may be able to communicate headache pain associated with a cavernous malformation. Some people experience a pain they describe as brief, cold, and sharp going through their head. Others have intense ongoing pain. Headache, like seizure, often accompanies cavernous malformation even if there is no new bleeding.

Your child may exhibit new and unusual irritability, similar to what you might notice when they are becoming ill with influenza or other more serious contagious illness. The irritability may go on for days without evidence of other symptoms. In the absence of any of the other warning signs, this may not indicate a hemorrhage, but it is something to note.

Your child may have a new onset sleep disturbance, waking up with head discomfort or projectile vomiting. A preschool age child may not be able to tell you about head discomfort, but may wake up multiple times over the night. Pressure from a cavernous malformation bleed is greater when a child is sleeping because gravity is not helping to move blood away from the head, making frequent awakenings common.

A child who had previously not experienced seizure may have a seizure or those with seizure disorders may experience a worsening that can't be attributed to outgrowing medication doses.

Many people who have cavernous malformation hemorrhages experience vision problems or dizziness as an initial symptom. Your child may complain of seeing double or having blurry vision. They may become so dizzy that they can not walk. Some anti-seizure medications have these symptoms as side effects. It is important to rule this out.

A child may be able to communicate to you that they are experiencing tingling or numbness in a part of their body, most often in arms or legs. You may also notice speech problems—difficulty finding words, slurred speech, or difficulty understanding oral instructions.

Should my child have any medication restrictions?

As with adults, children with cavernous malformations should not be given aspirin or other non-steroidal anti-inflammatory drugs (NSAIDs) such as ibuprofen or Naprosyn products. These products reduce the ability of blood to clot, worsening any bleed that might occur. For aspirin, this effect lasts long after the aspirin has left the child's system. For the same reason, some physicians advise against the use of valproic acid (Depakote or Depakene) as an anti-seizure medication for patients with cavernous malformations. Other drugs that have drug thinning properties such as warfarin (Coumadin) or heparin should never be used.

Some controversy exists regarding the safety of many of the medications used to treat attention deficit/hyperactivity disorder (ADHD) because most increase blood pressure and heart rate, if only slightly. High blood pressure is thought to be associated with increased cavernous malformation bleeding, but the impact of the small blood pressure increase caused by prescription stimulant use is not known.

What are the symptoms of a seizure disorder?

While most of us think of a seizure as a very dramatic event in which a person becomes unconscious, falls to the ground, and engages in a few minutes of jerking movements, a seizure can be quite subtle. There are two classes of seizure—general and focal. All seizures caused by cavernous malformations begin as focal seizures, but some may generalize from there.

A focal seizure can be either a partial motor or partial complex seizure. With either, there is no loss of consciousness. A child may have jerking in a single body part that is not in their conscious control, may have odd mouth movements like lip smacking, may pick at clothing, or may have odd movements. In some cases, a child may be overwhelmed by a sudden strong feeling that comes on without explanation.

Generalized seizures include tonic-clonic seizures (also known as grand mal) and absence seizures. With tonic-clonic seizure, there is a loss of consciousness and a loss of body control. The child will not be able to stand, will exhibit strong jerking movements, and may lose bladder control. With absence seizure, there is a loss of consciousness, but no loss of body control. These are often called stop and stare seizures because a child may simply stop their activity and stare into space for thirty seconds or more.

Can my child be treated with anti-seizure medication?

Yes, children are treated with anti-seizure medication. A number of common anti-seizure medications are approved for use in children and are available in liquid, sprinkle, or chewable form.

Most anti-seizure medications are designed to be most effective for one or two specific types of seizure. Your child's doctor should discuss with you the medication options for your child. Every anti-seizure medication has side effects. Your child may need to try several medications before finding the one that is effective and has a tolerable number of side effects. Side effects tend to be worst when first starting a medication, during periods when the dosage is being increased, and during the times of the day when the blood concentration of the medication is at its peak. Common side effects include sedation, nausea and stomach distress, dizziness, vision problems, attention problems, mood disturbance, and balance or coordination problems. Not every anti-epileptic medication causes every side effect. Other more severe side effects are possible. It is important to discuss the possibility of side effects, both minor and severe, with your child's doctor before beginning treatment.

Should my child have any activity restrictions?

If your child has seizures as a result of cavernous malformations, she or he may be advised about a number of activity restrictions.

Table 34.1. Activity Restrictions for Children with Cavernous Malformations with or without Epilepsy

No or Very Little Risk: No extra supervision needed	Moderate Risk: May need supervision or help during a seizure	High Risk: Avoid
Jogging	Climbing a tree or jungle gym: Always have a spotter underneath; avoid being upside down	Mountain or rock climbing
Aerobics	Swimming: Always swim with a buddy and/or lifeguard	Bungee jumping
Cross-country skiing	Horseback riding: Wear a helmet	Scuba diving
Dancing	Bike and scooter riding: Wear a helmet	Skydiving
Hiking	Canoeing: Wear a life vest and helmet	Caving
Golf	Ice-skating or hockey: Wear a helmet	Boxing
Ping-pong	Tennis	Hang gliding or surfing/windsurfing
Bowling	Gymnastics: Always have a spotter underneath; avoid being upside down	Solo flying
Baseball: wear a helmet	Rollerblading, skate boarding: Wear a helmet	
Field hockey: wear a helmet	Football: There is concern about the level of contact those with cavernous malformations	
Most track and field events	Soccer: Restrict heading the ball	

Table 34.1 lists the comparative risks of activities for children with epilepsy and can be found in "A Guide for Parents of Children with Epilepsy" produced by Shire Richwood, a pharmaceutical company. We have adapted some entries to make this table appropriate for children with cavernous malformations whether or not they have epilepsy.

Although head trauma has not been shown to be associated with cavernous malformation hemorrhage, most physicians recommend that children with cavernous malformations stay away from contact sports. Children should also be diligent about wearing a helmet in other situations in which there is an increased chance of head injury, such as skateboarding, biking, scooter riding, or inline skating. Many physicians also encourage helmet use while snowboarding or skiing.

It is unwise to allow your child to spend extended periods upside down. This can increase blood volume and venous pressure in the brain. Following this restriction may limit participation in gymnastics or in the use of some playground equipment.

Cavernous malformations run in our family. When should I have my child tested for the illness?

This is a very individual decision, but physicians often recommend to their patients that children be screened before school age. Some parents have their children screened in infancy because sedation is sometimes easier with babies, babies won't remember the MRI, and parents can be relieved of the worry if the child doesn't have the illness. Some parents wait until their child is old enough to lie still for the MRI without sedation. Others never have their child screened unless there are symptoms because they want their kids to have as normal a childhood as possible.

Screening as early as possible and at minimum before school age is recommended for several reasons. First, children who are identified with cavernous malformations can be monitored, and in some cases, a cavernous malformation can be removed before it causes irreparable damage or death. Second, early identification can allow parents to work with a school system to create a plan in case of a medical emergency. Cavernous malformations may play a role in learning or behavior problems a child might experience. Knowing whether a child has the condition can help in making decisions about how to address these problems. Third, parents are better prepared to make informed decisions about a child's participation in activities such as contact sports. Fourth, teachers may notice symptoms of neurological deficit before parents notice them. Knowing the diagnosis and what to watch for can help a teacher to become an extra set of eyes for your family.

Clinical diagnostic blood testing is available for three genetic mutations that can cause the illness. This means that a family will be able to submit a child's blood or cheek swab sample to a lab rather than have the child undergo an MRI to determine if there is a mutation. The affected parent should have genetic testing first to determine the specific mutation before submitting the child's sample.

How is an MRI for a child different from that for an adult?

Children who are unable to remain still for the 30–60 minutes required for an MRI will require some kind of sedation before the procedure. Your child will either be sedated to the level of sedation analgesia, also known as conscious sedation or twilight sleep, or to the deeper level induced by general anesthesia. Most hospitals will try sedation analgesia first, but some children become agitated by or are unable to tolerate the medications used for sedation analgesia. If this is the case, subsequent MRIs are performed using general anesthesia.

My child seems tired most of the time. What could be causing this?

There are a number of factors that may be causing your child to be fatigued:

1. Research has shown that fatigue is a common long-term after effect of stroke and of mild traumatic brain injury. There is no reason to believe that this would not be the case for cavernous malformation hemorrhage. The mechanism behind the fatigue is not understood, but the fatigue itself can feel debilitating to those who experience it. Making sure your child gets enough rest at night and has opportunity for rest during the day is essential. A 504 plan to address fatigue at school may be needed. If your child has difficulty sleeping at night, another common after effect of brain trauma, it would be wise to consult his neurologist for suggestions.

2. Children with seizure disorders that emanate from the parietal lobe or with cavernous malformations in the pons have a lower quality of sleep than children without seizure disorders.

This means that even if a child has what appears to be sufficient sleep, the lower quality of their sleep will make them feel less rested.

3. Most anti-seizure medications have sedation as a side effect. If your child seems debilitated by this, speak to his neurologist to see if there might be an alternative medication.

4. Children with even mild muscle weakness or decreased coordination resulting from a cavernous malformation bleed often have reduced physical stamina. It simply requires more energy to use legs that feel heavy or that won't do what the child asks of them.

Chapter 35

Hydrocephalus

The term hydrocephalus is derived from the Greek words *hydro* meaning water and *cephalus* meaning head. As the name implies, it is a condition in which the primary characteristic is excessive accumulation of fluid in the brain. Although hydrocephalus was once known as water on the brain, the water is actually cerebrospinal fluid (CSF)—a clear fluid that surrounds the brain and spinal cord. The excessive accumulation of CSF results in an abnormal widening of spaces in the brain called ventricles. This widening creates potentially harmful pressure on the tissues of the brain.

The ventricular system is made up of four ventricles connected by narrow passages. Normally, CSF flows through the ventricles, exits into cisterns (closed spaces that serve as reservoirs) at the base of the brain, bathes the surfaces of the brain and spinal cord, and then reabsorbs into the bloodstream. CSF has three important life-sustaining functions: 1) to keep the brain tissue buoyant, acting as a cushion or shock absorber; 2) to act as the vehicle for delivering nutrients to the brain and removing waste; and 3) to flow between the cranium and spine and compensate for changes in intracranial blood volume (the amount of blood within the brain). The balance between production and absorption of CSF is critically important. Because CSF is made continuously, medical conditions that block its normal flow or absorption will result in an over-accumulation of CSF. The resulting pressure of the fluid against brain tissue is what causes hydrocephalus.

Excerpted from "Hydrocephalus," National Institute of Neurological Disorders and Stroke (NINDS), NIH Publication No. 08–385, updated February 10, 2010.

Hydrocephalus may be congenital or acquired: Congenital hydrocephalus is present at birth and may be caused by either events or influences that occur during fetal development, or genetic abnormalities. Acquired hydrocephalus develops at the time of birth or at some point afterward. This type of hydrocephalus can affect individuals of all ages and may be caused by injury or disease.

Hydrocephalus may also be communicating or non-communicating: Communicating hydrocephalus occurs when the flow of CSF is blocked after it exits the ventricles. This form is called communicating because the CSF can still flow between the ventricles, which remain open. Non-communicating hydrocephalus—also called "obstructive" hydrocephalus—occurs when the flow of CSF is blocked along one or more of the narrow passages connecting the ventricles. One of the most common causes of hydrocephalus is aqueductal stenosis.

There are two other forms of hydrocephalus which do not fit exactly into the categories mentioned and primarily affect adults: hydrocephalus ex-vacuo and normal pressure hydrocephalus. Hydrocephalus ex-vacuo occurs when stroke or traumatic injury cause damage to the brain. In these cases, brain tissue may actually shrink. Normal pressure hydrocephalus can happen to people at any age, but it is most common among the elderly. It may result from a subarachnoid hemorrhage, head trauma, infection, tumor, or complications of surgery. However, many people develop normal pressure hydrocephalus even when none of these factors are present for reasons that are unknown.

The number of people who develop hydrocephalus or who are currently living with it is difficult to establish since there is no national registry or database of people with the condition. However, experts estimate that hydrocephalus affects approximately one in every 500 children. The causes of hydrocephalus are still not well understood.

Symptoms of hydrocephalus vary with age, disease progression, and individual differences in tolerance to the condition. For example, an infant's ability to compensate for increased CSF pressure and enlargement of the ventricles differs from an adult's. The infant skull can expand to accommodate the buildup of CSF because the sutures (the fibrous joints that connect the bones of the skull) have not yet closed.

In infancy, the most obvious indication of hydrocephalus is often a rapid increase in head circumference or an unusually large head size. Other symptoms may include vomiting, sleepiness, irritability, downward deviation of the eyes (also called sunsetting), and seizures.

Older children and adults may experience different symptoms because their skulls cannot expand to accommodate the buildup of CSF. Symptoms may include headache followed by vomiting, nausea, papilledema (swelling of the optic disk which is part of the optic nerve), blurred or double vision, sunsetting of the eyes, problems with balance, poor coordination, gait disturbance, urinary incontinence, slowing or loss of developmental progress, lethargy, drowsiness, irritability, or other changes in personality or cognition including memory loss.

Symptoms of normal pressure hydrocephalus include, problems with walking, impaired bladder control leading to urinary frequency and/or incontinence, and progressive mental impairment and dementia. An individual with this type of hydrocephalus may have a general slowing of movements or may complain that his or her feet feel stuck. Because some of these symptoms may also be experienced in other disorders such as Alzheimer disease, Parkinson disease, and Creutzfeldt-Jakob disease, normal pressure hydrocephalus is often incorrectly diagnosed and never properly treated. Doctors may use a variety of tests, including brain scans, a spinal tap or lumbar catheter, intracranial pressure monitoring, and neuropsychological tests, to help them accurately diagnose normal pressure hydrocephalus and rule out any other conditions.

Treatment: Hydrocephalus is most often treated by surgically inserting a shunt system. This system diverts the flow of CSF from the central nervous system to another area of the body where it can be absorbed as part of the normal circulatory process.

A shunt is a flexible but sturdy plastic tube. A shunt system consists of the shunt, a catheter, and a valve. One end of the catheter is placed within a ventricle inside the brain or in the CSF outside the spinal cord. The other end of the catheter is commonly placed within the abdominal cavity, but may also be placed at other sites in the body such as a chamber of the heart or areas around the lung where the CSF can drain and be absorbed. A valve located along the catheter maintains one-way flow and regulates the rate of CSF flow.

A limited number of individuals can be treated with an alternative procedure called third ventriculostomy. In this procedure, a neuroendoscope—a small camera that uses fiber optic technology to visualize small and difficult to reach surgical areas—allows a doctor to view the ventricular surface. Once the scope is guided into position, a small tool makes a tiny hole in the floor of the third ventricle, which allows the CSF to bypass the obstruction and flow toward the site of resorption around the surface of the brain.

Possible complications: Shunt systems are not perfect devices. Complications may include mechanical failure, infections, obstructions, and the need to lengthen or replace the catheter. Generally, shunt systems require monitoring and regular medical follow up. When complications occur, the shunt system usually requires some type of revision. Some complications can lead to other problems such as over-draining or under-draining. When there is reason to suspect that a shunt system is not functioning properly (for example, if the symptoms of hydrocephalus return), medical attention should be sought immediately.

Prognosis: For individuals diagnosed with hydrocephalus, prognosis is difficult to predict, although there is some correlation between the specific cause of the hydrocephalus and the outcome. Prognosis is further complicated by the presence of associated disorders, the timeliness of diagnosis, and the success of treatment. The degree to which relief of CSF pressure following shunt surgery can minimize or reverse damage to the brain is not well understood.

Affected individuals and their families should be aware that hydrocephalus poses risks to both cognitive and physical development. However, many children diagnosed with the disorder benefit from rehabilitation therapies and educational interventions and go on to lead normal lives with few limitations. Early diagnosis and treatment improves the chance of a good recovery.

Chapter 36

Stroke

Chapter Contents

Section 36.1

Stroke Basics

Excerpted from "Stroke: Challenges, Progress, and Promise,"
National Institute of Neurological Disorders and Stroke (NINDS),
NIH Publication No. 09–6451, February 2009.

The effects of stroke manifest themselves rapidly. The five most common symptoms of stroke are:

- sudden weakness or numbness of the face or limbs, especially on one side of the body;

- sudden confusion or difficulty speaking or understanding speech;

- sudden trouble seeing in one or both eyes;

- sudden trouble walking, dizziness, or loss of balance or coordination; and

- sudden severe headache with no known cause.

The exact symptoms depend on where in the brain's vascular system the blockage or rupture has occurred. Strokes that predominantly affect one hemisphere of the brain are common. Since each hemisphere controls the opposite side of the body, a stroke in the left hemisphere will cause motor and sensory deficits on the right side of the body, and vice versa.

The long-term outcomes after a stroke vary considerably and depend partly on the type of stroke and the age of the affected person. Although most stroke survivors regain their functional independence, 15–30% will have a permanent physical disability. Some will experience a permanent decline in cognitive function known as post-stroke or vascular dementia. Unfortunately, many stroke survivors face a danger of recurrent stroke in the future. About 20% of people who experience a first-ever stroke between ages 40 and 69 will have another stroke within five years.

Ischemic Stroke and Transient Ischemic Attack

Ischemic strokes make up about 80% of all strokes. Just as a heart attack occurs when there is insufficient blood flow to the heart, an ischemic stroke (sometimes called a brain attack) occurs when there is a sudden interruption in blood flow to one or more regions of the brain. Like all cells in the body, neurons and other brain cells require oxygen and glucose delivered through the blood in order to function and survive. A few minutes of oxygen deprivation, called ischemia, is enough to kill millions of neurons. Moreover, ischemia can provoke inflammation, swelling (edema), and other processes that can continue to cause damage for hours to days after the initial insult.

Obstructive blood clots are the most common cause of ischemic stroke. Clotting (or coagulation) is a vital function that helps prevent bleeding when a blood vessel is damaged, but clots can also obstruct normal blood flow. When a clot forms in association with the wall of a blood vessel and grows large enough to impair blood flow, it is called a thrombus; a clot that breaks off the vessel wall and travels through the blood is an embolus. A cardioembolic stroke is caused by a clot that originates in the heart. Cardiac emboli are most likely to form in people with heart conditions such as atrial fibrillation (AF, an irregular heartbeat), heart failure, stenosis, or infections within the valves of the heart. They also may occur post-heart attack.

Another contributor to ischemic stroke is chronic atherosclerosis, which is a buildup of fatty deposits and cellular debris (plaque) on the inside of the blood vessel wall. As atherosclerotic plaques grow, they cause narrowing of the blood vessel (a condition called stenosis). Atherosclerosis can also activate cells involved in clotting.

Immediately after an ischemic stroke, the brain usually contains an irreversibly damaged core of tissue and an area of viable but at-risk tissue called the ischemic penumbra. Restoring normal blood flow—a process known as reperfusion—is essential to rescuing the penumbra. The longer reperfusion is delayed, the more cells in the penumbra will die. The region of brain tissue that is finally damaged is called an infarct.

If a stroke were a storm, a transient ischemic attack (TIA), or mini-stroke, would be an ominous thunderclap. Symptoms of a TIA are similar to those of a full-blown stroke but resolve within 24 hours, typically in less than one hour. Still, the short-lived nature of TIAs does not mean that they leave the brain unharmed. In about 40–50% of people who have experienced a TIA, a tiny dot of infarct can be seen by brain imaging.

Even when there is no sign of brain infarction, a TIA is both a warning and an opportunity for intervention. While someone who has experienced a full-blown stroke has a 2–7% risk of having another stroke within the next 90 days; the 90-day risk of stroke following a

TIA is 10–20%. In many cases, TIAs may be caused by an unstable clot that could create a more permanent blockage within the brain's blood supply at any moment. Fortunately, there are a variety of treatments that can reduce the risk of stroke following a TIA, including medications to lower blood pressure and inhibit blood clotting. If necessary, surgical procedures can clear away plaque in the arteries that supply the brain, or a procedure called stenting can be used to widen the arteries. Severe strokes could be avoided if more people sought medical attention after a TIA.

Hemorrhagic Stroke

An intracerebral hemorrhage occurs when a blood vessel ruptures within the brain. Several conditions can render blood vessels in the brain prone to rupture and bleeding. Chronic hypertension and a condition known as cerebral amyloid angiopathy can weaken the blood vessel wall. Poor blood clotting ability due to blood disorders or blood-thinning medications like warfarin further increase the risk of bleeding. Finally, structural abnormalities that can form in blood vessels

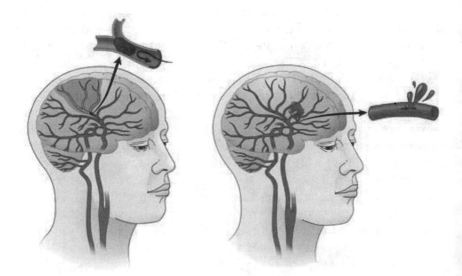

Figure 36.1. *Ischemic Stroke and Hemorrhagic Stroke. An ischemic stroke occurs when a blood vessel supplying the brain becomes blocked, as by a clot (L). A hemorrhagic stroke occurs when a blood vessel bursts, leaking blood into the brain (R).*

during brain development also a play a role. For instance, an arteriovenous malformation (AVM) is a tangled mass of thin-walled cerebral blood vessels in the brain. AVMs are thought to be present from birth in 1% or less of the population.

Cerebral amyloid angiopathy (CAA) refers to a buildup of protein deposits known as amyloid on the inside wall of blood vessels. It is a major contributing factor to intracerebral hemorrhage in older people and is sometimes associated with small ischemic infarctions and vascular cognitive impairment. CAA is regarded as a disease of aging. It is rarely observed in individuals under age 50, but is seen in about 50% of individuals over age 90.

A subarachnoid hemorrhage is the rupture of a blood vessel located within the subarachnoid space—a fluid-filled space between layers of connective tissue (meninges) that surround the brain. The first sign of a subarachnoid hemorrhage is typically a severe headache with a split-second onset and no known cause. Neurologists call this a thunderclap headache and it demands immediate medical attention. The rupture may occur in an AVM, but typically it occurs at a site where a blood vessel has weakened and bulged, called an aneurysm. Aneurysms affect as much as 1% of the population, and are sometimes hereditary. National Institute of Neurological Disorders and Stroke (NINDS)-funded studies have shown that the risk that an aneurysm will rupture is related to its size and shape, its location, and the person's age. The risk is increased by smoking.

Unlike other tissues in the body, neural tissue normally is shielded from direct contact with blood by the blood-brain barrier, which is a tightly sealed network of cellular and extracellular components that lines blood vessels in the brain. The blood-brain barrier is permeable to oxygen and other nutrients in the blood, but generally impermeable to red and white blood cells, and large molecules. During a hemorrhagic stroke, these cells and molecules are released en masse into the delicate environment that surrounds neurons. Meanwhile, the accumulation of blood, known as a hematoma, can cause an increase in intracranial pressure that further impairs normal blood flow and damages the brain by compression.

Vascular cognitive impairment: Even in the absence of a clinically obvious stroke or TIA, impaired blood flow in the brain may eventually lead to vascular cognitive impairment (VCI). At one extreme, VCI includes vascular dementia, but it also refers to a gradual decline in mental function caused by multiple strokes, some silent, over time. It is often associated with a more diffuse small vessel disease, caused by narrowing of small-diameter blood vessels that supply limited territories within the brain. Clinically, VCI may resemble Alzheimer disease (AD) and many older individuals with dementia meet the diagnostic criteria for both diseases. However, while AD primarily affects memory, VCI appears to primarily affect the brain's executive function—the ability to plan activities from getting dressed in the morning to negotiating a business deal.

Stroke Diagnostics and Brain Imaging

When a stroke is suspected, a physician will carry out a detailed assessment of the individual's signs and symptoms. One common assessment tool is the National Institutes of Health (NIH) Stroke Scale, developed by NINDS. This is a checklist of questions and tasks that scores an individual's level of alertness and ability to communicate and perform simple movements. Other common diagnostic procedures include blood tests and an electrocardiogram to check for cardiac abnormalities that might have contributed to the stroke.

Brain imaging techniques play an important role in stroke diagnosis, in the evaluation of individuals with stroke for clinical trials, and to a growing extent, assessment of stroke risk. Several imaging techniques can be used to generate visual slices of the brain or even three-dimensional reconstructions. This in-depth look at the brain helps to: rule out other potential neurological conditions such as a brain tumor, differentiate ischemic from hemorrhagic stroke, identify which blood vessels have been damaged, and determine the extent and location of the infarct.

Stroke Risk Factors

Given that stroke is caused by blockage or rupture of a blood vessel, it should be no surprise that similar modifiable risk factors contribute to stroke and cardiovascular disease, including hypertension, smoking, diabetes, high cholesterol, and lack of physical activity. It is possible to dramatically reduce these risks through healthier lifestyle choices or medications (such as blood pressure-lowering drugs).

Hypertension causes a two-fold to four-fold increase in the risk of stroke before age 80. Hypertension promotes atherosclerosis and causes mechanical damage to the walls of blood vessels. Blood pressure medications can reduce the risk of stroke by 30–40%. Early treatment is essential. Among older people with normal blood pressure, prior mid-life hypertension increases stroke risk up to 92%. Guidelines from the Centers for Disease Control and Prevention recommend a target blood pressure of less than 140/90 mm Hg.

Cigarette smoking causes about a two-fold increase in the risk of ischemic stroke and up to a four-fold increase in the risk of hemorrhagic stroke. Smoking promotes atherosclerosis and aneurysm formation, and stimulates blood clotting factors. Stroke risk decreases significantly two years after quitting smoking and is at the level of nonsmokers by five years.

Having diabetes, in terms of stroke and cardiovascular disease risk, is the equivalent of aging 15 years. In diabetes, glucose is not efficiently taken up by the body's cells and accumulates in the blood instead, where it can damage the vascular system. Hypertension is common among diabetics and accounts for much of their increased stroke risk. Blood pressure medications, dietary changes, and weight loss can lower stroke risk. Controlling blood sugar appears to reduce the risk of recurrent stroke.

Physical inactivity and obesity: Waist-to-hip ratio equal to or above the median (mid-value for the population) increases the risk of ischemic stroke three-fold. Obesity is associated with hypertension, diabetes, and heart disease. While no clinical studies have tested the effects of exercise or weight loss on stroke risk, both tend to reduce hypertension and boost cardiovascular health.

Atrial fibrillation (AF) affects fewer than 1% of people under age 60, but is more prevalent in older people. It is responsible for one in four strokes after age 80, and is associated with high mortality and disability. AF refers to irregular contraction of the atrium—the chamber where blood enters the heart. AF can lead to blood stagnation and increased clotting. Warfarin, a blood-thinning medication, can reduce the risk of stroke in people with AF. People under age 60 with AF and no other stroke risk factors may benefit from aspirin. Importantly, pacemakers have no effect on the risk of stroke associated with AF.

Cholesterol imbalance: High-density lipoprotein (HDL) cholesterol is generally considered protective against ischemic stroke. Low-density lipoprotein (LDL) cholesterol, when present in excess, is considered harmful. Because LDL delivers cholesterol to cells throughout the body, excess LDL can cause cholesterol to build up in blood vessels, leading to atherosclerosis. HDL sends cholesterol to the liver to be eliminated. Clinical trials have shown that cholesterol-lowering drugs known as statins reduce the risk of stroke. However, some studies point to only a weak association between stroke and cholesterol, and there is speculation that statins reduce stroke risk by acting through some unknown mechanism.

Stroke in Infants and Children

Compared to stroke in the adult brain, stroke in the young, growing brain is associated with unique symptoms, risk factors, and outcomes—and with more uncertainty in all three of these areas. Although stroke is often considered a disease of aging, the risk of stroke in childhood is actually highest during the perinatal period, which encompasses the last few months of fetal life and the first few weeks after birth. Because the incidence of childhood stroke is relatively low, parents and doctors often mistakenly attribute these symptoms to other causes, leading to delays in diagnosis. Moreover, the time of onset is usually unknown for strokes during the perinatal period.

Investigators know less about the risk of childhood stroke than they know about the risk of adult stroke. However, well-documented risk factors include congenital (inborn) heart abnormalities, head trauma, and blood-clotting disorders. An important risk factor for African American children is sickle cell disease. Strokes during the perinatal period have been associated with premature birth, maternal infections, maternal drug abuse, prior infertility treatments, and maternal health conditions such as autoimmune disease and preeclampsia (a potentially serious combination of hypertension and kidney problems that affects about 6% of pregnant women).

The outcome of stroke in the very young is difficult to predict. A stroke during fetal development may lead to cerebral palsy—a permanent problem with body movement and muscle coordination that appears in infancy or early childhood. A stroke that occurs during infancy or childhood can also cause permanent disability. Generally, outcomes are worse in children under age one and in those who experience decreased consciousness or seizures. Fortunately, the developing brain is also known for its remarkable capacity to replace lost nerve cells and fix damaged connections between them. Healthy areas of the brain are often still pliable enough to compensate for damaged areas. A child with serious deficits immediately after a stroke can make an impressive recovery.

Stroke in Adults

From ages 55–75, the annual incidence and short-term risk of stroke are higher in men than in women. However, because women generally live longer than men, their lifetime risk of stroke is higher and they account for a larger number (about 61%) of stroke deaths each year.

Many studies show that the age-adjusted incidence of stroke is about twice as high in African Americans and Hispanic Americans as in Caucasians. Moreover, several studies have found that, on average, African and Hispanic Americans tend to experience stroke at younger ages than Caucasians. The stroke mortality rate is higher in African Americans than in Caucasians or Hispanics. The incidence of the various stroke subtypes also varies considerably in different ethnic groups.

Stroke mortality is unusually high in people living in a cluster of Southeastern states—Alabama, Arkansas, Georgia, Louisiana, Mississippi, North Carolina, South Carolina, and Tennessee—known as the stroke belt. Although clearly influenced by differences in the prevalence of known stroke risk factors, the basis for these ethnic and geographic trends is not fully understood. For example, higher rates of hypertension and diabetes explain some, but not all, of the increased stroke risk among African Americans and residents of the Stroke Belt. Socioeconomic disadvantages in income and education level also appear to play a role. However, within a given geographic area, the most disadvantaged groups do not necessarily have the highest stroke risk. Finally, the relatively high percentage of African Americans living in stroke belt states does not explain the stroke belt's existence, since Caucasians living there also have an increased risk of stroke.

Section 36.2

Stroke Treatment and Rehabilitation

Excerpted from "Stroke: Hope through Research,"
National Institute of Neurological Disorders and Stroke (NINDS),
NIH Publication No. 99–2222, updated February 10, 2010.

Medication

Medication or drug therapy is the most common treatment for stroke. The most popular classes of drugs used to prevent or treat stroke are antithrombotics (antiplatelet agents and anticoagulants) and thrombolytics.

Antithrombotics prevent the formation of blood clots that can become lodged in a cerebral artery and cause strokes. Antiplatelet drugs prevent clotting by decreasing the activity of platelets, blood cells that contribute to the clotting property of blood. These drugs reduce the risk of blood-clot formation, thus reducing the risk of ischemic stroke. In the context of stroke, physicians prescribe antiplatelet drugs mainly for prevention. The most widely known and used antiplatelet drug is aspirin. Other antiplatelet drugs include clopidogrel, ticlopidine, and dipyridamole.

Anticoagulants reduce stroke risk by reducing the clotting property of the blood. The most commonly used anticoagulants include warfarin (also known as Coumadin®), heparin, and enoxaparin (also known as Lovenox). The National Institute of Neurological Disorders and Stroke (NINDS) has sponsored several trials to test the efficacy of anticoagulants versus antiplatelet drugs. The Stroke Prevention in Atrial Fibrillation (SPAF) trial found that, although aspirin is an effective therapy for the prevention of a second stroke in most patients with atrial fibrillation, some patients with additional risk factors do better on warfarin therapy. Another study, the Trial of Org 10127 in Acute Stroke Treatment (TOAST), tested the effectiveness of low-molecular weight heparin (Org 10172) in stroke prevention. TOAST showed that heparin anticoagulants are not generally effective in preventing recurrent stroke or improving outcome.

Thrombolytic agents are used to treat an ongoing, acute ischemic stroke caused by an artery blockage. These drugs halt the stroke by dissolving the blood clot that is blocking blood flow to the brain. Recombinant tissue plasminogen activator (rt-PA) is a genetically engineered form of t-PA, a thrombolytic substance made naturally by the body. It can be effective if given intravenously within three hours of stroke symptom onset, but it should be used only after a physician has confirmed that the patient has suffered an ischemic stroke. Thrombolytic agents can increase bleeding and therefore must be used only after careful patient screening. The NINDS rt-PA Stroke Study showed the efficacy of t-PA and in 1996 led to the first Food and Drug Administration (FDA)-approved treatment for acute ischemic stroke. Other thrombolytics are currently being tested in clinical trials.

Neuro-protectants are medications that protect the brain from secondary injury caused by stroke. Although no neuro-protectants are FDA-approved for use in stroke at this time, many are in clinical trials. There are several different classes of neuro-protectants that show promise for future therapy, including glutamate antagonists, antioxidants, apoptosis inhibitors, and many others.

Surgery

Surgery can be used to prevent stroke, to treat acute stroke, or to repair vascular damage or malformations in and around the brain. There are two prominent types of surgery for stroke prevention and treatment: carotid endarterectomy and extracranial/intracranial (EC/IC) bypass.

Carotid endarterectomy is a surgical procedure in which a doctor removes fatty deposits (plaque) from the inside of one of the carotid arteries, which are located in the neck and are the main suppliers of blood to the brain. As mentioned earlier, the disease atherosclerosis is characterized by the buildup of plaque on the inside of large arteries, and the blockage of an artery by this fatty material is called stenosis. The NINDS has sponsored two large clinical trials to test the efficacy of carotid endarterectomy: the North American Symptomatic Carotid Endarterectomy Trial (NASCET) and the Asymptomatic Carotid Atherosclerosis Trial (ACAS). These trials showed that carotid endarterectomy is a safe and effective stroke prevention therapy for most people with greater than 50% stenosis of the carotid arteries when performed by a qualified and experienced neurosurgeon or vascular surgeon.

Currently, the NINDS is sponsoring the Carotid Revascularization Endarterectomy versus Stenting Trial (CREST), a large clinical trial designed to test the effectiveness of carotid endarterectomy versus a newer surgical procedure for carotid stenosis called stenting. The procedure involves inserting a long, thin catheter tube into an artery in the leg and threading the catheter through the vascular system into the narrow stenosis of the carotid artery in the neck. Once the catheter is in place in the carotid artery, the radiologist expands the stent with a balloon on the tip of the catheter. The CREST trial will test the effectiveness of the new surgical technique versus the established standard technique of carotid endarterectomy surgery.

Extracranial/intracranial (EC/IC) bypass surgery is a procedure that restores blood flow to a blood-deprived area of brain tissue by rerouting a healthy artery in the scalp to the area of brain tissue affected by a blocked artery. The NINDS-sponsored EC/IC Bypass Study tested the ability of this surgery to prevent recurrent strokes in stroke patients with atherosclerosis. The study showed that, in the long run, EC/IC does not seem to benefit these patients. The surgery is still performed occasionally for patients with aneurysms, some types of small artery disease, and certain vascular abnormalities.

Clipping: One useful surgical procedure for treatment of brain aneurysms that cause subarachnoid hemorrhage is a technique called clipping. Clipping involves clamping off the aneurysm from the blood vessel, which reduces the chance that it will burst and bleed.

Detachable coil: A new therapy that is gaining wide attention is the detachable coil technique for the treatment of high-risk intracranial aneurysms. A small platinum coil is inserted through an artery in the thigh and threaded through the arteries to the site of the aneurysm. The coil is then released into the aneurysm, where it evokes an immune response from the body. The body produces a blood clot inside the aneurysm, strengthening the artery walls and reducing the risk of rupture. Once the aneurysm is stabilized, a neurosurgeon can clip the aneurysm with less risk of hemorrhage and death to the patient.

Rehabilitation Therapy

Stroke is the number one cause of serious adult disability in the United States. Stroke disability is devastating to the stroke patient and family, but therapies are available to help rehabilitate post-stroke patients.

414

Physical therapy: For most stroke patients, physical therapy (PT) is the cornerstone of the rehabilitation process. A physical therapist uses training, exercises, and physical manipulation of the stroke patient's body with the intent of restoring movement, balance, and coordination. The aim of PT is to have the stroke patient relearn simple motor activities such as walking, sitting, standing, lying down, and the process of switching from one type of movement to another.

Occupational therapy: Another type of therapy involving relearning daily activities is occupational therapy (OT). OT also involves exercise and training to help the stroke patient relearn everyday activities such as eating, drinking, dressing, bathing, cooking, reading and writing, and toileting. The goal of OT is to help the patient become independent or semi-independent.

Speech therapy: Speech and language problems arise when brain damage occurs in the language centers of the brain. Due to the brain's great ability to learn and change (called brain plasticity), other areas can adapt to take over some of the lost functions. Speech language pathologists help stroke patients relearn language and speaking skills, including swallowing, or learn other forms of communication. Speech therapy is appropriate for any patients with problems understanding speech or written words, or problems forming speech. A speech therapist helps stroke patients help themselves by working to improve language skills, develop alternative ways of communicating, and develop coping skills to deal with the frustration of not being able to communicate fully. With time and patience, a stroke survivor should be able to regain some, and sometimes all, language and speaking abilities.

Talk therapy: Many stroke patients require psychological or psychiatric help after a stroke. Psychological problems, such as depression, anxiety, frustration, and anger, are common post-stroke disabilities. Talk therapy, along with appropriate medication, can help alleviate some of the mental and emotional problems that result from stroke. Sometimes it is also beneficial for family members of the stroke patient to seek psychological help as well.

Section 36.3

Preventing Stroke

Know Your Blood Pressure

Have your blood pressure checked at least annually. If it is elevated, work with your doctor to keep it under control. High blood pressure (hypertension) is a leading cause of stroke. You can check your blood pressure at your doctor's office, at health fairs, at home with an automatic blood pressure machine, or at your local pharmacy or supermarket. If the higher number (your systolic blood pressure) is consistently above 120 or if the lower number (your diastolic blood pressure) is consistently over 80, talk to your doctor. If your doctor decides that you have high blood pressure, she or he may recommend some changes in your diet, regular exercise, or medicine. Blood pressure drugs have improved. Once you and your doctor find the right medicine for you, it will almost never cause side effects or interfere with your quality of life.

Find Out If You Have Atrial Fibrillation

Atrial fibrillation (AF) is an irregular heartbeat that changes how your heart works and allows blood to collect in the chambers of your heart. This blood, which is not moving through your body, tends to clot. The beating of your heart can move one of these blood clots into your blood stream, and can cause a stroke. Your doctor can diagnose AF by carefully taking your pulse. AF can be confirmed or ruled out with an electrocardiogram (ECG) (a recording of the electrical activity of the heart) which can probably be done in your doctor's office. If you have AF, your doctor may choose to lower your risk for stroke by prescribing medicines called blood thinners. Aspirin and warfarin (Coumadin®) are the most commonly prescribed treatments.

If You Smoke, Stop

Smoking doubles the risk for stroke. If you stop smoking today, your risk for stroke will immediately begin to drop. Quitting smoking today can significantly reduce your risk of stroke from this factor.

If You Drink Alcohol, Do So in Moderation

Studies now show that drinking up to two alcoholic drinks per day can reduce your risk for stroke by about half. More alcohol than this each day can increase your risk for stroke by as much as three times and can also lead to liver disease, accidents and more. If you drink, we recommend no more than two drinks each day, and if you don't drink, don't start.

Remember that alcohol is a drug and it can interact with some drugs. It's a good idea to ask your doctor or pharmacist if any of the medicines you are taking could interact with alcohol.

Find Out If You Have High Cholesterol

Cholesterol is a soft, waxy fat (lipid) in the bloodstream and in all body cells. Know your cholesterol number. If your total cholesterol level (low-density lipoprotein [LDL] plus high-density lipoprotein [HDL]) is over 200, talk to your doctor. You may be at increased risk for stroke.

LDL, known as the bad cholesterol, is the form that builds up and causes plaque which may narrow arteries and limit or stop blood flow. LDL can be inherited from your family members or be a result of your body chemistry. It can also be the result of a diet high in saturated fats, lack of exercise, or diabetes. HDL is the good cholesterol that sweeps the blood and removes plaque.

Lowering your cholesterol (if elevated) may reduce your risk for stroke. High cholesterol can be controlled in many individuals with diet and exercise. Some individuals with high cholesterol may require medicine.

If You Are Diabetic

Follow your doctor's advice carefully to control your diabetes. Often, diabetes may be controlled through careful attention to what you eat. Work with your doctor and your dietitian (a health care professional who helps promote good health through proper eating) to develop a healthy eating program that fits your lifestyle. Your doctor can prescribe life-style changes and medicine that can help control your diabetes. Having diabetes puts you at an increased risk for stroke; by controlling your diabetes, you may lower your risk for stroke.

Exercise

Include exercise in your daily activities. A brisk walk for as little as 30 minutes a day can improve your health in many ways, and may reduce your risk for stroke. Try walking with a friend; this will make it more likely that you'll make it a habit. If you don't enjoy walking, choose another exercise or activity that you do enjoy, such as biking, swimming, golf, tennis, dance, or aerobics. Make time each day to take care of yourself by exercising.

Enjoy a Lower Sodium (Salt), Lower Fat Diet

By cutting down on sodium and fat in your diet, you may be able to lower your blood pressure and, most importantly, lower your risk for stroke. Work towards a balanced diet each day with plenty of fruits, vegetables, grains, and a moderate amount of protein (meat, fish, eggs, milk, nuts, tofu, and some beans). Adding fiber, such as whole grain bread and cereal products; raw, unpeeled fruits and vegetables; and dried beans, to the diet can reduce cholesterol levels by 6–19%.

Circulation Problems

Circulation is movement of the blood through the heart and blood vessels. Ask your doctor if you have circulation problems which increase your risk for stroke. Strokes can be caused by problems with your heart (pump), arteries and veins (tubes), or the blood which flows through them. Together, they are your circulation. Your doctor can check to see if you have problems in the circulation supplying blood to your brain.

Fatty deposits—caused by atherosclerosis (a hardening or buildup of cholesterol plaque and other fatty deposits in the arteries) or other diseases—can block the arteries which carry blood from your heart to your brain. These arteries, located on each side of your neck, are called carotid and vertebral arteries. This kind of blockage, if left untreated, can cause stroke. You can be tested for this problem by your doctor. Your doctor can listen to your arteries just as she or he listens to your heart, or look at x-rays called ultrasound or magnetic resonance images (MRI).

If you have blood problems such as sickle cell disease, severe anemia (lower than normal number of red blood cells), or other diseases, work with your doctor to manage these problems. Left untreated, these can cause stroke.

Circulation problems can usually be treated with medicines. If your doctor prescribes aspirin, warfarin (Coumadin®), ticlopidine (Ticlid®), clopidogrel (Plavix®), dipyridamole (Aggrenox®), or other medicine for circulation problems, take it exactly as prescribed. Occasionally, surgery is necessary to correct circulation problems such as a blocked artery.

Symptoms

If you have any stroke symptoms, seek immediate medical attention. These include:

- sudden numbness or weakness of face, arm or leg—especially on one side of the body;
- sudden confusion, trouble speaking or understanding;
- sudden trouble seeing in one or both eyes;
- sudden trouble walking, dizziness, loss of balance or coordination;
- sudden severe headache with no known cause.

If you have experienced any of these symptoms, you may have had a transient ischemic attack (TIA) or mini-stroke. Ask your doctor if you can lower your risk for stroke by taking aspirin, or by other means. If you think someone may be having a stroke, act F.A.S.T. and do this simple test:

Table 36.1. Act F.A.S.T.

Face	Ask the person to smile.
	Does one side of the face droop?
Arms	Ask the person to raise both arms.
	Does one arm drift downward?
Speech	Ask the person to repeat a simple sentence.
	Are the words slurred? Can he or she repeat the sentence correctly?
Time	If the person shows any of these symptoms, time is important.
	Call 911 or get to the hospital fast. Brain cells are dying.

Part Six

Brain Tumors

Chapter 37

Benign and Tumor-Associated Brain Cysts

Just like a cyst elsewhere in your body, a cyst in the brain is a sphere filled with fluid, similar to a miniature balloon filled with water. Cysts may contain fluid, blood, minerals, or tissue. Although cysts tend to be benign growths, they are sometimes found in parts of the brain that control vital functions, or they may be found inside malignant tumors.

The symptoms associated with a cyst in the brain depend on where the cyst is located. Each part of the brain controls a function somewhere in the body. Some parts of the brain are relatively silent, allowing a cyst to grow quite large before it causes symptoms. Other parts of the brain control functions such as swallowing, dexterity, or balance; a cyst growing in those locations may be noticed sooner than other locations. We offer extensive information about each part of the brain, what it controls, and what you might see when a tumor or cyst is present.

Computed tomography (CT) and magnetic resonance imaging (MRI) scans are used to diagnose brain cysts. CT scans show the detail of the skull bones, and provides a visual image of mineral content in or around these masses. MRI scans complement CT scanning by providing a picture of the location of the cyst in relation to the blood vessels and vital structures of the brain. When a cyst is found in the brain, there is usually only one; however, multiple tiny cysts may be found inside a malignant tumor. On a scan, a cyst has well-defined edges, as opposed to malignant tumors which have irregular borders.

There are specific types of cysts. They are named for the type of tissue from which they arise and for their contents. The most common cysts found in the brain are arachnoid, colloid, dermoid, epidermoid, and pineal cysts.

Arachnoid cyst (also called leptomeningeal cyst): An arachnoid cyst is an enlarged sphere containing cerebrospinal fluid. Arachnoid cysts are found in the subarachnoid space—the space between the arachnoid and pia mater layers of the meninges. Those layers form a membrane-like covering around the brain and spinal cord. Arachnoid cysts are thought to represent a duplication or split in these normal membranes, which creates a localized pouch of trapped cerebrospinal fluid. Arachnoid cysts can occur in both adults and children, but are most often found in infants and adolescents. They affect more males than females. Arachnoid cysts tend to be located in the area of the Sylvian fissure (a deep fold which separates the frontal, temporal and parietal lobes of the brain), the cerebellopontine angle (the corner at which the upper parts of the brain meet the lower parts), the cisterna magna (a fluid-containing space near the brain stem), or the suprasellar region (the area above the sella—a bony pouch near the center of the skull).

Treatment for an arachnoid cyst may be watchful waiting, or it may be surgery. If the cyst is small and is not causing problems, your doctor may suggest watching the cyst for a while to see if it grows. During that time, it is important to keep your appointments for follow-up scans on a regular basis, as these cysts may slowly continue to enlarge. After each scan, your doctor will compare the new scan to the old scan to monitor the size of the cyst. Some arachnoid cysts never enlarge.

If the cyst is causing symptoms or is located in a part of the brain where continued growth would cause a problem, your doctor may suggest surgery to remove the cyst. The usual procedure is to drain and attempt to remove the entire cyst, including its outermost lining. Sometimes, when this is not feasible, the surgeon will open the cyst wall to drain the contents into the normal cerebrospinal fluid pathways. If the cyst is blocking the flow of cerebrospinal fluid through the brain, a shunt may be used to help move the fluid and open these passageways. If the fluid in the cyst is aspirated through a needle, without the cyst wall being addressed, the fluid generally reaccumulates rapidly.

Colloid cyst: Although scientists are not sure exactly which cells give rise to colloid cysts, they do agree that this type of cyst begins during the embryonic formation of the central nervous system. These grape-like spheres contain a thick, gelatinous substance called colloid. As the colloid filling of the sphere increases, the size of the cyst increases. These cysts may quietly sit in the brain during childhood, not making their presence known until the adult years when they finally reach a large enough size to cause symptoms. In addition to the colloid filling, they may also contain blood, minerals, or cholesterol crystals.

Colloid cysts are typically found growing along the roof of the third ventricle (a space in the center of the brain which holds spinal fluid) or in the choroid plexus (the lining of the third ventricle). Cysts in these locations may block the flow of fluid through the brain, causing a fluid backup called hydrocephalus. As the fluid builds up in the ventricles, increased pressure occurs and causes headaches. Other symptoms may include confusion, difficulty walking, and brief interruption of consciousness.

Continued, untreated pressure from a cyst in this location may cause brain herniation or sudden death. For that reason, the first goal of therapy for a colloid cyst will be to relieve the pressure buildup. A shunt may be used to drain fluid, or surgery may be done to remove or drain the cyst. Removing the entire cyst can be challenging because of its location on or near the third ventricle. Some surgeons are exploring the use of endoscopes for operating in the ventricles; others are exploring computer-assisted surgical navigation tools for tumor removal in this area. The best treatment is still under discussion and study.

Dermoid cyst (also called dermoid): Dermoid cysts most likely form during the very early weeks of fetal growth. As an embryo is developing, the neural tube—the cells which eventually form the brain and spine—separate from the cells destined to become the skin and bones of the face, nose, and vertebrae. A dermoid cyst results when cells predestined for the face become entrapped in the brain or the spinal cord. Consequently, the inside of a dermoid cyst often contains hair follicles, bits of cartilage, or glands which produce skin oils and fats. On very rare occasions, a dermoid cyst may spontaneously open, releasing these oils into the brain or spinal cord. This event can cause a situation called chemical meningitis, in which the released contents irritate the meninges.

Dermoid cysts located in the brain are relatively rare; more often, they are found in the ovaries, spine, face, neck, or scalp. Outside the brain, they are sometimes referred to as sebaceous cysts. In the brain, these benign masses tend to be located in the posterior fossa (the lower back portion of the brain) or the neighboring meninges (the thin membranes which form the covering of the brain and spinal cord).

Dermoid cysts in the brain tend to be found in children under ten years old. In older children and young adults, they are usually located at the lower end of the spine. The cavity of the fourth ventricle and the base of the brain, under the surface of the frontal lobes, are also common sites.

The standard treatment for a dermoid cyst is surgical removal. If the lining of the cyst (the complete outer wall of the sphere) is unable to be completely removed, it will likely regrow. But that growth may be very slow, and it could be years before symptoms again return.

Epidermoid cyst (also called epidermoid, or epidermoid tumor): Epidermoid cysts, also referred to as epidermoid tumors, develop in the same manner as dermoid cysts. These masses arise when embryonic cells meant to be skin, hair, or nail tissue become entrapped in the cells forming the brain and spinal cord. The distinction between dermoid cysts and epidermoids is that epidermoid cysts do not contain hair or sebaceous glands. These cysts contain a thick yellow substance that may also contain hair, skin oils, or cholesterol crystals. As with dermoid cysts, on very rare occasions, an epidermoid cyst may spontaneously open, releasing these contents into the brain or spinal cord. Epidermoid cysts are benign masses, occurring more frequently in the brain than in the spine. They are most often found in middle-aged adults. These cysts tend to be located near the cerebellopontine angle (the area where the top part of the brain meets the brain stem), near the pituitary gland, or along the skull where they may actually grow through the skull bone.

Standard treatment of epidermoid cysts is surgical removal. If the complete cyst (including the sac-like lining of the cyst) is able to be removed, the cyst may be considered cured. If the complete lining cannot be removed, however, the cyst may begin to grow. Regrowth tends to occur slowly, often with years passing before symptoms again return. There are a few, albeit extremely rare, cases of these benign tumors transforming themselves into squamous cell cancer. If this were to occur, surgery and radiation therapy may be suggested.

Pineal cysts: Cysts in the pineal gland are found in 1–4% of people undergoing MRI for other causes. Why they develop remains unclear. They may be developmental in origin, or they may arise when the pineal gland begins the normal process of shrinkage following puberty. It is rare for pineal cysts to cause neurologic problems. When this does occur, problems arise either because there has been increased cerebrospinal fluid production or bleeding into the cyst. Symptoms may include headache and difficulty looking upwards; if hydrocephalus (blockage of fluid pathways in the brain) occurs, patients may experience sleepiness, confusion, trouble walking, and double vision. Most patients with asymptomatic pineal cysts (cysts not causing symptoms) will never experience cyst enlargement or the development of symptoms. Pineal cysts are rarely associated with underlying tumors, and typically an associated tumor is readily identified with MRI scanning. Some doctors obtain repeat scans of pineal cysts over time to make sure there is no associated tumor or cyst enlargement. Once it has been determined that there is no associated tumor, some doctors continue to recommend periodic scans to look for cyst growth. Others advocate getting further scans if, and only if, the person develops symptoms.

Tumor-associated cysts: The cysts already discussed are generally not considered neoplasms or tumors because they originate as developmental abnormalities. Both benign and malignant tumors, however, may be associated with cysts (sometimes known as tumor cysts). When a cyst is associated with an underlying tumor, the tumor is usually obvious because CT or MRI scan shows a nodule or lump adjoining the cyst. Certain benign tumors—including hemangioblastomas, pilocytic astrocytomas, and gangliogliomas—are commonly associated with cysts and are usually treated with surgery. Malignant tumors may also be associated with cysts; these tumors may require radiation and/or chemotherapy in addition to surgery, when feasible.

Frequently Asked Questions about Cysts

I've been told to wait to see if my cyst grows. Should I worry about this?

Very often, cysts do not produce any symptoms and do not enlarge over time. If a cyst is not causing symptoms and is not thought to be associated with a tumor, that patient might never develop a problem from the cyst. An operation to remove the cyst might carry a greater risk than living with the cyst. Your doctor can help you weigh the risks of watching and waiting with the risks of undergoing surgery.

Can my cyst explode if it isn't removed?

Cysts rarely produce explosive symptoms; much more commonly, a gradual increase in fluid inside a cyst leads to progressive symptoms. As mentioned, some cysts (such as dermoids and epidermoids) contain fluid that if released may be irritating to the brain or meninges. On the rare occasions that such cysts spontaneously burst and release their contents, patients may experience fever, headache, or neck stiffness.

How can the doctors tell this is a cyst, and not some type of cancerous brain tumor?

A CT, or particularly, an MRI scan of a cyst generally shows no solid or nodular components which could suggest an associated malignant tumor. Sometimes, when a cyst appears benign but the doctor cannot be 100% certain, repeated radiological studies over time will be recommended. A malignant tumor would be expected to grow over time, whereas a benign cyst might not.

What is the difference between a cyst and a tumor? Why are epidermoid cysts also called epidermoid tumors?

The term cyst refers to a fluid-filled structure, whereas a tumor consists of a mass of abnormal cells with abnormal growth potential. Cysts not associated with tumors typically have a very thin rim surrounding the fluid. When a tumor has an associated cyst, there is generally a mass, or at least a thickening of the rim, visible on CT or MRI scan. Since the growth rate of the skin cells in an epidermoid cyst is generally the same as that of normal skin, from a technical standpoint, epidermoids are more accurately classified as cysts than tumors.

It appears that surgery may, or may not, be suggested. What are the guidelines a neurosurgeon uses to make this decision?

There are no rigorous guidelines. If the cyst is causing symptoms, or it is a size that it is likely soon to cause symptoms, surgery will generally be recommended. If the cyst is associated with an undiagnosed tumor, this may be grounds for surgery. If a cyst is asymptomatic (the patient has no symptoms) and the neurosurgeon believes growth potential is low, the surgeon may recommend observation with surveillance brain scanning.

Is radiation therapy ever used to treat a cyst?

In general, radiation is used to kill dividing cells. The fluid inside a cyst does not contain dividing cells, and the cells forming the walls of most cysts (including arachnoid, colloid, dermoid, epidermoid, and pineal cysts) are not dividing. Targeting the fluid or the cyst walls would therefore not be of use. If the cyst is associated with a tumor, radiation is sometimes directed (usually from outside the body) at the tumor plus or minus the cyst wall. Rarely, in tumor-associated cysts such as craniopharyngiomas, particles emitting radiation may be injected into the cyst fluid to deliver a very high dose of radiation to the cells comprising the wall of the cyst.

What are the odds of a cyst regrowing?

It depends on what is causing the cyst. In general, if the wall of the cyst is completely removed, the chance of cyst recurrence is quite low. If the cyst is drained but the wall is left intact, the odds of fluid reaccumulating are much higher.

Can cysts be prevented?

There is nothing specifically to be done to prevent development of cysts.

What does it mean when a cyst is an incidental finding?

This means that the cyst is unlikely to be causing any symptoms, and the cyst is unrelated to what the doctor who ordered the brain scan was looking for.

Can a cyst affect your white blood cell count?

As a general rule, it would not.

Can you tell a cyst from a tumor on MRI?

A cyst may be part of a tumor, or it may exist without a tumor. Sometimes it is easy to tell if a cyst is associated with a tumor, particularly if there is a lump of excess, abnormal tissue next to a cyst. Sometimes it is very clear that a cyst is not associated with a tumor. Occasionally, it is hard to be sure—even with an MRI.

Chapter 38

Primary Brain Tumors

The brain directs the things we choose to do (like walking and talking) and the things our body does without thinking (like breathing). The brain is also in charge of our senses (sight, hearing, touch, taste, and smell), memory, emotions, and personality. The three major parts of the brain control different activities:

Cerebrum: The cerebrum uses information from our senses to tell us what is going on around us and tells our body how to respond. It controls reading, thinking, learning, speech, and emotions. The cerebrum is divided into the left and right cerebral hemispheres. The right hemisphere controls the muscles on the left side of the body. The left hemisphere controls the muscles on the right side of the body.

Cerebellum: The cerebellum controls balance for walking and standing, and other complex actions.

Brain stem: The brain stem connects the brain with the spinal cord. It controls breathing, body temperature, blood pressure, and other basic body functions.

Tumor Grades and Types

When most normal cells grow old or get damaged, they die, and new cells take their place. Sometimes, this process goes wrong. New cells form

This chapter includes excerpts from "What You Need to Know about Brain Tumors," National Cancer Institute (NCI), NIH Publication No. 09–1558, Fe bruary 2009.

431

when the body doesn't need them, and old or damaged cells don't die as they should. The buildup of extra cells often forms a mass of tissue called a growth or tumor. Primary brain tumors can be benign or malignant.

Benign brain tumors do not contain cancer cells:

- Usually, benign tumors can be removed, and they seldom grow back.

- Benign brain tumors usually have an obvious border or edge. Cells from benign tumors rarely invade tissues around them. They don't spread to other parts of the body. However, benign tumors can press on sensitive areas of the brain and cause serious health problems.

- Unlike benign tumors in most other parts of the body, benign brain tumors are sometimes life threatening.

- Benign brain tumors may become malignant.

Malignant brain tumors (also called brain cancer) contain cancer cells:

- Malignant brain tumors are generally more serious and often are a threat to life.

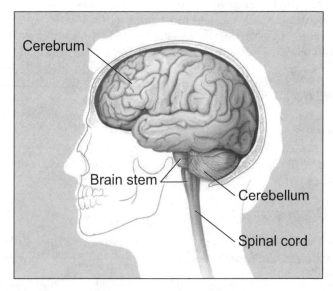

Figure 38.1. *Major Parts of the Brain*

- They are likely to grow rapidly and crowd or invade the nearby healthy brain tissue.

- Cancer cells may break away from malignant brain tumors and spread to other parts of the brain or to the spinal cord. They rarely spread to other parts of the body.

Tumor Grade

Doctors group brain tumors by grade. The grade of a tumor refers to the way the cells look under a microscope:

- Grade I: The tissue is benign. The cells look nearly like normal brain cells, and they grow slowly.

- Grade II: The tissue is malignant. The cells look less like normal cells than do the cells in a Grade I tumor.

- Grade III: The malignant tissue has cells that look very different from normal cells. The abnormal cells are actively growing (anaplastic).

- Grade IV: The malignant tissue has cells that look most abnormal and tend to grow quickly.

Cells from low-grade tumors (grades I and II) look more normal and generally grow more slowly than cells from high-grade tumors (grades III and IV).

Over time, a low-grade tumor may become a high-grade tumor. However, the change to a high-grade tumor happens more often among adults than children.

Types of Primary Brain Tumors

There are many types of primary brain tumors. Primary brain tumors are named according to the type of cells or the part of the brain in which they begin. For example, most primary brain tumors begin in glial cells. This type of tumor is called a glioma.

Adults: Common Types of Tumors

Astrocytoma: The tumor arises from star-shaped glial cells called astrocytes. It can be any grade. In adults, an astrocytoma most often arises in the cerebrum.

- Grade I or II astrocytoma: It may be called a low-grade glioma.

- Grade III astrocytoma: It's sometimes called a high-grade or an anaplastic astrocytoma.

- Grade IV astrocytoma: It may be called a glioblastoma or malignant astrocytic glioma.

Meningioma: The tumor arises in the meninges. It can be grade I, II, or III. It's usually benign (grade I) and grows slowly.

Oligodendroglioma: The tumor arises from cells that make the fatty substance that covers and protects nerves. It usually occurs in the cerebrum. It's most common in middle-aged adults. It can be grade II or III.

Children: Common Types of Tumors

Medulloblastoma: The tumor usually arises in the cerebellum. It's sometimes called a primitive neuroectodermal tumor. It is grade IV.

Grade I or II astrocytoma: In children, this low-grade tumor occurs anywhere in the brain. The most common astrocytoma among children is juvenile pilocytic astrocytoma. It's grade I.

Ependymoma: The tumor arises from cells that line the ventricles or the central canal of the spinal cord. It's most commonly found in children and young adults. It can be grade I, II, or III.

Brain stem glioma: The tumor occurs in the lowest part of the brain. It can be a low-grade or high-grade tumor. The most common type is diffuse intrinsic pontine glioma.

Risk Factors

When you're told that you have a brain tumor, it's natural to wonder what may have caused your disease. But no one knows the exact causes of brain tumors. Doctors seldom know why one person develops a brain tumor and another doesn't. Researchers are studying whether people with certain risk factors are more likely than others to develop a brain tumor. A risk factor is something that may increase the chance of getting a disease.

Studies have found the following risk factors for brain tumors:

- Ionizing radiation: Ionizing radiation from high-dose x-rays (such as radiation therapy from a large machine aimed at the head) and other sources can cause cell damage that leads to a tumor. People exposed to ionizing radiation may have an increased risk of a brain tumor, such as meningioma or glioma.

- Family history: It is rare for brain tumors to run in a family. Only a very small number of families have several members with brain tumors.

Researchers are studying whether using cell phones, having had a head injury, or having been exposed to certain chemicals at work or to magnetic fields are important risk factors. Studies have not shown consistent links between these possible risk factors and brain tumors, but additional research is needed.

Symptoms

The symptoms of a brain tumor depend on tumor size, type, and location. Symptoms may be caused when a tumor presses on a nerve or harms a part of the brain. Also, they may be caused when a tumor blocks the fluid that flows through and around the brain, or when the brain swells because of the buildup of fluid.

These are the most common symptoms of brain tumors:

- Headaches (usually worse in the morning)
- Nausea and vomiting
- Changes in speech, vision, or hearing
- Problems balancing or walking
- Changes in mood, personality, or ability to concentrate
- Problems with memory
- Muscle jerking or twitching (seizures or convulsions)
- Numbness or tingling in the arms or legs

Most often, these symptoms are not due to a brain tumor. Another health problem could cause them. If you have any of these symptoms, you should tell your doctor so that problems can be diagnosed and treated.

Diagnosis

If you have symptoms that suggest a brain tumor, your doctor will give you a physical exam and ask about your personal and family health history. You may have one or more of the following tests:

Neurologic exam: Your doctor checks your vision, hearing, alertness, muscle strength, coordination, and reflexes. Your doctor also examines your eyes to look for swelling caused by a tumor pressing on the nerve that connects the eye and the brain.

Magnetic resonance imaging (MRI): A large machine with a strong magnet linked to a computer is used to make detailed pictures of areas inside your head.

Computed tomography (CT) scan: An x-ray machine linked to a computer takes a series of detailed pictures of your head. You may receive contrast material by injection into a blood vessel in your arm or hand.

Angiogram: Dye injected into the bloodstream makes blood vessels in the brain show up on an x-ray. If a tumor is present, the x-ray may show the tumor or blood vessels that are feeding into the tumor.

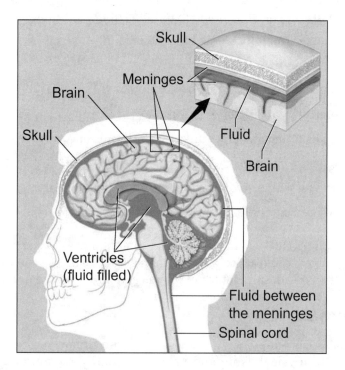

Figure 38.2. *The Brain and Nearby Structures*

Spinal tap: Your doctor may remove a sample of cerebrospinal fluid (the fluid that fills the spaces in and around the brain and spinal cord).

Biopsy: The removal of tissue to look for tumor cells is called a biopsy. A biopsy can show cancer, tissue changes that may lead to cancer, and other conditions. A biopsy is the only sure way to diagnose a brain tumor, learn what grade it is, and plan treatment. However, if the tumor is in the brain stem or certain other areas, the doctor may use MRI, CT, or other imaging tests to learn about the brain tumor.

Treatment

People with brain tumors have several treatment options. The options are surgery, radiation therapy, and chemotherapy. Many people get a combination of treatments. The choice of treatment depends mainly on the type and grade of brain tumor, its location in the brain, its size, and your age and general health. For some types of brain cancer, the doctor also needs to know whether cancer cells were found in the cerebrospinal fluid.

Your doctor can describe your treatment choices, the expected results, and the possible side effects. Because cancer therapy often damages healthy cells and tissues, side effects are common. Before treatment starts, ask your health care team about possible side effects and how treatment may change your normal activities. You and your health care team can work together to develop a treatment plan that meets your medical and personal needs.

You may want to talk with your doctor about taking part in a clinical trial, a research study of new treatment methods. Your doctor may refer you to a specialist, or you may ask for a referral.

Editor's note: For further information about treatments for brain tumors, please refer to Chapters 8–14 in *Part II: Diagnosing and Treating Brain Disorders* of this book.

Second Opinion

Before starting treatment, you might want a second opinion about your diagnosis and treatment plan. Some people worry that the doctor will be offended if they ask for a second opinion. Usually the opposite is true. Most doctors welcome a second opinion. And many health insurance companies will pay for a second opinion if you or your doctor requests it. Some companies require a second opinion.

If you get a second opinion, the doctor may agree with your first doctor's diagnosis and treatment plan. Or the second doctor may suggest another approach. Either way, you'll have more information and perhaps a greater sense of control. You can feel more confident about the decisions you make, knowing that you've looked at your options.

It may take some time and effort to gather your medical records and see another doctor. In many cases, it's not a problem to take several weeks to get a second opinion. The delay in starting treatment usually won't make treatment less effective. To make sure, you should discuss this delay with your doctor. Some people with a brain tumor need treatment right away.

There are many ways to find a doctor for a second opinion. You can ask your doctor, a local or state medical society, a nearby hospital, or a medical school for names of specialists. Also, you can request a consultation with specialists at the National Institutes of Health Clinical Center in Bethesda, Maryland, toll-free at 866-251-9686.

Care during Treatment

Nutrition: It's important for you to take care of yourself by eating well. You need the right amount of calories to maintain a good weight. You also need enough protein to keep up your strength. Eating well may help you feel better and have more energy.

Sometimes, especially during or soon after treatment, you may not feel like eating. You may be uncomfortable or tired. You may find that foods don't taste as good as they used to. In addition, the side effects of treatment (such as poor appetite, nausea, vomiting, or mouth blisters) can make it hard to eat well. Your doctor, a registered dietitian, or another health care provider can suggest ways to deal with these problems.

Supportive care: A brain tumor and its treatment can lead to other health problems. You may receive supportive care to prevent or control these problems. You can have supportive care before, during, and after cancer treatment. It can improve your comfort and quality of life during treatment. Your health care team can help you with swelling of the brain, seizures, fluid buildup in the skull, and emotional distress.

Many people with brain tumors receive supportive care along with treatments intended to slow the progress of the disease. Some decide not to have antitumor treatment and receive only supportive care to manage their symptoms.

Rehabilitation: Can be a very important part of the treatment plan. The goals of rehabilitation depend on your needs and how the tumor has affected your ability to carry out daily activities. Some people may never regain all the abilities they had before the brain tumor and its treatment. But your health care team makes every effort to help you return to normal activities as soon as possible.

Follow-up care: You'll need regular checkups after treatment for a brain tumor. For example, for certain types of brain tumors, checkups may be every three months. Checkups help ensure that any changes in your health are noted and treated if needed. If you have any health problems between checkups, you should contact your doctor.

Your doctor will check for return of the tumor. Also, checkups help detect health problems that can result from cancer treatment. Checkups may include careful physical and neurologic exams, as well as MRI or CT scans. If you have a shunt, your doctor checks to see that it's working well.

Taking Part in Cancer Research

Cancer research has led to real progress in the detection and treatment of brain tumors. Continuing research offers hope that in the future even more people with brain tumors will be treated successfully. Doctors all over the country are conducting many types of clinical trials (research studies in which people volunteer to take part). Clinical trials are designed to find out whether new approaches are safe and effective. Doctors are trying to find better ways to care for adults and children with brain tumors. They are testing new drugs and combining drugs with radiation therapy. They are also studying how drugs may reduce the side effects of treatment.

Even if the people in a trial do not benefit directly, they may still make an important contribution by helping doctors learn more about brain tumors and how to control them. Although clinical trials may pose some risks, doctors do all they can to protect their patients. If you're interested in being part of a clinical trial, talk with your doctor.

Chapter 39

Metastatic Brain Tumors

Definition: A metastatic brain tumor is brain cancer that has spread from another part of the body.

Causes

Many tumor or cancer types can spread to the brain, the most common being lung cancer, breast cancer, melanoma, kidney cancer, bladder cancer, certain sarcomas, testicular and germ cell tumors, and a number of others. Some types of cancers only spread to the brain infrequently, such as colon cancer, or very rarely, such as prostate cancer.

Brain tumors can directly destroy brain cells, or they may indirectly damage cells by producing inflammation, compressing other parts of the brain as the tumor grows, inducing brain swelling, and causing increased pressure within the skull.

Metastatic brain tumors are classified depending on the exact site of the tumor within the brain, type of tissue involved, original location of the tumor, and other factors. Infrequently, a tumor can spread to the brain, yet the original site or location of the tumor is unknown. This is called cancer of unknown primary (CUP) origin.

Metastatic brain tumors occur in about one-fourth of all cancers that metastasize (spread through the body). They are much more common than primary brain tumors. They occur in approximately 10–30% of adult cancers.

Symptoms

- Changes in sensation of a body area
- Decreased coordination, clumsiness, falls
- Emotional instability, rapid emotional changes
- Fever (sometimes)
- General ill feeling
- Headache—recent, persistent, and a new type for the person
- Lethargy
- Memory loss, impaired judgment, calculating deficiencies
- Personality changes
- Pupils of eyes are a different size
- Seizures—new for the person
- Speech difficulties
- Vision changes—double vision, decreased vision
- Vomiting—with or without nausea
- Weakness of a body area

Note: Specific symptoms vary. The symptoms commonly seen with most types of metastatic brain tumor are those caused by increased pressure in the brain.

Exams and Tests

An examination reveals neurologic changes that are specific to the location of the tumor. Signs of increased pressure within the skull are also common. Some tumors may not show symptoms until they are very large. Then, they suddenly cause rapid decline in the person's neurologic functioning.

The original (primary) tumor may already be known, or it may be discovered after an examination of tumor tissues from the brain indicates that it is a metastatic type of tumor.

- A computed tomography (CT) scan or magnetic resonance image (MRI) of the brain can confirm the diagnosis of brain tumor and identify the location of the tumor. MRI is usually better for finding tumors in the brain.

- Cerebral angiography is occasionally performed. It may show a space-occupying mass, which may or may not be highly vascular (filled with blood vessels).

- A chest x-ray, mammogram, CT scans of the chest, abdomen, and pelvis, and other tests are performed to look for the original site of the tumor.

- An electroencephalogram (EEG) may reveal abnormalities.

- An examination of tissue removed from the tumor during surgery or CT scan-guided biopsy is used to confirm the exact type of tumor. If the primary tumor can be located outside of the brain, the primary tumor is usually biopsied rather than the brain tumor.

- A lumbar puncture (spinal tap) is sometimes also performed to test the cerebral spinal fluid.

Treatment

Treatment depends on the size and type of the tumor, the initial site of the tumor, and the general health of the person. The goals of treatment may be relief of symptoms, improved functioning, or comfort.

Radiation to the whole brain is often used to treat tumors that have spread to the brain, especially if there is more than one tumor.

Surgery may be used for metastatic brain tumors when there is a single lesion and when there is no cancer elsewhere in the body. Some may be completely removed. Tumors that are deep or that infiltrate brain tissue may be debulked (removing much of the tumor's mass to reduce its size). Surgery may reduce pressure and relieve symptoms in cases when the tumor cannot be removed.

Chemotherapy for brain metastases is not as helpful as surgery or radiation for many types of cancer.

Medications for some symptoms of a brain tumor may include the following:

- Corticosteroids such as dexamethasone to reduce brain swelling

- Osmotic diuretics such as urea or mannitol to reduce brain swelling

- Anticonvulsants such as phenytoin to reduce seizures

- Pain medication

- Antacids or antihistamines to control stress ulcers

When multiple metastases (widespread cancer) are discovered, treatment may focus primarily on relief of pain and other symptoms. Comfort measures, safety measures, physical therapy, occupational therapy, and other interventions may improve the patient's quality of life. Legal advice may be helpful in forming advanced directives, such as power of attorney, in cases where continued physical or intellectual decline is likely.

Outlook (Prognosis)

In general, the probable outcome is fairly poor. For many people with metastatic brain tumors, the cancer spreads to other areas of the body. Death often occurs within two years.

Possible Complications

- Brain herniation (fatal)

- Loss of ability to function or care for self

- Loss of ability to interact

- Permanent, progressive, profound neurologic losses

When to contact a medical professional: Call your health care provider if you develop a persistent headache that is new or different for you. Call your provider or go to the emergency room if you or someone else suddenly develops stupor, vision changes, or speech impairment, or has seizures that are new or different.

References

Nguyen TD, Abrey LE. Brain metastases: old problem, new strategies. *Hematol Oncol Clin North Am.* 2007;21(2):369–388.

Nguyen TD, DeAngelis LM. Brain metastases. *Neurol Clin.* 2007;25(4):1173–1192.

Peak S, Abrey LE. Chemotherapy and the treatment of brain metastases. *Hematol Oncol Clin North Am.* 2006;20(6):1287–1295.

Chapter 40

Pituitary Tumors

The pituitary gland is a bean-sized organ located in the midline at the base of the brain, just behind the bridge of the nose, in a bony pouch called the sella turcica.

The pituitary itself is known as the master gland because it helps to control the secretion of hormones from a number of other glands and organs in the body. These include the thyroid, the adrenals, testes, and ovaries. The pituitary gland releases hormones into the blood stream, where they are carried to distant glands or organs in the body. Those distant glands release other hormones which, in turn, feed back to the brain through the bloodstream. Once back in the brain, hormones cause the hypothalamus (a part of the brain near the pituitary) to

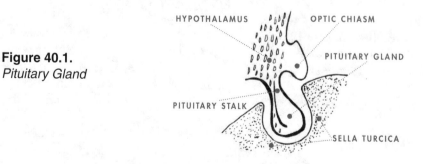

Figure 40.1.
Pituitary Gland

HYPOTHALAMUS   OPTIC CHIASM

PITUITARY GLAND

PITUITARY STALK

SELLA TURCICA

signal the pituitary gland to secrete more hormones or slow down hormone production, depending on the needs of the body. A stem-like stalk connects the pituitary gland to the hypothalamus and it is through this stalk that the hypothalamus sends signals to control the activity of the pituitary gland.

The medical term for pituitary tumors is pituitary adenoma—*adeno* means gland, *oma* means tumor. Most pituitary adenomas develop in the front two-thirds of the pituitary gland. That area is called the adenohypophysis, or the anterior pituitary. Pituitary tumors rarely develop in the rear one-third of the pituitary gland, called the neurohypophysis or the posterior pituitary. The tumors are almost always benign and are very treatable. Some tumors can be treated effectively with medications while others require surgery. Because the pituitary gland is important in the function of other glands in the body, treating a pituitary tumor requires an active coordinated multi-disciplinary health care approach, support, and follow-up care.

Incidence

Pituitary tumors account for 9–12% of all primary brain tumors, making them the third most common primary brain tumor in adults following meningiomas and the gliomas. Abnormalities including small tumors and benign cysts within the pituitary are quite common. Although

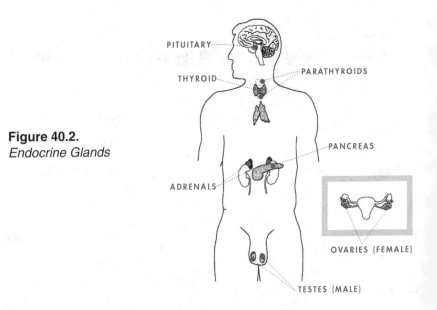

Figure 40.2.
Endocrine Glands

exact statistics are not yet available on these tumors (registries only recently began counting pituitary tumors in their data) it is estimated that 20–25% of the general population may have small, symptomless pituitary tumors. It appears that 10% of the general population will have an abnormality big enough to see on magnetic resonance imaging (MRI). These abnormalities most often do not cause symptoms and generally do not require medical or surgical therapy.

Pituitary tumors can be found in every age group, but their incidence tends to increase with age. Functioning (also called secreting) tumors most frequently occur in younger adults. Non-functioning (non-secreting) tumors tend to occur in older adults. Women are diagnosed with pituitary tumors slightly more often than men. This may be due to the tumors' interference with the female menstrual cycle, which sometimes makes symptoms more obvious.

Causes

Pituitary tumors, similar to tumors located elsewhere in the body, develop from one single abnormal cell that multiplies into many abnormal cells, eventually forming a tumor. Stimulation from the hypothalamus may also contribute to tumor growth. If your doctor determines you have a tumor, the next step is learning the type of pituitary tumor.

Types of Tumors

Pituitary tumors may be classified and named by the hormones they secrete, if any; their size; and the appearance of the tumor cells under a microscope.

Hormones: Some pituitary tumors inappropriately secrete excessive amounts of a particular hormone. These are known by several names including functioning adenomas, hormonally active adenomas, and secretory adenomas. Functioning or secreting tumors may cause the pituitary gland to ignore the signals from the hypothalamus, allowing the pituitary gland to secrete excessive amounts of hormones such as prolactin (PRL), growth hormone (GH), adrenocorticotropic hormone (ACTH), or thyroid-stimulating hormone (TSH).

Sometimes these tumors secrete more than one type of hormone. Other pituitary tumors do not over-secrete any active hormone at all and may even cause a slow down or a stoppage in hormone production (a condition called hypopituitarism). These tumors are commonly called nonfunctioning adenomas (NFAs).Other names for these nonsecreting tumors include hormonally inactive or non-secretory adenomas.

Size: Pituitary tumors are also classified by their size. Tumors appearing to be less than ten millimeters (mm), or about three-quarters inch, in diameter on an MRI scan are called microadenomas. Those larger than ten mm are called macroadenomas.

Microscopic appearance: If your tumor is surgically removed, it will be examined by a pathologist—a doctor specially trained to look at tumor cells using a microscope. The pathologist will examine the sample of tumor tissue, and provide a report to your doctor. The pathology report describes the hormone content, structure, and the cells that gave rise to your tumor. It usually takes about a week for your doctor to receive the surgical pathology report. All of this information is then used to determine your tumor type, form a treatment plan, and predict the possible future activity of the tumor.

Symptoms

Since almost 70% of pituitary tumors are functional, or secreting, tumors the most common symptoms are related to excess hormone production. Lack of menstrual periods (amenorrhea), production of breast milk without pregnancy (galactorrhea), excessive growth (acromegaly or gigantism), Cushing syndrome, or a hyperactive thyroid may be clues to the presence of a tumor in this gland. Headache, vision changes, sleep and eating disorders, and excessive thirst and urination (diabetes insipidus) may also be noted.

Do you think you have a pituitary tumor?

If you have symptoms causing you concern, begin by making an appointment to see your family doctor or your primary care physician. Explain your symptoms, and be a good historian. How long have you been experiencing the symptoms? Have they changed any since your symptoms first began? Share your concerns and your medical history. Your doctor can order a few basic tests (blood work and/or a scan) that will help determine the next step. There are many diseases that can cause hormone-related symptoms; not all of them are tumors. Your primary care physician can help you sort through your symptoms, and make the appropriate referrals if necessary. An endocrinologist may be very helpful in clarifying the diagnosis and managing medical therapy.

Diagnosis

If your doctor suspects you have a tumor, several tests are available that can help determine the diagnosis. Special blood tests can determine your hormone levels and whether the pituitary gland is the source of any excess hormone.

Following a neurological exam and endocrine screening (blood hormone levels), an MRI scan with contrast dye is used to obtain images of the pituitary gland, the sella and the area around it. In some circumstances, scans of the chest or abdomen may be necessary to verify that the hormone imbalances are caused by the pituitary gland. An ophthalmologist—a doctor specializing in visual problems—may examine your eyes if the tumor affects your eyesight, and impairs peripheral vision.

Sometimes, pituitary tumors are found incidentally. This usually means the tumor was seen on an MRI scan ordered for another, unassociated medical reason such as a sports-related accident. These symptomless tumors require careful evaluation, but may not always need immediate treatment.

Specific Tumors

Prolactinomas, or prolactin-producing adenomas: Prolactinomas represent about 30–40% of all pituitary tumors, making them the most common of these tumors. Prolactinomas are most often found in women of childbearing age. In men, prolactinomas are more frequent

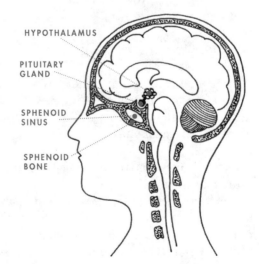

Figure 40.3.
Lateral View of the Brain

HYPOTHALAMUS

PITUITARY GLAND

SPHENOID SINUS

SPHENOID BONE

in the fourth and fifth decade of life. About half of these tumors are microadenomas, which are small tumors.

In women, high prolactin levels may cause menstruation to stop (amenorrhea) or inappropriate production of breast milk (galactorrhea) may develop. In men, prolactin-secreting tumors may cause a decreased sex drive and impotence. Men also tend to develop larger tumors which may cause headaches or vision problems.

Growth hormone-producing adenomas: These tumors represent about 20% of pituitary adenomas. Growth hormone-producing tumors are more common in men than in women. Often macroadenomas, these tumors may extend toward the cavernous sinus, an area of the brain located next to the pituitary. Mixed prolactin and growth hormone-secreting tumors are not uncommon.

Growth hormone-secreting tumors may cause gigantism in children and adolescents. In adults who have reached their full height, the hands, feet, and lower jaw become enlarged. This is called acromegaly. Excessive growth hormone can aggravate other medical conditions such as diabetes mellitus, hypertension, and heart disease.

Adrenocorticotrophic hormone (ACTH)-producing adenomas: These tumors represent about 16% of the pituitary adenomas. They are much more common in women than in men. ACTH (adrenocorticotropic hormone) stimulates the adrenal gland to make and secrete glucocorticoids, which are natural steroids. Excess glucocorticoids cause Cushing disease. Some of the symptoms of Cushing disease are a moon-shaped face, excess hair growth on the body, bruising, menstrual irregularities, and high blood pressure.

Other hypersecreting pituitary adenomas: This group represents less than 1% of pituitary adenomas. Some of these tumors excrete increased amounts of thyrotropin (thyroid-stimulating hormone).Others may secrete follicle stimulating hormone/luteinizing hormone (which controls the ovaries and testes) or alpha subunit (a glycoprotein hormone).

Non-secreting tumors: Also called non-functioning tumors, these represent about 25% of the pituitary adenomas. Null cell adenomas, oncocytomas, silent corticotroph adenomas, and gonadotroph adenomas fall into this group. These tumors grow slowly and generally cause minimal symptoms. They may be sizable before their presence is suspected. When they expand outside the sella turcica, they may press on the nearby optic nerves causing vision loss and headache. Such tumors can also compress the pituitary gland itself so it cannot produce and deliver its normal output of hormones. Called hypopituitarism, this symptom is associated with general weakness and fatigue, a pale complexion, loss of sexual function, and apathy.

Pituitary carcinoma: Cancers, or true malignancies of the tissue of the pituitary gland, are very rare. Instead, a pituitary carcinoma is usually defined as a tumor that begins in the pituitary gland and then metastasizes, or spreads, within the brain or outside the central nervous system. These tumors are generally macroadenomas which are resistant to therapy, recur locally and ultimately metastasize to the spinal canal or other organs of the body. The majority of pituitary carcinomas are functional tumors, secreting prolactin or ACTH.

Treatment

Treatment of a pituitary tumor depends on the hormonal activity of the tumor, the size and location of the tumor, as well as the age and overall health of the person with the tumor. The goals of treatment may be to remove the tumor, to reduce or control tumor size, and to re-balance hormone levels.

Surgery: If your doctor recommends surgery, the goal will be to remove as much tumor as possible. A transsphenoidal approach—literally meaning across the sphenoid sinus—is the most common. During this surgery, extremely small instruments, microscopes and endoscopes are used to remove the tumor from within the nose (endonasal) or under the lip and above the teeth (sublabial). Less often, a craniotomy may be done, during which a portion of the skull bone is temporarily removed to gain access to the pituitary gland. Some surgeons use endoscopes (a long, thin tube-like instrument) to reach the tumor.

Your neurosurgeon will speak with you about the surgery planned for your tumor, the risks and benefits of the procedure, and your follow-up care. The American Brain Tumor Association offers a free publication, titled *Surgery*, which explains the different surgical tools available, how procedures are planned, and questions to ask your physician about the procedure recommended for you. If you would like a copy, please call 800-886-2282.

Radiation therapy or radiosurgery: Radiation therapy is often used as a second, or adjuvant, treatment for pituitary tumors. It may be given in addition to surgery or drug therapy. Radiation therapy may be used to treat tumors that have regrown, or it may be used for aggressive tumors. The goal of radiation therapy for pituitary tumors is to reduce or control tumor size; however, it may take several months or longer before the effects of this treatment cause a change in your hormone levels or your MRI scan. There are several different types of radiation therapy; your doctor will decide which is best for your tumor. Conventional external beam radiation is standard radiation given five days a week for five or six weeks. Stereotactic radiosurgery is focused radiation therapy.

The Gamma Knife, LINAC (modified linear accelerators), CyberKnife, and proton beam radiation are all forms of stereotactic radiosurgery. Conformal photon radiation, also known as intensity-modulated radiation therapy, shapes radiation beams to the contours of the tumor. If your doctor thinks your tumor would be best treated with radiation, he or she can initiate an appropriate referral, and can speak with you about the type of therapy suggested and the effects of that particular treatment.

Drug therapy: There are several drugs used to treat pituitary tumors. The drug chosen will depend on the hormone functions of the tumor.

Dopamine agonists, such as bromocriptine (Parlodel) or cabergoline, are used to control the production of prolactin. The drugs reduce tumor size by reducing the amount of prolactin made by the pituitary gland. Most people with prolactin-secreting tumors require long-term therapy to control the size of their tumor; generally, if the medication is stopped prolactin levels begin to increase. In a small percent of people with very small tumors, treatment may be stopped after a year or so to see if the tumor regrows. Those with very high prolactin levels may find that drug therapy decreases their hormone levels but does not relieve all of their symptoms. In these situations, the drug successfully lowers the prolactin level but the level may still be higher than normal, thus causing symptoms.

Somatostatin analogues such as octreotide (Sandostatin or Sandostatin LAR, or Lanreotide) can reduce growth hormone levels and relieve the associated symptoms. These drugs may also be used to control the production of thyroid-stimulating hormone in thyrotrophic tumors. Dopamine agonists, such as those listed, can be given to treat growth-hormone secreting tumors, but their effect is primarily relief of symptoms rather than reduction of hormone levels to normal.

A growth hormone receptor antagonist drug called pegvisomant is highly effective in normalizing a protein called IGF-1, found in elevated levels in people with acromegaly, but is not yet in general use. New drugs are being tested in research studies called clinical trials; information about those trials can be found through your endocrinologist.

Ketoconazole (Nizoral) is used to treat ACTH secreting tumors that produce Cushing disease. This drug lowers cortisol (natural steroid) production, but generally does not reduce the size of the tumor or inhibit its activity, and is not suitable for long-term treatment.

Follow-Up Care

Once you recover from surgery or radiation therapy, or begin medical treatment, your doctors will determine a schedule for follow-up MRI scans and endocrine testing. These are used to monitor the effectiveness of therapy, assure normal hormonal balance, and watch for possible tumor re-growth.

Many people with pituitary tumors are followed regularly by an endocrinologist—a physician specially trained in the treatment of disorders of the hormone-producing glands. Hormone imbalances can be caused by the tumor itself, or may result from the treatment necessary to control the tumor. The endocrinologist will monitor your hormone blood levels, outline a treatment plan, and make drug adjustments when needed. The endocrinologist becomes an active member of your health care team, working closely with your neurosurgeon and your primary care physician.

Although pituitary tumors are almost always benign, they can recur, and therefore periodic follow-up MRI scans are necessary. Your doctor will tell you how often those scans should be done. If you do not know when your next MRI should be scheduled, call your doctor's office to ask.

Chapter 41

Childhood Brain Tumors

A childhood brain or spinal cord tumor is a disease in which abnormal cells form in the tissues of the brain or spinal cord. There are many types of childhood brain and spinal cord tumors. The tumors are formed by the abnormal growth of cells and may begin in different areas of the brain or spinal cord. Tumors may be benign (noncancerous) or malignant (cancerous).

Brain and spinal cord tumors are a common type of childhood cancer. Although cancer is rare in children, brain and spinal cord tumors are the third most common type of childhood cancer, after leukemia and lymphoma. Brain tumors can occur in both children and adults. Treatment for children is usually different than treatment for adults.

Types of Childhood Brain Tumors

There are different types of childhood brain tumors. Childhood brain tumors are named based on the type of cell they formed in and where the tumor first formed in the central nervous system (CNS).

Astrocytomas: Childhood astrocytomas are tumors that form in cells called astrocytes. They can be low-grade or high-grade tumors. The grade of the tumor describes how abnormal the cancer cells look

This chapter is excerpted from "Childhood Brain and Spinal Cord Tumors Treatment Overview (PDQ®): Patient Version." PDQ® Cancer Information Summary. National Cancer Institute; Bethesda, MD. Updated October 15, 2009. Available at: http://www.cancer.gov. Accessed January 7, 2010.

under a microscope and how quickly the tumor is likely to grow and spread. High-grade astrocytomas are fast-growing, malignant tumors. Low-grade astrocytomas are slow-growing tumors that are less likely to be malignant.

Atypical teratoid/rhabdoid tumor: Childhood atypical teratoid/rhabdoid tumors are fast-growing tumors that often form in the cerebellum. They may also form in other parts of the brain and in the spinal cord.

Brain stem glioma: Childhood brain stem gliomas form in the brain stem (the part of the brain connected to the spinal cord).

Central nervous system (CNS) embryonal tumor: Childhood CNS embryonal tumors form in brain and spinal cord cells when the fetus is beginning to develop. They include the following types of tumors:

- CNS atypical teratoid/rhabdoid tumors

- Ependymoblastoma

- Medulloblastoma

- Medulloepithelioma

- Pineal parenchymal tumors

- Pineoblastoma

- Supratentorial primitive neuroectodermal tumors (SPNET)

CNS germ cell tumor: Childhood CNS germ cell tumors form in germ cells, which are cells that develop into sperm or ova (eggs). There are different types of childhood germ cell tumors. These include germinomas, embryonal yolk sac carcinomas, choriocarcinomas, and teratomas. A mixed germ cell tumor has two types of germ cell tumors in it. Germ cell tumors can be either benign or malignant.

Germ cell brain tumors usually form in the center of the brain, near the pineal gland. The pineal gland is a tiny organ in the brain that makes melatonin, which is a substance that helps control the sleeping and waking cycle. Germ cell tumors can spread to other parts of the brain and spinal cord.

Craniopharyngioma: Childhood craniopharyngiomas are tumors that usually form just above the pituitary gland. The pituitary gland is found in the center of the brain behind the back of the nose. It is about the size of a pea and controls many important body functions including growth. Craniopharyngiomas rarely spread, but may affect important areas of the brain, such as the pituitary gland.

Ependymoma: Childhood ependymomas are slow-growing tumors formed in cells that line the fluid-filled spaces in the brain and spinal cord.

Medulloblastoma: Childhood medulloblastomas form in the cerebellum.

Supratentorial primitive neuroectodermal tumor: Childhood supratentorial primitive neuroectodermal tumors (SPNET) form in immature cells in the cerebrum.

Cause and Symptoms

The cause of most childhood brain tumors is unknown. The symptoms of childhood brain and spinal cord tumors are not the same in every child. Headaches and other symptoms may be caused by childhood brain tumors. Other conditions may cause the same symptoms. A doctor should be consulted if any of the following problems occur:

- Morning headache or headache that goes away after vomiting
- Frequent nausea and vomiting
- Vision, hearing, and speech problems
- Loss of balance and trouble walking
- Unusual sleepiness or change in activity level
- Unusual changes in personality or behavior
- Seizures
- Increase in the head size (in infants)

In addition to these symptoms of brain tumors, some children are unable to reach certain growth and development milestones such as sitting up, walking, and talking in sentences.

Diagnosis

Tests that examine the brain are used to detect (find) childhood brain tumors. The following tests and procedures may be used:

457

Physical exam and history: An exam of the body to check general signs of health, including checking for signs of disease, such as lumps or anything else that seems unusual. A history of the patient's health habits and past illnesses and treatments will also be taken.

Neurological exam: A series of questions and tests to check the brain, spinal cord, and nerve function. The exam checks a person's mental status, coordination, and ability to walk normally, and how well the muscles, senses, and reflexes work. This may also be called a neuro exam or a neurologic exam.

Serum tumor marker test: A procedure in which a sample of blood is examined to measure the amounts of certain substances released into the blood by organs, tissues, or tumor cells in the body. Certain substances are linked to specific types of cancer when found in increased levels in the blood. These are called tumor markers.

MRI (magnetic resonance imaging) with gadolinium: A procedure that uses a magnet, radio waves, and a computer to make a series of detailed pictures of the brain and spinal cord. A substance called gadolinium is injected into a vein. The gadolinium collects around the cancer cells so they show up brighter in the picture. This procedure is also called nuclear magnetic resonance imaging (NMRI).

CT scan (CAT scan): A procedure that makes a series of detailed pictures of areas inside the body, taken from different angles. The pictures are made by a computer linked to an x-ray machine. A dye may be injected into a vein or swallowed to help the organs or tissues show up more clearly. This procedure is also called computed tomography, computerized tomography, or computerized axial tomography.

Angiogram: A procedure to look at blood vessels and the flow of blood in the brain. A contrast dye is injected into the blood vessel. As the contrast dye moves through the blood vessel, x-rays are taken to see if there are any blockages.

PET scan (positron emission tomography scan): A procedure to find malignant tumor cells in the body. A small amount of radioactive glucose (sugar) is injected into a vein. The PET scanner rotates around the body and makes a picture of where glucose is being used in the body. Malignant tumor cells show up brighter in the picture because they are more active and take up more glucose than normal cells do.

Most childhood brain tumors are diagnosed and removed in surgery: If doctors think there might be a brain tumor, a biopsy may be done to remove a sample of tissue. For tumors in the brain, the biopsy is done by removing part of the skull and using a needle to remove a sample of tissue. A pathologist views the tissue under a microscope to look for cancer cells. If cancer cells are found, the doctor may remove as much tumor as safely possible during the same surgery. The pathologist checks the cancer cells to find out the type and grade of brain tumor. The grade of the tumor is based on how abnormal the cancer cells look under a microscope and how quickly the tumor is likely to grow and spread.

The following tests may be done on the sample of tissue that is removed:

- Immunohistochemistry study: A laboratory test in which a substance such as an antibody, dye, or radioisotope is added to a sample of cancer tissue to test for certain antigens. This type of study is used to tell the difference between different types of cancer.

- Light and electron microscopy: A laboratory test in which cells in a sample of tissue are viewed under regular and high-powered microscopes to look for certain changes in the cells.

- Cytogenetic analysis: A laboratory test in which cells in a sample of tissue are viewed under a microscope to look for certain changes in the chromosomes.

Some childhood brain and spinal cord tumors are diagnosed by imaging tests. Sometimes a biopsy or surgery cannot be done safely because of where the tumor formed in the brain or spinal cord. These tumors are diagnosed based on the results of imaging tests and other procedures.

Prognosis: Certain factors affect prognosis (chance of recovery). The prognosis (chance of recovery) depends on the whether there are any cancer cells left after surgery; the type of tumor; the location of the tumor; the child's age; and whether the tumor has just been diagnosed or has recurred (come back).

Stages of Childhood Brain and Spinal Cord Tumors

In childhood brain tumors, treatment options are based on several factors. Staging is the process used to find how much cancer there is and if cancer has spread within the brain, spinal cord, or to other parts of the body. It is important to know the stage in order to plan cancer treatment. In childhood brain tumors, there is no standard staging system. Instead, the plan for cancer treatment depends on several factors including: the type of tumor and where the tumor formed in the brain, whether the tumor is newly diagnosed or recurrent, the grade of the tumor, and the tumor risk group.

The information from tests and procedures done to detect (find) childhood brain tumors is used to determine the tumor risk group. After the tumor is removed in surgery, some of the tests used to detect childhood brain and spinal cord tumors are repeated to help determine the tumor risk group. This is to find out how much tumor remains after surgery. Other tests and procedures may be done to find out if cancer has spread include lumbar puncture, bone scan, chest x-ray, and bone marrow aspiration.

The three ways that cancer spreads in the body are through tissue, the lymph system, and the blood. When cancer cells break away from the primary (original) tumor and travel through the lymph or blood to other places in the body, another (secondary) tumor may form. This process is called metastasis. The secondary (metastatic) tumor is the same type of cancer as the primary tumor. For example, if breast cancer spreads to the bones, the cancer cells in the bones are actually breast cancer cells. The disease is metastatic breast cancer, not bone cancer.

Recurrent Childhood Brain Tumors

A recurrent childhood brain tumor is one that has recurred (come back) after it has been treated. Childhood brain tumors may come back in the same place or in another part of the brain. Sometimes they may come back in another part of the body. The tumor may come back many years after first being treated. Diagnostic and staging tests and procedures, including biopsy, may be done to confirm the tumor has recurred.

Treatment Option Overview

Different types of treatment are available for children with brain tumors. Some treatments are standard (the currently used treatment), and some are being tested in clinical trials. A treatment clinical trial is a research study meant to help improve current treatments or obtain information on new treatments for patients with cancer. When clinical trials show that a new treatment is better than the standard treatment, the new treatment may become the standard treatment. Because cancer in children is rare, taking part in a clinical trial should be considered. Clinical trials are taking place in many parts of the country. Some clinical trials are open only to patients who have not started treatment.

Children with brain tumors should have their treatment planned by a team of health care providers who are experts in treating childhood brain and spinal cord tumors. Treatment will be overseen by a pediatric oncologist, a doctor who specializes in treating children with cancer. The pediatric oncologist works with other health care providers who are experts in treating children with brain tumors and who specialize in certain areas of medicine.

Symptoms caused by treatment may begin during or right after treatment. Some cancer treatments cause side effects months or years after treatment has ended. These are called late effects. Late effects of cancer treatment may include physical problems; changes in mood, feelings, thinking, learning, or memory; and second cancers (new types of cancer). Some late effects may be treated or controlled. It is important to talk with your child's doctors about the effects cancer treatment can have on your child.

Three types of standard treatment are surgery, radiation therapy, and chemotherapy. New types of treatment are being tested in clinical trials. One of these is high-dose chemotherapy with stem cell transplant which is a way of giving high doses of chemotherapy and replacing blood-forming cells destroyed by cancer treatment.

Clinical trial: Patients may want to think about taking part in a clinical trial. For some patients, taking part in a clinical trial may be the best treatment choice. Clinical trials are part of the cancer research process. Clinical trials are done to find out if new cancer treatments are safe and effective or better than the standard treatment. Many of today's standard treatments for cancer are based on earlier clinical trials. Patients who take part in a clinical trial may receive the standard treatment or be among the first to receive a new treatment. Patients who take part in clinical trials also help improve the way cancer will be treated in the future. Even when clinical trials do not lead to effective new treatments, they often answer important questions and help move research forward.

Patients can enter clinical trials before, during, or after starting their cancer treatment. Some clinical trials only include patients who have not yet received treatment. Other trials test treatments for patients

461

whose cancer has not gotten better. There are also clinical trials that test new ways to stop cancer from recurring (coming back) or reduce the side effects of cancer treatment.

Clinical trials are taking place in many parts of the country.

Follow-up care: Some of the tests that were done to diagnose the cancer or to find out the stage of the cancer may be repeated. Some tests will be repeated in order to see how well the treatment is working. Decisions about whether to continue, change, or stop treatment may be based on the results of these tests. This is sometimes called re-staging.

Some of the tests will continue to be done from time to time after treatment has ended. The results of these tests can show if your condition has changed or if the cancer has recurred (come back). These tests are sometimes called follow-up tests or check-ups.

Chapter 42

Living with a Brain Tumor

Chapter Contents

Section 42.1

Managing Fatigue

"Conquering Fatigue," © 2008 American Brain Tumor Association
(www.abta.org). Reprinted with permission.

When you have a brain tumor, the words "I'm tired" have a profound meaning. Your fatigue may be unlike anything you've ever experienced. You may rest and sleep for a significant period of time and yet still feel exhausted. You actually may feel worse after a nap or night's rest. In fact, the exhaustion may be so persistent that it interferes with your ability to adequately function, affecting your quality of life and perhaps that of your family.

Fortunately, fatigue has come to the forefront of brain tumor treatment. It is a symptom that can be managed. By working with your doctor and healthcare team to identify how the fatigue is affecting you and its potential cause or causes, and by following important steps to help you conserve and improve energy, you may be able to minimize your fatigue and more effectively adapt to your new abilities.

Determine How the Fatigue Affects You

A brain tumor and related treatment can cause physical, mental, and social exhaustion.

- Physical fatigue affects your stamina, strength, and endurance. You may have energy but not strength, or strength but not stamina. You may feel strong in the morning, but lose energy as the day continues. This physical exhaustion may occur in addition to other physical changes or limitations caused by the brain tumor.

- Mental fatigue limits your ability to focus, remember, and block out noise and distraction. In addition, you may feel easily overwhelmed or have difficulty making decisions. As all of these challenges directly affect your ability to solve problems, set goals, and accomplish tasks on your own terms. Fatigue can also be extremely frustrating, causing irritability and impatience.

- Social fatigue can cause you to avoid friends or social outings. While family relationships and roles often change after a brain tumor diagnosis, social fatigue may cause you to avoid friends for fear of not having enough energy to fully participate in an outing or event, or cause concern about not finding the right word during a conversation. In these situations, you may find it easier to avoid social contact and communication altogether. That solution can be isolating.

Identify the Possible Causes of Your Fatigue

It's critical to review all possible causes of fatigue with your doctor and health care team, including:

The brain tumor itself can cause physical and mental fatigue, which may or may not diminish over time.

Related treatment—surgery, radiation, chemotherapy, steroids, and other cancer-related drugs (especially those with sedative properties)—all may cause or exacerbate your exhaustion. With radiation, the fatigue may build then slowly diminish. In contrast, exhaustion from chemotherapy often comes and goes, and is more consistent. In addition, chemotherapy may exacerbate or cause mental exhaustion affecting your memory, and ability to focus and solve problems. Some chemotherapy can cause a drop in red blood cell counts (anemia) which also causes fatigue. A drop in white cell counts can cause infection, which can also be linked to fatigue.

Other conditions—such as diabetes, heart disease, or respiratory issues—also may cause fatigue. It's not unusual for patients and medical staff to focus so intently on the cancer that they inadvertently overlook the treatment of other conditions. Other possible causes of fatigue can include dehydration, especially in warmer months; and a hormone or electrolyte imbalance either from a nutritional deficiency or medication. A lack of exercise and mobility or prolonged bed rest also may cause or contribute to profound fatigue, as can sleep disruption caused by medication or changes in melatonin.

Medications, or medication interactions, may cause or contribute to your fatigue. Check with your pharmacist to review your prescriptions; a lower dosage or alternative medication may reduce fatigue.

465

Depression is sometimes blamed for mental fatigue. If you experience ongoing feelings of hopelessness, shame, anxiety, and guilt, you indeed may be depressed. In addition, a profound loss of motivation or interest in activities that used to bring you joy—gardening, spending time with grandchildren, and so forth—are red flags for depression and signal the need for a formal evaluation. Call your doctor, nurse, or social worker for resources to manage depression.

Suggestions for Conquering Fatigue

Conserve energy: If you are frequently exhausted, you may find yourself trying to do everything during the days or times when have energy. Instead, try to optimize, conserve, and plan your energy use. A daily journal can help you determine your energy pattern. During low-energy periods, ask for help from neighbors and friends, and only focus on completing tasks and activities that are truly a personal priority. During high-energy periods, choose one or two activities—don't try to do it all.

Get enough sleep: When possible, maintain a regular sleep schedule: go to bed and wake up at approximately the same time every day. Exercising, avoiding caffeine and alcohol, and keeping stress and distractions out of the bedroom, can also improve your sleep patterns and limit fatigue.

Keep moving: Exercise or keep moving whenever it is physically possible for you to do so. Choose activities that are easy for you, such as walking, swimming, seated yoga, or other low-impact exercises. Even sitting and lifting weights along with a television exercise program can be beneficial.

Know your limitations: To optimally manage your fatigue you need to acknowledge your physical and emotional limitations. Develop an exercise routine that reflects your new physical abilities. For example, if you easily become dizzy or weak, do not exercise in a place or on an apparatus where you could easily fall. Choose group activities so someone will always be around for safety and socialization. If your energy levels are unpredictable, choose to associate with friends and family members who are flexible and willing to put your needs first.

Rethink expectations: To make the most of your new energy level, you will need to rethink your goals. Initially you may need to mourn the loss of your former self and adjust to your new normal. There may be days, months and weeks when you feel like you have no purpose. During these times, take a break and do something that you enjoy: Sit by the pool, work in your garden, or water your flowers. Continue your pursuit of enjoyment and leisure.

Use nature to restore energy: Nature can be the simplest, most effective way to restore energy. As often as possible, go outside to explore and tap into the fascination and restorative powers of nature.

Section 42.2

Cognitive Changes

"Cognitive Retraining," © 2006 American Brain Tumor Association (www.abta.org). Reprinted with permission.

Becoming Well through Cognitive Retraining

When we use the word cognitive, we mean our thinking, reasoning, and perceptual abilities. Cognitive rehabilitation has two parts: restoring the actual cognitive skill and learning to use strategies to compensate for the impaired ability.

The first part of cognitive retraining—restoring skills—is sometimes compared to rebuilding a weakened muscle. Exercises used in retraining programs may actually rebuild cognitive skills such as attention, concentration, memory, organization, perception, judgment, and problem solving. These exercises can include computer programs designed to improve visual-perceptual skills (our ability to correctly interpret what we see), reaction time, memory, and attention. A large chalk board or a practice grocery store shelf can be used to practice visual scanning and visual attention skills. Workbooks and puzzle books can help with reasoning, mathematical skills, memory, and visual-perceptual skills. These items can be found at teachers' stores or large discount stores such as K-Mart or Wal-Mart. It is important that the materials selected are neither too difficult nor too easy. Strategic games, such as Uno are also an excellent way to work on a variety of cognitive skills while interacting with others.

The therapy setting itself offers many opportunities to practice cognitive skills. Therapists can develop personalized tasks that require thinking on your feet and more closely simulate your real life situations. For example, for those who prepare meals, therapy may include using the program facility's kitchen to practice following a simple recipe or to plan, in sequence, a more complex meal.

For those whose jobs require organizational skills, the therapist may suggest using a checklist format to complete complex tasks or using the copy machine to practice planning skills and problem solving skills. One of our favorite activities involves patients organizing and ordering lunch from a local restaurant. This works on the skills required making and following a plan of action, the ability to keep track of details, and staying focused on a cognitive task. Another good way to work on memory is to ask the patient to relay a message, later in the day, to another therapist.

These are just a small sample of the activities and exercises available to rebuild cognitive skills. Working with a therapist allows selected tasks to be supervised and tailored to each patient's needs, strengths, and functional levels.

The second component of cognitive retraining is learning to use strategies, compensatory techniques, or tools to cope with weaker areas. Strategies are designed for each patient using his or her areas of strength to compensate for weaker skill areas. Learning to use these tools not only compensates for impaired ability, but may help to rebuild the skill itself. For example, using a checklist may actually improve attention skills. The following strategies are some of the other tools we find helpful for our patients.

Memory strategies: Take written notes and make certain that notes contain accurate, complete information. Including who, what, where, when, and why, helps to ensure that notes have all the critical data. Refer to your notes regularly. Use association, visualization, repetition, rehearsal, and categorization to help with recall. Use a daily planner system to keep track of all information. It is too complicated to try and locate information that is recorded in several different places. Use a daily or weekly pill box to keep track of medication. Arrange items in an organized fashion and place them in strategic, easy-to-see locations. Consider using a tape recorder to record lengthy and important conversations.

Attention strategies: Organizing your environment will help you maintain control. Use a self-talking technique to stay on track. For example, ask yourself "Am I wandering?" or "What should I be doing right now?" To improve your attention while listening to someone, make constant eye contact with the speaker, ask the speaker to slow down, request clarification or repetition, take notes, and ask the speaker to provide the information in an alternate way—such as in writing or with pictures. Make a checklist for lengthy tasks and check off each item as it is completed. Be sure to double check all work. Avoid fatigue: when activities start to become overwhelming or frustrating, stop and take a mental break. Reduce distractions as much as possible, turn off the radio or television, or close the door.

Problem solving strategies: List several solutions to a given situation, and then list the pros and cons before deciding upon the best option. Ask yourself, "What else could I do?" and consider asking for someone else's opinion. Review the steps needed to solve the problem. Evaluate the success of the outcome.

Organization strategies: Make a checklist. If a task is large or complex break it down into smaller parts and make a checklist for each part. Make a verbal or written pre-plan. Prepare the work area with necessary materials. Eliminate clutter. Spend time making a daily plan using your planner system. Most people like to plan their day early in the morning when things tend to be quiet. Remember to prioritize tasks and pace yourself. Plan to work on more demanding tasks when your energy level is highest. Make and use to-do lists.

Strategies for impulsiveness: Give yourself permission to take the time to think through tasks. Complete one task before beginning another, and use your checklist. Pause and think before acting (count to five or ten). If you become confused by a task, take a time-out before you become frustrated.

An important part of therapy is training and education of caregivers. It is important that those who spend the most time with the patient understand these cognitive strategies and encourage their use. Consistent practice of learned strategies is critical to becoming proficient in their use. Patience is the key word. It takes time for the brain to heal, and it takes time to learn new ways to do familiar things. The results are worth the effort.

If you are interested in learning more, speak with your doctor. He or she can make a referral to a rehabilitation facility offering these programs, or refer you to an individual practitioner in your area.

Section 42.3

Returning to Work

"Returning to Work," © 2009 American Brain Tumor Association
(www.abta.org). Reprinted with permission.

Due to innovations in surgery, new chemotherapies, and localized radiation techniques, more and more brain tumor survivors are choosing to work during treatment, or return to work soon after. While working with a brain tumor can present its share of challenges, there are strategies that may help you maintain your productivity.

Depending on the location or type of brain tumor, different skills and functions may change. Therefore, it is important that you take an honest inventory of your ability to do the following:

1. Remember information.

2. Organize, multi-task, and problem-solve.

3. Make decisions.

4. Focus on details.

5. Function and process information.

If difficulties with some of these functions are affecting you or your loved ones work productivity, the following tips may help:

1. Keep work-related goals realistic and reflective of any changes you may be experiencing in terms of memory, attention, judgment, organization, and processing speed. Revisit your goals often to make sure they are feasible and manageable.

2. Seek out professional help from a social worker, career counselor, or neuropsychologist. A neuropsychologist can perform testing to help determine if there are limitations in these areas. He or she can also provide compensation strategies which can help you to stay organized and work more efficiently.

3. Consider vocational rehabilitation services. Vocational services can be a great resource for help with a job search, resume

writing, career exploration, skills assessment, and career counseling. For more information, contact the Department of Rehabilitation Services in your state.

4. Get some advice from fellow brain tumor survivors on how you can adapt to changes and cope with work productivity issues. Networking with others through in-person, telephone, and online support groups can provide rich information and wonderful support.

5. Reduce stress levels. Try exercise (even mild exercise will help), get enough sleep, learn meditation, or use deep breathing, or other various stress management techniques. If you are less stressed out at work, you will perform better.

6. Try slowing down, which can help to reduce errors on the job. Think things through one step at a time. Take your time. Try not to multi-task until you can successfully manage one task at a time.

7. If you feel comfortable disclosing your personal health care information, discuss your needs with your supervisor and co-workers. Also, consider requesting reasonable accommodations for your work environment.

8. Be informed. Know your rights as an employee and what you are entitled to, but make sure to be very cautious especially in the current economic environment.

9. Do something you enjoy to help improve your mood. Try a recreational activity or hobby to help boost your energy and self-esteem. If you feel better about yourself, you will perform better.

10. Talk with your doctor about any changes in your mood or attention span to see if there are any medications or additional resources that may be of help to you.

Most of all, it is important to remain optimistic. Through your own efforts, you can adapt to many of the work-related challenges you may experience. Just remember, to be patient and realistic of what you can expect from yourself.

Part Seven

Degenerative Brain Disorders

Chapter 43

Dementias

Chapter Contents

Section 43.1

Dementia Types, Causes, and Treatments

Text in this section is excerpted from "Dementia: Hope through Research," National Institute of Neurological Disorders and Stroke (NINDS), updated February 12, 2010.

Dementia is not a specific disease. It is a descriptive term for a collection of symptoms that can be caused by a number of disorders that affect the brain. People with dementia have significantly impaired intellectual functioning that interferes with normal activities and relationships. They also lose their ability to solve problems and maintain emotional control, and they may experience personality changes and behavioral problems such as agitation, delusions, and hallucinations. While memory loss is a common symptom of dementia, memory loss by itself does not mean that a person has dementia. Doctors diagnose dementia only if two or more brain functions—such as memory, language skills, perception, or cognitive skills including reasoning and judgment—are significantly impaired without loss of consciousness.

There are many disorders that can cause dementia. Some, such as Alzheimer disease (AD), lead to a progressive loss of mental functions. But other types of dementia can be halted or reversed with appropriate treatment. With AD and many other types of dementia, disease processes cause many nerve cells to stop functioning, lose connections with other neurons, and die. In contrast, normal aging does not result in the loss of large numbers of neurons in the brain.

Different Kinds of Dementia

Dementing disorders can be classified many different ways. These classification schemes attempt to group disorders that have particular features in common, such as whether they are progressive or what parts of the brain are affected. Some frequently used classifications include the following:

Cortical dementia: The brain damage primarily affects the brain's cortex, or outer layer. Cortical dementias tend to cause problems with memory, language, thinking, and social behavior.

Subcortical dementia: Affects parts of the brain below the cortex. Subcortical dementia tends to cause changes in emotions and movement in addition to problems with memory.

Progressive dementia: Gets worse over time, gradually interfering with more and more cognitive abilities.

Primary dementia: Dementia such as AD that does not result from any other disease.

Secondary dementia: Occurs as a result of a physical disease or injury.

Some types of dementia fit into more than one of these classifications. For example, AD is considered both a progressive and a cortical dementia.

Alzheimer disease is the most common cause of dementia in people aged 65 and older.

Vascular dementia is the second most common cause of dementia, after AD. It accounts for up to 20% of all dementias and is caused by brain damage from cerebrovascular or cardiovascular problems—usually strokes.

Lewy body dementia (LBD) is one of the most common types of progressive dementia. LBD usually occurs sporadically, in people with no known family history of the disease.

Frontotemporal dementia (FTD), sometimes called frontal lobe dementia, describes a group of diseases characterized by degeneration of nerve cells—especially those in the frontal and temporal lobes of the brain. Experts believe FTD accounts for 2–10% of all cases of dementia.

Other conditions that can cause dementia include reactions to medications, metabolic problems and endocrine abnormalities, nutritional deficiencies, infections, subdural hematomas, poisoning, brain tumors, anoxia, and heart and lung problems.

Causes of Dementia

All forms of dementia result from the death of nerve cells and/or the loss of communication among these cells. The human brain is a very complex and intricate machine and many factors can interfere with its functioning. Researchers have uncovered many of these factors, but they have not yet been able to fit these puzzle pieces together in order to form a complete picture of how dementias develop.

Many types of dementia, including AD, Lewy body dementia, Parkinson dementia, and Pick disease, are characterized by abnormal structures called inclusions in the brain. Because these inclusions, which contain abnormal proteins, are so common in people with dementia, researchers suspect that they play a role in the development of symptoms. However, that role is unknown, and in some cases the inclusions may simply be a side effect of the disease process that leads to the dementia.

Genes clearly play a role in the development of some kinds of dementia. However, in AD and many other disorders, the dementia usually cannot be tied to a single abnormal gene. Instead, these forms of dementia appear to result from a complex interaction of genes, lifestyle factors, and other environmental influences.

Treatment

While treatments to reverse or halt disease progression are not available for most of the dementias, patients can benefit to some extent from treatment with available medications and other measures, such as cognitive training.

Drugs to specifically treat AD and some other progressive dementias are now available and are prescribed for many patients. Although these drugs do not halt the disease or reverse existing brain damage, they can improve symptoms and slow the progression of the disease. This may improve the patient's quality of life, ease the burden on caregivers, and delay admission to a nursing home. Many researchers are also examining whether these drugs may be useful for treating other types of dementia.

Many people with dementia, particularly those in the early stages, may benefit from practicing tasks designed to improve performance in specific aspects of cognitive functioning. For example, people can sometimes be taught to use memory aids, such as mnemonics, computerized recall devices, or note taking.

Behavior modification—rewarding appropriate or positive behavior and ignoring inappropriate behavior—also may help control unacceptable or dangerous behaviors.

478

Section 43.2

Alzheimer Disease

Excerpted from "Alzheimer's Disease Fact Sheet," National Institute on Aging (NIA), NIH Publication No. 08–6423, updated September 19, 2009.

Alzheimer disease (AD) is an irreversible, progressive brain disease that slowly destroys memory and thinking skills, and eventually even the ability to carry out the simplest tasks. In most people with AD, symptoms first appear after age 60. AD is the most common cause of dementia among older people. Dementia is the loss of cognitive functioning—thinking, remembering, and reasoning—to such an extent that it interferes with a person's daily life and activities. According to recent estimates, as many as 2.4 to 4.5 million Americans are living with AD.

Changes in the Brain in AD

Although we still don't know what starts the AD process, we do know that damage to the brain begins as many as 10–20 years before any problems are evident. Tangles begin to develop deep in the brain, in an area called the entorhinal cortex, and plaques form in other areas. As more and more plaques and tangles form in particular brain areas, healthy neurons begin to work less efficiently. Then, they lose

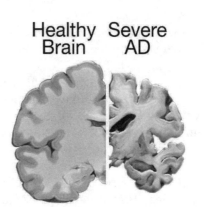

Healthy Severe
Brain   AD

Figure 43.1. *Healthy Brain and Severe Alzheimer Disease*

their ability to function and communicate with each other, and eventually they die. This damaging process spreads to a nearby structure, called the hippocampus, which is essential in forming memories. As the death of neurons increases, affected brain regions begin to shrink. By the final stage of AD, damage is widespread and brain tissue has shrunk significantly.

Very Early Signs and Symptoms

Memory problems are one of the first signs of AD. Some people with memory problems have a condition called amnestic mild cognitive impairment (MCI). People with this condition have more memory problems than normal for people their age, but their symptoms are not as severe as those with AD. More people with MCI, compared with those without MCI, go on to develop AD. Other changes may also signal the very early stages of AD. For example, recent research has found links between some movement difficulties and MCI. Researchers also have seen links between some problems with the sense of smell and cognitive problems.

Mild AD: As AD progresses, memory loss continues and changes in other cognitive abilities appear. Problems can include getting lost, trouble handling money and paying bills, repeating questions, taking longer to complete normal daily tasks, poor judgment, and mood and personality changes. People often are first diagnosed in this stage.

Moderate AD: In this stage, damage occurs in areas of the brain that control language, reasoning, sensory processing, and conscious thought. Memory loss and confusion increase, and people begin to have problems recognizing family and friends. They may be unable to learn new things, carry out tasks that involve multiple steps (such as getting dressed), or cope with new situations. They may have hallucinations, delusions, and paranoia, and may behave impulsively.

Severe AD: By the final stage, plaques and tangles have spread throughout the brain and brain tissue has shrunk significantly. People with severe AD cannot communicate and are completely dependent on others for their care. Near the end, the person may be in bed most or all of the time as the body shuts down.

Causes: Scientists don't yet fully understand what causes AD, but it is clear that it develops because of a complex series of events that

Preclinical AD

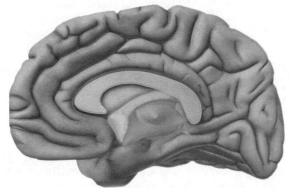

Mild to Moderate AD

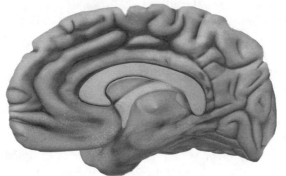

Severe AD

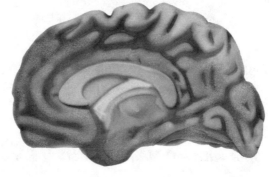

Figure 43.2. *As Alzheimer disease progresses, neurofibrillary tangles spread throughout the brain. Plaques also spread throughout the brain, starting in the neocortex. By the final stage, damage is widespread and brain tissue has shrunk significantly.*

take place in the brain over a long period of time. It is likely that the causes include genetic, environmental, and lifestyle factors. Because people differ in their genetic make-up and lifestyle, the importance of these factors for preventing or delaying AD differs from person to person.

Scientists are conducting studies to learn more about plaques, tangles, and other features of AD. They can now visualize plaques by imaging the brains of living individuals. They are also exploring the very earliest steps in the disease process. Findings from these studies will help them understand the causes of AD.

One of the great mysteries of AD is why it largely strikes older adults. Research on how the brain changes normally with age is shedding light on this question. For example, scientists are learning how age-related changes in the brain may harm neurons and contribute to AD damage. These age-related changes include inflammation and the production of unstable molecules called free radicals.

A nutritious diet, exercise, social engagement, and mentally stimulating pursuits can all help people stay healthy. New research suggests the possibility that these factors also might help to reduce the risk of cognitive decline and AD.

Early diagnosis is beneficial for several reasons. Having an early diagnosis and starting treatment in the early stages of the disease can help preserve function for months to years, even though the underlying AD process cannot be changed. Having an early diagnosis also helps families plan for the future, make living arrangements, take care of financial and legal matters, and develop support networks. In addition, an early diagnosis can provide greater opportunities for people to get involved in clinical trials. In a clinical trial, scientists test drugs or treatments to see which are most effective and for whom they work best.

AD is a complex disease, and no single magic bullet is likely to prevent or cure it. That's why current treatments focus on several different aspects including: helping people maintain mental function; managing behavioral symptoms; and slowing, delaying, or preventing AD.

Helping People with AD Maintain Mental Function

Four medications are approved by the U.S. Food and Drug Administration to treat AD. Donepezil (Aricept®), rivastigmine (Exelon®), and galantamine (Razadyne®) are used to treat mild to moderate AD (donepezil can be used for severe AD as well). Memantine (Namenda®) is used to treat moderate to severe AD. These drugs may help maintain thinking, memory, and speaking skills, and help with certain behavioral problems. However, these drugs don't change the underlying disease process and may help only for a few months to a few years.

Slowing, Delaying, or Preventing AD

AD research has developed to a point where scientists can look beyond treating symptoms to think about addressing the underlying disease process. In ongoing AD clinical trials, scientists are looking at many possible interventions, such as cardiovascular treatments, antioxidants, immunization therapy, cognitive training, and physical activity.

Supporting Families and Caregivers

Caring for a person with AD can have high physical, emotional, and financial costs. The demands of day-to-day care, changing family roles, and difficult decisions about placement in a care facility can be hard to handle. Researchers are learning a lot about AD caregiving, and studies are helping experts develop new ways to support caregivers.

Some AD caregivers have found that participating in an AD support group is a critical lifeline. These support groups allow caregivers to find respite, express concerns, share experiences, get tips, and receive emotional comfort. There are a growing number of groups for people in the early stage of AD and their families. Support networks can be especially valuable when caregivers face the difficult decision of whether and when to place a loved one in a nursing home.

Section 43.3

Vascular Dementia

Vascular dementia is widely considered the second most common type of dementia. It develops when impaired blood flow to parts of the brain deprives cells of food and oxygen. The diagnosis may be clearest when symptoms appear soon after a single major stroke blocks a large blood vessel and disrupts the blood supply to a significant portion of the brain. This situation is sometimes called post-stroke dementia.

There is also a form in which a series of very small strokes, or infarcts, block small blood vessels. Individually, these strokes do not cause major symptoms, but over time their combined effect becomes noticeable. This type is referred to as vascular cognitive impairment (VCI) or multi-infarct dementia.

Symptoms of vascular dementia can vary, depending on the specific brain areas deprived of blood. Impairment may occur in steps, where there is a fairly sudden, noticeable change in function, rather than the slow, steady decline usually seen in Alzheimer disease.

The person may have a past history of heart attacks. High blood pressure, high cholesterol, hardening of the arteries, diabetes, or other risk factors for heart disease are often present.

Symptoms of Vascular Dementia

- Memory problems may or may not be a prominent symptom, depending on whether brain regions important in memory are affected.

- Confusion, which may get worse at night.

- Difficulty concentrating, planning, communicating, and following instructions.

- Reduced ability to carry out daily activities.

- Physical symptoms associated with strokes, such as sudden weakness, difficulty speaking, or confusion.

- Magnetic resonance imaging (MRI) of the brain may show characteristic abnormalities associated with vascular damage.

Treatment of Vascular Dementia

Because vascular dementia is closely tied to diseases of the heart and blood vessels, many experts consider it the most potentially treatable form.

- Monitoring of blood pressure, weight, blood sugar, and cholesterol should begin early in life. Managing these risk factors, avoiding smoking and excess alcohol, and treating underlying diseases of the heart and blood vessels could play a major role in preventing later cognitive decline for many individuals. In some cases, active management of these factors in older adults who develop vascular dementia may help symptoms from getting worse.

- Once vascular dementia develops, there are no drugs currently approved by the U.S. Food and Drug Administration (FDA) to treat it.

- Most of the drugs used to treat cognitive symptoms of Alzheimer disease have also been shown to help individuals with vascular dementia to about the same extent they help those with Alzheimer. However, in March 2006, Eisai Co. Ltd., manufacturer of donepezil (Aricept), reported that in a clinical trial of donepezil for vascular dementia, a significantly greater number of deaths occurred in study participants receiving donepezil than in those taking the placebo.

Section 43.4

Lewy Body Dementia

You Are Not Alone

The word dementia is very frightening to everyone. Simply stated, it means "a decline in mental functions that affects daily living." In Lewy body dementia (LBD), dementia is the primary symptom and a component of the disease. When you live with dementia, you and those around you will have to adapt to your changing abilities. This section will help you understand your diagnosis and prepare for the changes ahead.

You don't have to face Lewy body dementia alone. The Lewy Body Dementia Association is here to educate, assist, and support you and your family as you begin your journey with this unique form of dementia. Since 2003, LBDA has grown to national recognition as a leader in LBD issues. You will find more in-depth information on the Lewy Body Dementia Association's website at www.lbda.org, including: educational resources on LBD; medical research updates; discussion forums to exchange practical tips for living with LBD, to offer support, or simply to lend an ear; lists of local LBD support groups; and links to related organizations.

Understanding Lewy Body Dementia

Lewy body dementia is not a rare disease. It affects an estimated 1.3 million individuals and their families in the United States alone. Because LBD symptoms may closely resemble other more commonly known diseases like Alzheimer and Parkinson, it is currently widely under-diagnosed.

LBD is an umbrella term for two related diagnoses. It refers to both Parkinson disease dementia and dementia with Lewy bodies. The earliest symptoms differ, but reflect the same underlying biological changes in the brain. Over time, people with both diagnoses will develop very similar cognitive, physical, sleep, and behavioral symptoms.

LBD is a multi-system disease and usually requires a comprehensive treatment approach with a collaborative team of physicians from varying specialties. Early diagnosis and treatment may extend your quality of life and independence. Many people with LBD enjoy significant lifestyle improvement with a comprehensive treatment approach, and some may even experience little change from year to year.

Some people with LBD are extremely sensitive, or may react negatively, to certain medications used to treat Alzheimer or Parkinson disease, as well as certain over-the-counter medications.

LBD Symptoms and Treatments

Dementia is the primary symptom and includes problems with memory, problem solving, planning, and abstract or analytical thinking. Cholinesterase inhibitors, medications originally developed for Alzheimer, are the standard treatment today for cognitive LBD symptoms.

Cognitive fluctuations involve unpredictable changes in concentration and attention from day to day.

Parkinson-like symptoms include rigidity or stiffness, shuffling gait, tremor and slowness of movement. Sometimes a Parkinson's medication called levodopa is prescribed for these symptoms.

Hallucinations are seeing or hearing things that are not really present. If the hallucinations are not disruptive, they may not need to be treated further. However, if they are frightening or dangerous, your physician may recommend a cautious trial use of a newer antipsychotic medication. Dementia medications called cholinesterase inhibitors have also been shown to be effective in treating hallucinations and other psychiatric symptoms of LBD. *Warning:* Up to 50% of LBD patients treated with any antipsychotic medication may experience severe neuroleptic sensitivity, including worsening cognition, heavy sedation, increased or possibly irreversible parkinsonism, or symptoms resembling neuroleptic malignant syndrome (NMS), which can be fatal. NMS causes severe fever, muscle rigidity and breakdown that can lead to kidney failure.

Rapid eye movement (REM) sleep behavior disorder (RBD) involves acting out dreams, sometimes violently. This symptom appears in some people years before any changes in cognition. Some sleep partners have reported being physically injured when the disorder was left untreated. RBD can be responsive to treatment by melatonin or clonazepam.

Severe sensitivity to neuroleptics is common in LBD. Neuroleptics, also known as antipsychotics, are medications used to treat hallucinations or other serious mental disorders. While traditional antipsychotic medications, for example, haloperidol and thioridazine HCL are commonly prescribed for individuals with Alzheimer disease for disruptive behavior, these medications can affect the brain of an individual with LBD differently, sometimes causing severe side effects. For this reason, traditional antipsychotic medications like haloperidol should be avoided. Some newer atypical antipsychotic medications like risperidone may also be problematic for someone with LBD. Some LBD experts prefer quetiapine. If quetiapine is not tolerated or is not helpful, clozapine should be considered, but requires ongoing blood tests to assure a rare but serious blood condition does not develop. Hallucinations must be treated very conservatively, using the lowest doses possible under careful observation for side effects.

Other Common Lewy Body Dementia Symptoms Not Required for Diagnosis

These symptoms also need to be monitored and treated:

Significant changes in the autonomic nervous system, including temperature regulation, blood pressure and digestion. Dizziness, fainting, sensitivity to heat and cold, sexual dysfunction, early urinary incontinence, or constipation are common LBD symptoms.

Repeated falls attributed to dizziness, fainting, or the effects of parkinsonism on posture and balance.

Excessive daytime sleepiness or transient loss of consciousness. Sleep disorders are common in LBD, but are often undiagnosed. If you experience these symptoms, consult with a sleep specialist to identify and treat all sleep disorders.

Other mood disorders and psychiatric symptoms such as depression, delusions (false beliefs), or hallucinations in other senses, like touch or smell. Your doctor may recommend treating depression with classes of antidepressants called selective serotonin reuptake inhibitors (SSRI) or serotonin-norepinephrine reuptake inhibitors (SNRI).

Certain Medications May Worsen Your Condition

Speak with your doctor about possible side effects. The following drugs may cause sedation, motor impairment, or confusion:

- Benzodiazepines, tranquilizers like diazepam and lorazepam
- Anticholinergics (antispasmodics), such as oxybutynin and glycopyrrolate
- Some surgical anesthetics
- Older antidepressants
- Certain over-the-counter medications, including diphenhydramine and dimenhydrinate

Some medications, like anticholinergics, amantadine, and dopamine agonists, which help relieve parkinsonian symptoms, might increase confusion, delusions, or hallucinations.

Note: Be sure to meet with your anesthesiologist in advance of any surgery to discuss medication sensitivities and risks unique to LBD. People with LBD often respond to certain anesthetics and surgery with acute states of confusion or delirium and may have a sudden significant drop in functional abilities, which may or may not be permanent. Possible alternatives to general anesthesia include a spinal or regional block. These methods are less likely to result in postoperative confusion. If you are told to stop taking all medications prior to surgery, consult with your doctor to develop a plan for careful withdrawal.

Not All Treatments Include Taking Medications

- Physical therapy includes cardiovascular, strengthening, flexibility exercises, gait training, and general physical fitness programs.
- Speech therapy may improve low voice volume, poor enunciation, muscular strength, and swallowing difficulties.
- Occupational therapy helps maintain skills and promotes functional ability and independence. Music and aromatherapy may reduce anxiety and improve mood.
- Individual and family psychotherapy may be useful for learning strategies to manage emotional and behavioral symptoms and

to help make plans that address individual and family concerns about the future.

• Support groups may be helpful for caregivers and persons with LBD to identify practical solutions to day-to-day frustrations and to obtain emotional support from others.

What is the long-term prognosis for someone with Lewy body dementia?

The prognosis is different for each person and may be affected by your general health or the existence of unrelated illnesses. Because LBD progresses at varying rates for each individual, it is not possible to determine how long someone may live with the disease.

The average duration of LBD is typically five to eight years after the onset of obvious LBD symptoms, but may range from two to twenty years. It is important to remember that this is a disorder that progresses gradually over years, not days or months.

Some families must make the decision whether or not to inform a person with LBD about the diagnosis. Those decisions may depend on the cognitive ability and temperament of the individual with LBD. While some people may find a dementia diagnosis distressing, a recent study indicates that most individuals actually find some relief in knowing the diagnosis and in understanding how this relates to their changing abilities. A correct diagnosis can also lead to an optimum treatment plan.

What if I haven't received a diagnosis yet?

Sometimes early dementia symptoms can be vague, making it hard to identify. It may even take several years for enough symptoms to develop to point to a specific type of dementia.

Some types of dementia are reversible and may be caused by an interaction of certain medications, a vitamin deficiency, or a curable illness. If you are experiencing changes in your memory or cognitive abilities, please consult with a doctor to identify the cause so you can begin treatment immediately.

Unfortunately, for many types of dementia, there are no known cures. These types of dementia mainly affect older adults, though some people are diagnosed with early-onset dementia as early as their forties. Getting an early and accurate diagnosis along with appropriate treatment is very important, since people often respond very differently to certain medications.

Other Common Types of Dementia

Alzheimer disease patients experience a progressive loss of recent memory; problems with language, calculation, abstract thinking, and judgment; depression or anxiety; personality and behavioral changes; and disorientation to time and place.

Vascular dementia is caused by a series of small strokes that deprive the brain of vital oxygen. Symptoms, such as disorientation in familiar locations; walking with rapid, shuffling steps; incontinence; laughing or crying inappropriately; difficulty following instructions; and problems handling money may appear suddenly and worsen with additional strokes. High blood pressure, cigarette smoking, and high cholesterol are some of the risk factors for stroke that may be controlled to prevent vascular dementia.

Frontotemporal dementia (FTD) includes several disorders with a variety of symptoms. The most common signs of FTD include changes in personality and behavior, such as inappropriate or compulsive behavior, euphoria, apathy, decline in personal hygiene, and a lack of awareness concerning these changes. Some forms of FTD involve language and speech symptoms or movement changes.

Do I have to see a special kind of doctor to find out what type of dementia I have?

Family physicians are a great, first-step resource if you are experiencing any cognitive, emotional, or physical changes. However, neurologists generally possess the specialized knowledge necessary to diagnose specific types of dementia or movement disorders, as do geriatric psychiatrists and neuropsychologists. However, these specialists may require a referral from your primary care physician. Geriatricians, who specialize in treating older adults, are also usually familiar with the different forms of dementia. If you have access to a hospital affiliated with a medical school, the hospital may have a clinic specializing in dementia or movement disorders where you may find a high level of diagnostic and treatment capability.

What information will the doctor need to make an accurate diagnosis and provide the best treatment?

Most people know to tell their doctors about any memory or other cognitive problems they are experiencing. However, since the symptoms of LBD and other types of dementia go far beyond cognitive issues, be sure to tell your doctor about any memory, cognitive, emotional, behavioral, movement, cardiac, digestive, or sleep problems you are having. Bring someone close to you with you, such as a spouse or an adult child, to discuss any changes they have observed. Also, tell your doctor about all of your current medications, including prescriptions, over-the-counter drugs, vitamins, and herbal supplements, since certain medications can worsen your symptoms.

The doctor may perform physical and neurological exams, run blood tests to rule out other diseases, do a brief mental status test, and order one or more types of brain scans that provide images of your brain or brain functioning. Ask your doctor for a referral for a complete neuropsychological examination. This is an assessment of thinking abilities, including memory, attention, word-finding, and visual-spatial skills. Neuropsychological exams are much more extensive and sensitive than routine office tests of mental status and can help differentiate among LBD, Alzheimer disease, the usually mild changes associated with normal aging, and other neurological conditions.

LBD Is a Family Disease, Affecting Both the Patient and Primary Caregiver

Unfortunately, LBD is not an easy disease with which to live. It affects both the person with LBD and their entire family. Here are a few things you can do today to start preparing for the challenges ahead.

- Share your diagnosis with those closest to you, so you can stand together to face LBD.

- Become a knowledgeable partner with your doctor. Learn everything you can about LBD symptoms, treatment options, and caregiving.

- Fill out and carry the LBD Medical Alert Wallet Card, and present it any time you are hospitalized, require emergency medical care, or meet with your doctors.

- Subscribe to a medical alert bracelet service to provide important medical information to emergency care providers.

- Identify local resources that provide information or assistance before you need it, including your local Area Agency on Aging office.

- Consult with an attorney who specializes in elder law about your legal and financial situation during the early stage of LBD.

- Contact national organizations including the Administration on Aging, Family Caregiver Alliance, or National Alliance for Caregiving for additional information on caregiving.

Section 43.5

Memory Loss and Early Dementia

Excerpted from "New Research Illuminates Memory Loss and Early Dementia," National Institute on Aging (NIA), Spring 2009.

"Recent research has greatly enhanced our understanding of how memories are formed and what really happens in the brain when memory loss occurs," says Dr. Marcelle Morrison-Bogorad, director of the National Institute on Aging (NIA) Division of Neuroscience. "These findings are helping us focus on the very earliest stages, when normal aging may be giving way to a disease process such as Alzheimer disease (AD). Knowing more about these early events will help us understand what may trigger the AD process and will contribute to improved diagnosis and effective treatments."

Is It Forgetfulness or a Memory Disorder?

Studies have shown that the aging brain is much more adaptable than once thought. For example, as adults age, they improve in some cognitive areas, such as vocabulary and other forms of verbal knowledge. The brain also continues to develop new neurons (nerve cells) in certain regions, even late in life. Pathways used by neurons to transmit signals can reroute themselves to bypass obstructions and maintain essential communications.

However, studies of memory and cognition have found that healthy people also may lose some cognitive function as they get older. They may have more difficulty learning new information, remembering things, or doing tasks like planning or making decisions. These minor declines in memory and cognitive ability may occur because the brain, like other parts of the body, changes with age.

For some people, the brain changes that come with age are minimal and result in occasional memory lapses, such as forgetting keys or blanking out on a person's name. Others experience progressive and significant declines in their ability to remember things, without having other problems characteristic of AD, such as difficulty processing and organizing information, problems with judgment and decision-making, personality changes, and psychiatric and behavioral problems.

Telling the Difference between Normal Forgetfulness and Memory Loss

Normal age-related memory loss:

- Sometimes misplaces keys, eyeglasses, or other items
- Momentarily forgets an acquaintance's name
- Occasionally has to search for a word
- Occasionally forgets to run an errand
- May forget an event from the distant past
- When driving, may momentarily forget where to turn, but quickly orients self
- Jokes about memory loss

Memory loss in mild cognitive impairment (MCI):

- Frequently misplaces items
- Frequently forgets people's names and is slow to recall them
- Has increasing difficulty finding desired words
- Begins to forget important events and appointments
- May forget recent events or newly learned information
- Becomes temporarily lost more often; may have trouble understanding and following a map
- Worries about memory loss; family, and friends notice lapses

Memory loss in Alzheimer disease:

- Forgets what an item is used for or puts it in an inappropriate place
- May not remember knowing a person

- Begins to lose language skills and may withdraw from social interaction

- Loses the sense of time; does not know what day it is

- Has seriously impaired recent memory and difficulty learning and remembering new information

- Becomes easily disoriented or lost in familiar places, sometimes for hours

- May have little or no awareness of cognitive problems

Source: Adapted from Rabins, P. Memory. In *The Johns Hopkins White Papers*. Baltimore: Johns Hopkins University, 2007.

Brain tissue reveals much: Scientists have learned that MCI has several subtypes. In the most common subtype, memory loss is the most prominent feature (other types of MCI feature other types of cognitive problems).

"We call the condition of memory impairment alone amnestic mild cognitive impairment (aMCI)," says Dr. Ronald Petersen, director of the National Institute on Aging (NIA)-funded Mayo Alzheimer's Disease Research Center, "Researchers are particularly interested in the brain changes and memory loss of aMCI, because more people with this condition go on to develop AD than do people without aMCI. We don't yet know for sure whether aMCI is a separate condition or a transitional stage between normal aging and AD."

In one of these studies, begun in 1988, Dr. Petersen and his colleagues followed a group of more than 270 people diagnosed with a MCI who participated in the Mayo Clinic Alzheimer's Disease Patient Registry. These volunteers were diagnosed with aMCI based on their concerns about memory loss, the results of memory and cognitive function tests, and the facts that they were able to carry out normal activities of daily living and did not have other signs of dementia.

Two recent studies with the same group of Mayo Clinic volunteers have significantly increased our knowledge about the damage to brain tissue in aMCI.

During the first study, 15 participants with aMCI died. After their deaths, the research team compared the brain tissue of these participants with that of 28 people who were cognitively healthy at the time of death and 28 people who had AD at the time of death. In the people with aMCI, the researchers found damage to brain tissue that suggested an intermediate stage. This damage included many neurofibrillary tangles in the temporal lobes, which could account for the memory loss, and some amyloid plaques in the cortex, but not enough to constitute a definition of AD.

Amyloid plaques and neurofibrillary tangles are considered two hallmarks of AD. The brain tissue of the healthy participants had few plaques and tangles, but plaques and tangles were very common in the brain tissue of those with AD.

In the second study, the Mayo research team examined the brain tissue of 34 people who were followed from their diagnosis of aMCI through dementia to death. In slightly more than 70% of the cases, those with aMCI went on to develop AD that could be confirmed by damage to brain tissue. In the remainder, dementia had another cause.

"These findings suggest that we can't definitively say that someone with aMCI has early AD," says Dr. Petersen. "aMCI may indeed be a transitional state. Following up these findings in other studies will help us learn more about aMCI and may even point to some useful therapeutic targets to prevent the possible development of AD."

The temporal lobe as puzzle solver: One of the great puzzles about aMCI is why, sometimes but not always, it leads to AD. Do people with this kind of memory loss who do not eventually develop AD have some special protective characteristics? Two research groups recently explored an approach for identifying individuals who are likely to progress from normal age-related forgetfulness to aMCI and from aMCI to AD.

As part of NIA's Alzheimer's Disease Cooperative Study, Dr. Charles DeCarli and colleagues at the University of California at Davis used magnetic resonance imaging (MRI) to measure how shrinkage (atrophy) of the temporal lobes of 187 study participants with MCI predicted development of AD over an 18-month period. The temporal lobes, which run along the sides of the brain, deal with the formation and storage of memories.

Moderate to marked atrophy, based on simple visual inspection of MRI, was associated with a more than twofold increase in the likelihood of progressing to AD. This was true even after the scientists took into account other factors, including age, education, sex, and cognitive abilities at the beginning of the study.

"These findings suggest that using MRI during evaluations for aMCI may help us identify people at higher risk of progressing to AD. Knowing this may help us start treatments earlier, when they may be most effective," says Dr. DeCarli.

Conclusion: We often take memory for granted. Its importance in how we define ourselves as human beings and as individuals becomes very evident when it begins to disappear. AD researchers are working on many fronts to learn more about what happens when memory loss occurs. Their findings may help in the development of drug and non-drug therapies to help people hold on to their memories for as long as possible.

Section 43.6

Body Fat Increases Risk of Dementia

Excerpted from "Connections Features: Is a Big Belly Bad for the Brain?," *Connections,* Spring 2009, National Institute on Aging (NIA).

Is a Big Belly Bad for the Brain? Examining Body Fat's Ties to Dementia

Belly fat may be bad for your brain. A number of recent studies, widely publicized in the media, have suggested that excess adipose tissue (body fat), particularly around the belly, during a person's midlife years may increase the risk of developing dementia, including Alzheimer disease (AD), during old age. AD is the most common type of dementia among older people.

Just how adipose tissue and its many chemical components may affect the brain is a complex story that researchers are eagerly investigating, with support from the National Institute on Aging (NIA). "We have two very serious public health burdens—Alzheimer disease and obesity—and if they interact so that one accentuates the other, then this is obviously a significant crisis," says Dr. Suzana Petanceska, a program director in the NIA's Division of Neuroscience. "This is very important to know because if metabolic abnormalities associated with obesity do indeed harm the brain, and we are able to understand how that happens, there is great potential for intervention."

"Several epidemiological studies already show an association between body mass index (BMI) and dementia," says Dr. Lenore Launer, chief of NIA's Neuroepidemiology Section of the Laboratory of Epidemiology, Demography, and Biometry. (BMI is a measurement of body fat relative to height and weight.) In support of these findings, there are also "a lot of interesting new experimental data on proteins such as leptin that are involved in obesity and may indeed be involved in the physiology of brain changes," Dr. Launer says. "It's an exciting area that needs to be explored."

The epidemiological evidence: At first, researchers did not consider obesity to be an independent risk factor for dementia—separate from the conditions obesity spawns, including diabetes and cardiovascular disease. Numerous studies have linked both diabetes and cardiovascular disease to dementia. In the early 2000s, researchers turned their attention to obesity itself as an independent threat to the brain.

With support from NIA, Dr. Deborah Gustafson, Associate Professor, Neuropsychiatric Epidemiology Unit, University of Gothenburg, Sweden, and her colleagues analyzed data on dementia incidence in 290 Swedish women who were age 70 at the beginning of the study. Women who developed dementia in their 80s had an average BMI at age 70 that was two units (kg/m^2) higher than that of women in their 80s who did not develop dementia. Imaging studies of women in another population study in Gothenburg showed that those with atrophy in their brains' temporal lobes were likely to have higher BMIs.

Since then, imaging studies have "convincingly demonstrated both generalized and regional brain atrophy and changes in white matter in association with obesity," writes Dr. William Jagust, a neurologist at the University of California, Berkeley, in the special issue on obesity and dementia of Current Alzheimer Research (April 2007).

Location, location, location: Research on the biology of fat has shown that there are several types of adipose tissue. Belly fat, also known as visceral fat, is the most damaging type. It wraps itself around organs, makes the abdomen protrude, and produces molecules that can pass into and interact with the brain. Compared with generalized obesity, excess visceral fat is a bigger risk factor for type 2 diabetes, insulin resistance, heart disease, stroke, and premature death, studies show. The fat that coats the hips and thighs, called subcutaneous fat, lies just below the skin and is benign in comparison.

In 2008, an NIA-funded study found that middle-aged people with large bellies are more likely than are their flat-bellied contemporaries to develop Alzheimer disease later in life. Epidemiologist Dr. Rachel A. Whitmer, Kaiser Permanente Division of Research, Oakland, CA, and her co-investigators analyzed epidemiological data collected on 6,583 Kaiser members, ages 40 to 45. Almost 16% of the entire group developed dementia.

How to measure belly fat: There are many ways to measure belly fat. Researchers may use large calipers to measure abdominal diameter, which is the distance from the back to the front of the belly. An abdominal diameter of more than 9.8 inches (25 centimeters [cm]) is considered obese. Scientists also may use imaging devices to get a thorough picture of belly fat. Another good tool for determining central obesity around the waist is a measuring tape. Central obesity is defined as more than 35 inches (89 cm) for women and more than 40 inches (102 cm) for men, but anything over 31.5 inches (80 cm) for women and over 37 inches (94 cm) for men may be a red flag of future health problems, says NIA's Dr. Petanceska.

Study participants in the top third for belly size had a threefold greater risk of dementia than participants in the bottom third had, even after researchers controlled for other factors, like diabetes, that increase a person's risk for developing Alzheimer disease. Some participants had a normal BMI and a large belly. They probably weighed less because they had little muscle in their arms and legs or had low bone density, Dr. Whitmer explains. But, they too were more likely than the flat-bellied participants were to develop dementia.

Effects of belly fat: "The more we understand about adipose tissue, the clearer it becomes that belly fat is its own disease-generating organism," says Dr. Launer. "Your fat is a very active endocrine organ that has a life of its own," Dr. Petanceska explains. As part of that life, it interacts with many other systems in the body. "How it interacts with the brain may profoundly inform us about brain aging and Alzheimers," she adds.

We normally associate the changes that belly fat initiates with aging, so some researchers suggest that fat may accelerate the aging process. For example, visceral fat increases a person's risk of developing insulin resistance, to which older people are more prone than are younger people. Insulin resistance is a condition in which the body cannot use insulin properly. This condition typically leads to high levels of insulin in the blood, yet low levels of insulin activity in the brain. NIA-funded studies, including work by Dr. Suzanne Craft, Veteran's Administration (VA) Puget Sound Healthcare System and the University of Washington, Seattle, indicate a correlation between insulin resistance and the risk of age-related memory impairment and Alzheimer disease.

Belly fat churns out a host of hormones, including cortisol and glucocorticoids known as stress hormones, which normally increase with age as well as during stress and are believed to affect cognition. The hippocampus, one of the main areas of the brain affected in AD, is rich in receptors for glucocorticoids. An elevated level of cortisol "has been linked to hippocampal atrophy in humans," writes Dr. Jagust.

The brains of AD patients show many signs of chronic inflammation. In addition, elevated levels of pro-inflammatory cytokines in the blood have been associated with a greater degree of age-related cognitive decline. Many of the substances produced by adipose tissue, known as adipokine, serve as mediators of inflammation (cytokines). The white adipose tissue that makes belly fat secretes cytokines that fuel and maintain a state of chronic inflammation, which is harmful to the body and may be one of the ways by which belly fat can accelerate brain aging and cause brain dysfunction.

Chapter 44

Amyotrophic Lateral Sclerosis (ALS)

Amyotrophic lateral sclerosis (ALS), sometimes called Lou Gehrig disease, is a rapidly progressive, invariably fatal neurological disease that attacks the nerve cells (neurons) responsible for controlling voluntary muscles. In ALS, both the upper motor neurons and the lower motor neurons degenerate or die, ceasing to send messages to muscles. Unable to function, the muscles gradually weaken, waste away, and twitch. Eventually the ability of the brain to start and control voluntary movement is lost. Individuals with ALS lose their strength and the ability to move their arms, legs, and body. When muscles in the diaphragm and chest wall fail, individuals lose the ability to breathe without ventilatory support. The disease does not affect a person's ability to see, smell, taste, hear, or recognize touch, and it does not usually impair a person's thinking or other cognitive abilities. However, several recent studies suggest that a small percentage of patients may experience problems with memory or decision-making, and there is growing evidence that some may even develop a form of dementia. The cause of ALS is not known, and scientists do not yet know why ALS strikes some people and not others.

Is there any treatment?

No cure has yet been found for ALS. However, the U.S. Food and Drug Administration (FDA) has approved the first drug treatment for

Excerpted from "Amyotrophic Lateral Sclerosis Information Page," National Institute of Neurological Disorders and Stroke (NINDS), February 10, 2010.

the disease—riluzole. Riluzole is believed to reduce damage to motor neurons and prolongs survival by several months, mainly in those with difficulty swallowing. Other treatments are designed to relieve symptoms and improve the quality of life for people with ALS. Drugs also are available to help individuals with pain, depression, sleep disturbances, and constipation. Individuals with ALS may eventually consider forms of mechanical ventilation (respirators).

What is the prognosis?

Regardless of the part of the body first affected by the disease, muscle weakness and atrophy spread to other parts of the body as the disease progresses. Individuals have increasing problems with moving, swallowing, and speaking or forming words. Eventually people with ALS will not be able to stand or walk, get in or out of bed on their own, or use their hands and arms. In later stages of the disease, individuals have difficulty breathing as the muscles of the respiratory system weaken. Although ventilation support can ease problems with breathing and prolong survival, it does not affect the progression of ALS. Most people with ALS die from respiratory failure, usually within 3–5 years from the onset of symptoms. However, about 10% of those individuals with ALS survive for ten or more years.

What research is being done?

The National Institute of Neurological Disorders and Stroke (NINDS) conducts research in its laboratories at the National Institutes of Health (NIH) and also supports additional research through grants to major medical institutions across the country. The goals of this research are to find the cause or causes of ALS, understand the mechanisms involved in the progression of the disease, and develop effective treatments.

Results of an NINDS-sponsored phase III randomized, placebo-controlled trial of the drug minocycline to treat ALS were reported in 2007. This study showed that people with ALS who received minocycline had a 25% greater rate of decline than those who received the placebo, according to the ALS functional rating scale (ALSFRS-R).

Chapter 45

Creutzfeldt-Jakob Disease

Creutzfeldt-Jakob disease (CJD) is a rare, degenerative, invariably fatal brain disorder. It affects about one person in every one million people per year worldwide; in the United States there are about 200 cases per year. CJD usually appears in later life and runs a rapid course. Typically, onset of symptoms occurs about age 60, and about 90% of patients die within one year. In the early stages of disease, patients may have failing memory, behavioral changes, lack of coordination, and visual disturbances. As the illness progresses, mental deterioration becomes pronounced and involuntary movements, blindness, weakness of extremities, and coma may occur.

There are three major categories of CJD:

- In sporadic CJD, the disease appears even though the person has no known risk factors for the disease. This is by far the most common type of CJD and accounts for at least 85% of cases.

- In hereditary CJD, the person has a family history of the disease and/or tests positive for a genetic mutation associated with CJD. About 5–10% of cases of CJD in the United States are hereditary.

- In acquired CJD, the disease is transmitted by exposure to brain or nervous system tissue, usually through certain medical

Excerpted from "Creutzfeldt-Jakob Disease Fact Sheet," National Institute of Neurological Disorders and Stroke (NINDS), NIH Publication No. 03–2760, updated December 18, 2009.

procedures. There is no evidence that CJD is contagious through casual contact with a CJD patient. Since CJD was first described in 1920, fewer than 1% of cases have been acquired CJD.

CJD belongs to a family of human and animal diseases known as the transmissible spongiform encephalopathies (TSEs). Spongiform refers to the characteristic appearance of infected brains, which become filled with holes until they resemble sponges under a microscope. CJD is the most common of the known human TSEs. Other human TSEs include kuru, fatal familial insomnia (FFI), and Gerstmann-Sträussler-Scheinker disease (GSS).

Symptoms

CJD is characterized by rapidly progressive dementia. Initially, patients experience problems with muscular coordination; personality changes, including impaired memory, judgment, and thinking; and impaired vision. People with the disease also may experience insomnia, depression, or unusual sensations. CJD does not cause a fever or other flu-like symptoms. As the illness progresses, the patients' mental impairment becomes severe. They often develop involuntary muscle jerks called myoclonus, and they may go blind. They eventually lose the ability to move and speak and enter a coma. Pneumonia and other infections often occur in these patients and can lead to death.

There are several known variants of CJD. These variants differ somewhat in the symptoms and course of the disease. For example, a variant form of the disease—called new variant or variant (nv-CJD, v-CJD), described in Great Britain and France—begins primarily with psychiatric symptoms, affects younger patients than other types of CJD, and has a longer than usual duration from onset of symptoms to death.

Diagnosis

There is currently no single diagnostic test for CJD. When a doctor suspects CJD, the first concern is to rule out treatable forms of dementia such as encephalitis (inflammation of the brain) or chronic meningitis. The only way to confirm a diagnosis of CJD is by brain biopsy or autopsy. This procedure may be dangerous for the patient, and the operation does not always obtain tissue from the affected part of the brain. Because a correct diagnosis of CJD does not help the patient, a brain biopsy is discouraged unless it is needed to rule out a treatable disorder.

Scientists are working to develop laboratory tests for CJD. One such test, developed at the National Institute of Neurological Disorders and Stroke (NINDS), is performed on a person's cerebrospinal fluid and detects a protein marker that indicates neuronal degeneration. This can help diagnose CJD in people who already show the clinical symptoms of the disease. This test is much easier and safer than a brain biopsy. The false positive rate is about 5–10%. Scientists are working to develop this test for use in commercial laboratories. They are also working to develop other tests for this disorder.

Treatment

There is no treatment that can cure or control CJD. Current treatment for CJD is aimed at alleviating symptoms and making the patient as comfortable as possible. Opiate drugs can help relieve pain if it occurs, and the drugs clonazepam and sodium valproate may help relieve myoclonus.

How is CJD transmitted?

CJD cannot be transmitted through the air or through touching or most other forms of casual contact. However, exposure to brain tissue and spinal cord fluid from infected patients should be avoided to prevent transmission of the disease through these materials.

In some cases, CJD has spread to other people from grafts of dura mater (a tissue that covers the brain), transplanted corneas, implantation of inadequately sterilized electrodes in the brain, and injections of contaminated pituitary growth hormone derived from human pituitary glands taken from cadavers. Doctors call these cases that are linked to medical procedures iatrogenic cases.

While there is no evidence that blood from people with sporadic CJD is infectious, studies have found that infectious prions from bovine spongiform encephalopathy (BSE) and v-CJD may accumulate in the lymph nodes (which produce white blood cells), the spleen, and the tonsils. These findings suggest that blood transfusions from people with v-CJD might transmit the disease. The possibility that blood from people with v-CJD may be infectious has led to a policy preventing people in the United States from donating blood if they have resided for more than three months in a country or countries where BSE is common.

How can people avoid spreading the disease?

To reduce the already very low risk of CJD transmission from one person to another, people should never donate blood, tissues, or organs if they have suspected or confirmed CJD, or if they are at increased risk because of a family history of the disease, a dura mater graft, or other factor.

Normal sterilization procedures such as cooking, washing, and boiling do not destroy prions. Caregivers, health care workers, and undertakers should take the following precautions when they are working with a person with CJD:

- Wash hands and exposed skin before eating, drinking, or smoking.

- Cover cuts and abrasions with waterproof dressings.

- Wear surgical gloves when handling a patient's tissues and fluids or dressing the patient's wounds.

- Avoid cutting or sticking themselves with instruments contaminated by the patient's blood or other tissues.

- Use face protection if there is a risk of splashing contaminated material such as blood or cerebrospinal fluid.

- Soak instruments that have come in contact with the patient in undiluted chlorine bleach for an hour or more, then use an autoclave (pressure cooker) to sterilize them in distilled water for at least one hour at 132–134 degrees Centigrade.

Chapter 46

Huntington Disease

What is Huntington disease?

Huntington disease (HD) results from genetically programmed degeneration of brain cells, called neurons, in certain areas of the brain. This degeneration causes uncontrolled movements, loss of intellectual faculties, and emotional disturbance. HD is a familial disease, passed from parent to child through a mutation in the normal gene. Each child of an HD parent has a 50–50 chance of inheriting the HD gene. If a child does not inherit the HD gene, he or she will not develop the disease and cannot pass it to subsequent generations. A person who inherits the HD gene will sooner or later develop the disease. Whether one child inherits the gene has no bearing on whether others will or will not inherit the gene. Some early symptoms of HD are mood swings; depression; and irritability or trouble driving, learning new things, remembering a fact, or making a decision. As the disease progresses, concentration on intellectual tasks becomes increasingly difficult and the patient may have difficulty feeding himself or herself and swallowing. The rate of disease progression and the age of onset vary from person to person. A genetic test, coupled with a complete medical history and neurological and laboratory tests, helps physicians diagnose HD. Presymptomatic testing is available for individuals who are at risk for carrying the HD gene. In 1–3% of individuals with HD, no family history of HD can be found.

"Huntington's Disease Information Page," National Institute of Neurological Disorders and Stroke (NIDNS), May 15, 2009.

Is there any treatment?

Physicians prescribe a number of medications to help control emotional and movement problems associated with HD. In August 2008 the U.S. Food and Drug Administration approved tetrabenazine to treat Huntington chorea (the involuntary writhing movements), making it the first drug approved for use in the United States to treat the disease. Most drugs used to treat the symptoms of HD have side effects such as fatigue, restlessness, or hyperexcitability. It is extremely important for people with HD to maintain physical fitness as much as possible, as individuals who exercise and keep active tend to do better than those who do not.

What is the prognosis?

At this time, there is no way to stop or reverse the course of HD. Now that the HD gene has been located, investigators are continuing to study the HD gene with an eye toward understanding how it causes disease in the human body.

What research is being done?

Scientific investigations using electronic and other technologies enable scientists to see what the defective gene does to various structures in the brain and how it affects the body's chemistry and metabolism. Laboratory animals are being bred in the hope of duplicating the clinical features of HD so that researchers can learn more about the symptoms and progression of HD. Investigators are implanting fetal tissue in rodents and nonhuman primates with the hope of understanding, restoring, or replacing functions typically lost by neuronal degeneration in individuals with HD. Related areas of investigation include excitotoxicity (over-stimulation of cells by natural chemicals found in the brain), defective energy metabolism (a defect in the mitochondria), oxidative stress (normal metabolic activity in the brain that produces toxic compounds called free radicals), tropic factors (natural chemical substances found in the human body that may protect against cell death).

Chapter 47

Multiple Sclerosis (MS)

What is multiple sclerosis?

An unpredictable disease of the central nervous system, multiple sclerosis (MS) can range from relatively benign to somewhat disabling to devastating, as communication between the brain and other parts of the body is disrupted. Many investigators believe MS to be an autoimmune disease—one in which the body, through its immune system, launches a defensive attack against its own tissues. In the case of MS, it is the nerve-insulating myelin that comes under assault. Such assaults may be linked to an unknown environmental trigger, perhaps a virus.

Most people experience their first symptoms of MS between the ages of 20 and 40; the initial symptom of MS is often blurred or double vision, red-green color distortion, or even blindness in one eye. Most MS patients experience muscle weakness in their extremities and difficulty with coordination and balance. These symptoms may be severe enough to impair walking or even standing. In the worst cases, MS can produce partial or complete paralysis. Most people with MS also exhibit paresthesias, transitory abnormal sensory feelings such as numbness, prickling, or pins and needles sensations. Some may also experience pain. Speech impediments, tremors, and dizziness are other frequent complaints. Occasionally, people with MS have hearing loss. Approximately half of all people with MS experience cognitive impairments such as difficulties

Excerpted from "Multiple Sclerosis Information Page," National Institute of Neurological Disorders and Stroke (NINDS), February 10, 2010.

with concentration, attention, memory, and poor judgment, but such symptoms are usually mild and are frequently overlooked. Depression is another common feature of MS.

Is there any treatment?

There is as yet no cure for MS. Many patients do well with no therapy at all, especially since many medications have serious side effects and some carry significant risks. However, three forms of beta interferon (Avonex, Betaseron, and Rebif) have now been approved by the U.S. Food and Drug Administration (FDA) for treatment of relapsing-remitting MS. Beta interferon has been shown to reduce the number of exacerbations and may slow the progression of physical disability. When attacks do occur, they tend to be shorter and less severe. The FDA also has approved a synthetic form of myelin basic protein, called copolymer I (Copaxone), for the treatment of relapsing-remitting MS. Copolymer I has few side effects, and studies indicate that the agent can reduce the relapse rate by almost one third. An immunosuppressant treatment, Novantrone (mitoxantrone), is approved by the FDA for the treatment of advanced or chronic MS.

One monoclonal antibody, natalizumab (Tysabri), was shown in clinical trials to significantly reduce the frequency of attacks in people with relapsing forms of MS and was approved for marketing by the FDA in 2004. However, in 2005 the drug's manufacturer voluntarily suspended marketing of the drug after several reports of significant adverse events. In 2006, the FDA again approved sale of the drug for MS but under strict treatment guidelines involving infusion centers where patients can be monitored by specially trained physicians.

While steroids do not affect the course of MS over time, they can reduce the duration and severity of attacks in some patients. Spasticity, which can occur either as a sustained stiffness caused by increased muscle tone or as spasms that come and go, is usually treated with muscle relaxants and tranquilizers such as baclofen, tizanidine, diazepam, clonazepam, and dantrolene. Physical therapy and exercise can help preserve remaining function, and patients may find that various aids—such as foot braces, canes, and walkers—can help them remain independent and mobile. Avoiding excessive activity and avoiding heat are probably the most important measures patients can take to counter physiological fatigue. If psychological symptoms of fatigue such as depression or apathy are evident, antidepressant medications may help. Other drugs that may reduce fatigue in some, but not all, patients include amantadine (Symmetrel), pemoline (Cylert), and the still-experimental drug aminopyridine. Although improvement of optic symptoms usually occurs even without treatment, a short course of treatment with intravenous methylprednisolone (Solu-Medrol) followed by treatment with oral steroids is sometimes used.

What is the prognosis?

A physician may diagnose MS in some patients soon after the onset of the illness. In others, however, doctors may not be able to readily identify the cause of the symptoms, leading to years of uncertainty and multiple diagnoses punctuated by baffling symptoms that mysteriously wax and wane. The vast majority of patients are mildly affected, but in the worst cases, MS can render a person unable to write, speak, or walk. MS is a disease with a natural tendency to remit spontaneously, for which there is no universally effective treatment.

What research is being done?

The National Institute of Neurological Disorders and Stroke (NINDS) and other institutes of the National Institutes of Health (NIH) conduct research in laboratories at the NIH and also support additional research through grants to major medical institutions across the country. Scientists continue their extensive efforts to create new and better therapies for MS. One of the most promising MS research areas involves naturally occurring antiviral proteins known as interferons. Beta interferon has been shown to reduce the number of exacerbations and may slow the progression of physical disability. When attacks do occur, they tend to be shorter and less severe. In addition, there are a number of treatments under investigation that may curtail attacks or improve function. Over a dozen clinical trials testing potential therapies are underway, and additional new treatments are being devised and tested in animal models.

Chapter 48

Parkinson Disease

Parkinson disease (PD) belongs to a group of conditions called motor system disorders, which are the result of the loss of dopamine-producing brain cells. The four primary symptoms of PD are tremor, or trembling in hands, arms, legs, jaw, and face; rigidity, or stiffness of the limbs and trunk; bradykinesia, or slowness of movement; and postural instability, or impaired balance and coordination. As these symptoms become more pronounced, patients may have difficulty walking, talking, or completing other simple tasks. PD usually affects people over the age of 50. Early symptoms of PD are subtle and occur gradually. In some people the disease progresses more quickly than in others. As the disease progresses, the shaking, or tremor, which affects the majority of PD patients may begin to interfere with daily activities. Other symptoms may include depression and other emotional changes; difficulty in swallowing, chewing, and speaking; urinary problems or constipation; skin problems; and sleep disruptions. There are currently no blood or laboratory tests that have been proven to help in diagnosing sporadic PD. Therefore, the diagnosis is based on medical history and a neurological examination. The disease can be difficult to diagnose accurately. Doctors may sometimes request brain scans or laboratory tests in order to rule out other diseases.

Is there any treatment?

At present, there is no cure for PD, but a variety of medications provide dramatic relief from the symptoms. Usually, patients are given

"Parkinson's Disease Information Page," National Institute of Neurological Disorders and Stroke (NINDS), February 12, 2010.

levodopa combined with carbidopa. Carbidopa delays the conversion of levodopa into dopamine until it reaches the brain. Nerve cells can use levodopa to make dopamine and replenish the brain's dwindling supply. Although levodopa helps at least three-quarters of parkinsonian cases, not all symptoms respond equally to the drug. Bradykinesia and rigidity respond best, while tremor may be only marginally reduced. Problems with balance and other symptoms may not be alleviated at all. Anticholinergics may help control tremor and rigidity. Other drugs, such as bromocriptine, pramipexole, and ropinirole, mimic the role of dopamine in the brain, causing the neurons to react as they would to dopamine. An antiviral drug, amantadine, also appears to reduce symptoms. In May 2006, the U. S. Food and Drug Administration (FDA) approved rasagiline to be used along with levodopa for patients with advanced PD or as a single-drug treatment for early PD.

In some cases, surgery may be appropriate if the disease doesn't respond to drugs. A therapy called deep brain stimulation (DBS) has now been approved by the FDA. In DBS, electrodes are implanted into the brain and connected to a small electrical device called a pulse generator that can be externally programmed. DBS can reduce the need for levodopa and related drugs, which in turn decreases the involuntary movements called dyskinesias that are a common side effect of levodopa. It also helps to alleviate fluctuations of symptoms and to reduce tremors, slowness of movements, and gait problems. DBS requires careful programming of the stimulator device in order to work correctly.

What is the prognosis?

PD is both chronic, meaning it persists over a long period of time, and progressive, meaning its symptoms grow worse over time. Although some people become severely disabled, others experience only minor motor disruptions. Tremor is the major symptom for some patients, while for others tremor is only a minor complaint and other symptoms are more troublesome. No one can predict which symptoms will affect an individual patient, and the intensity of the symptoms also varies from person to person.

What research is being done?

Scientists looking for the cause of PD continue to search for possible environmental factors, such as toxins, that may trigger the disorder, and study genetic factors to determine how defective genes play a role. Other scientists are working to develop new protective drugs that can delay, prevent, or reverse the disease.

Chapter 49

Progressive Supranuclear Palsy (PSP)

Progressive supranuclear palsy (PSP) is a rare brain disorder that causes serious and permanent problems with control of gait and balance. The most obvious sign of the disease is an inability to aim the eyes properly, which occurs because of lesions in the area of the brain that coordinates eye movements. Some patients describe this effect as a blurring. PSP patients often show alterations of mood and behavior, including depression and apathy as well as progressive mild dementia. It must be emphasized that the pattern of signs and symptoms can be quite different from person to person. The symptoms of PSP are caused by a gradual deterioration of brain cells in a few tiny but important places at the base of the brain, in the region called the brainstem. PSP is often misdiagnosed because some of its symptoms are very much like those of Parkinson disease, Alzheimer disease, and more rare neurodegenerative disorders, such as Creutzfeldt-Jakob disease. The key to establishing the diagnosis of PSP is the identification of early gait instability and difficulty moving the eyes, the hallmark of the disease, as well as ruling out other similar disorders, some of which are treatable. Although PSP gets progressively worse, no one dies from PSP itself.

Is there any treatment?

There is currently no effective treatment for PSP, although scientists are searching for better ways to manage the disease. In some

"Progressive Supranuclear Palsy Information Page," National Institute of Neurological Disorders and Stroke (NINDS), December 18, 2009.

patients the slowness, stiffness, and balance problems of PSP may respond to antiparkinsonian agents such as levodopa, or levodopa combined with anticholinergic agents, but the effect is usually temporary. The speech, vision, and swallowing difficulties usually do not respond to any drug treatment. Another group of drugs that has been of some modest success in PSP are antidepressant medications. The most commonly used of these drugs are Prozac, Elavil, and Tofranil. The anti-PSP benefit of these drugs seems not to be related to their ability to relieve depression. Non-drug treatment for PSP can take many forms. Patients frequently use weighted walking aids because of their tendency to fall backward. Bifocals or special glasses called prisms are sometimes prescribed for PSP patients to remedy the difficulty of looking down. Formal physical therapy is of no proven benefit in PSP, but certain exercises can be done to keep the joints limber. A surgical procedure, a gastrostomy, may be necessary when there are swallowing disturbances. This surgery involves the placement of a tube through the skin of the abdomen into the stomach (intestine) for feeding purposes.

What is the prognosis?

PSP gets progressively worse but is not itself directly life-threatening. It does, however, predispose patients to serious complications such as pneumonia secondary to difficulty in swallowing (dysphagia). The most common complications are choking and pneumonia, head injury, and fractures caused by falls. The most common cause of death is pneumonia. With good attention to medical and nutritional needs, however, most PSP patients live well into their 70s and beyond.

What research is being done?

Research is ongoing for Parkinson and Alzheimer diseases. Better understanding of those common, related disorders will go a long way toward solving the problem of PSP, just as studying PSP may help shed light on Parkinson and Alzheimer diseases.

Part Eight

Seizures and Neurological Disorders of Sleep

Chapter 50

What Is Epilepsy?

Epilepsy is a brain disorder in which clusters of nerve cells, or neurons, in the brain sometimes signal abnormally. Neurons normally generate electrochemical impulses that act on other neurons, glands, and muscles to produce human thoughts, feelings, and actions. In epilepsy, the normal pattern of neuronal activity becomes disturbed, causing strange sensations, emotions, and behavior, or sometimes convulsions, muscle spasms, and loss of consciousness. During a seizure, neurons may fire as many as 500 times a second, much faster than normal. In some people, this happens only occasionally; for others, it may happen up to hundreds of times a day.

More than two million people in the United States—about one in 100—have experienced an unprovoked seizure or been diagnosed with epilepsy. For about 80% of those diagnosed with epilepsy, seizures can be controlled with modern medicines and surgical techniques. However, about 25–30% of people with epilepsy will continue to experience seizures even with the best available treatment. Doctors call this situation intractable epilepsy. Having a seizure does not necessarily mean that a person has epilepsy. Only when a person has had two or more seizures is he or she considered to have epilepsy.

Epilepsy is not contagious and is not caused by mental illness or mental retardation. Some people with mental retardation may experience seizures, but seizures do not necessarily mean the person has

This chapter is excerpted from "Seizures and Epilepsy: Hope through Research," National Institute of Neurological Disorders (NINDS), NIH Publication No. 04–156, updated February 9, 2010.

or will develop mental impairment. Many people with epilepsy have normal or above-average intelligence. Seizures sometimes do cause brain damage, particularly if they are severe. However, most seizures do not seem to have a detrimental effect on the brain. Any changes that do occur are usually subtle, and it is often unclear whether these changes are caused by the seizures themselves or by the underlying problem that caused the seizures.

While epilepsy cannot currently be cured, for some people it does eventually go away. One study found that children with idiopathic epilepsy, or epilepsy with an unknown cause, had a 68–92% chance of becoming seizure-free by 20 years after their diagnosis. The odds of becoming seizure-free are not as good for adults or for children with severe epilepsy syndromes, but it is nonetheless possible that seizures may decrease or even stop over time. This is more likely if the epilepsy has been well-controlled by medication or if the person has had epilepsy surgery.

What causes epilepsy?

Epilepsy is a disorder with many possible causes. Anything that disturbs the normal pattern of neuron activity—from illness to brain damage to abnormal brain development—can lead to seizures.

Epilepsy may develop because of an abnormality in brain wiring, an imbalance of nerve signaling chemicals called neurotransmitters, or some combination of these factors. Researchers believe that some people with epilepsy have an abnormally high level of excitatory neurotransmitters that increase neuronal activity, while others have an abnormally low level of inhibitory neurotransmitters that decrease neuronal activity in the brain. Either situation can result in too much neuronal activity and cause epilepsy. One of the most-studied neurotransmitters that plays a role in epilepsy is gamma-aminobutyric acid (GABA) which is an inhibitory neurotransmitter. Research on GABA has led to drugs that alter the amount of this neurotransmitter in the brain or change how the brain responds to it. Researchers also are studying excitatory neurotransmitters such as glutamate.

In some cases, the brain's attempts to repair itself after a head injury, stroke, or other problem may inadvertently generate abnormal nerve connections that lead to epilepsy. Abnormalities in brain wiring that occur during brain development also may disturb neuronal activity and lead to epilepsy.

Research has shown that the cell membrane that surrounds each neuron plays an important role in epilepsy. Cell membranes are crucial for a neuron to generate electrical impulses. A disruption in any of these processes may lead to epilepsy. In some cases, epilepsy may result from changes in non-neuronal brain cells called glia. These cells regulate concentrations of chemicals in the brain that can affect neuronal signaling. About half of all seizures have no known cause. However, in other cases, the seizures are clearly linked to infection, trauma, or other identifiable problems.

What are the different kinds of seizures?

Doctors have described more than 30 different types of seizures. Seizures are divided into two major categories—focal seizures and generalized seizures. However, there are many different types of seizures in each of these categories.

Focal seizures, also called partial seizures, occur in just one part of the brain. About 60% of people with epilepsy have focal seizures. These seizures are frequently described by the area of the brain in which they originate. For example, someone might be diagnosed with focal frontal lobe seizures.

In a simple focal seizure, the person will remain conscious but experience unusual feelings or sensations that can take many forms. The person may experience sudden and unexplainable feelings of joy, anger, sadness, or nausea. He or she also may hear, smell, taste, see, or feel things that are not real.

In a complex focal seizure, the person has a change in or loss of consciousness. His or her consciousness may be altered, producing a dreamlike experience. People having a complex focal seizure may display strange, repetitious behaviors such as blinks, twitches, mouth movements, or even walking in a circle. These repetitious movements are called automatisms. More complicated actions, which may seem purposeful, can also occur involuntarily. Patients may also continue activities they started before the seizure began, such as washing dishes in a repetitive, unproductive fashion. These seizures usually last just a few seconds.

Some people with focal seizures, especially complex focal seizures, may experience auras—unusual sensations that warn of an impending seizure. These auras are actually simple focal seizures in which the person maintains consciousness. The symptoms an individual person has, and the progression of those symptoms, tend to be similar every time.

The symptoms of focal seizures can easily be confused with other disorders. For instance, the dreamlike perceptions associated with a complex focal seizure may be misdiagnosed as migraine headaches, which also may cause a dreamlike state. The strange behavior and sensations caused by focal seizures also can be is taken for symptoms of narcolepsy, fainting, or even mental illness. It may take many tests and careful monitoring by an experienced physician to tell the difference between epilepsy and other disorders.

Generalized seizures are a result of abnormal neuronal activity on both sides of the brain. These seizures may cause loss of consciousness, falls, or massive muscle spasms.

There are many kinds of generalized seizures. In absence seizures, the person may appear to be staring into space and have jerking or twitching muscles. These seizures are sometimes referred to as petit mal seizures, which is an older term. Tonic seizures cause stiffening of muscles of the body, generally those in the back, legs, and arms. Clonic seizures cause repeated jerking movements of muscles on both sides of the body. Myoclonic seizures cause jerks or twitches of the upper body, arms, or legs. Atonic seizures cause a loss of normal muscle tone. The affected person will fall down or may drop his or her head involuntarily. Tonic-clonic seizures cause a mixture of symptoms, including stiffening of the body and repeated jerks of the arms and/or legs as well as loss of consciousness. Tonic-clonic seizures are sometimes referred to by an older term: grand mal seizures.

Not all seizures can be easily defined as either focal or generalized. Some people have seizures that begin as focal seizures but then spread to the entire brain. Other people may have both types of seizures but with no clear pattern.

Society's lack of understanding about the many different types of seizures is one of the biggest problems for people with epilepsy. People who witness a non-convulsive seizure often find it difficult to understand that behavior which looks deliberate is not under the person's control. In some cases, this has led to the affected person being arrested or admitted to a psychiatric hospital. To combat these problems, people everywhere need to understand the many different types of seizures and how they may appear.

What are the different kinds of epilepsy?

Just as there are many different kinds of seizures, there are many different kinds of epilepsy. Doctors have identified hundreds of different epilepsy syndromes—disorders characterized by a specific set of symptoms that include epilepsy. Some of these syndromes appear to be hereditary. For other syndromes, the cause is unknown. Epilepsy syndromes are frequently described by their symptoms or by where in the brain they originate. People should discuss the implications of their type of epilepsy with their doctors to understand the full range of symptoms, the possible treatments, and the prognosis.

People with absence epilepsy have repeated absence seizures that cause momentary lapses of consciousness. These seizures almost always begin in childhood or adolescence, and they tend to run in families, suggesting that they may be at least partially due to a defective gene or genes. Some people with absence seizures have purposeless movements during their seizures, such as a jerking arm or rapidly blinking eyes. Others have no noticeable symptoms except for brief times when they are "out of it." Immediately after a seizure, the person can resume whatever he or she was doing. However, these seizures may occur so frequently that the person cannot concentrate in school or other situations. Childhood absence epilepsy usually stops when the child reaches puberty. Absence seizures usually have no lasting effect on intelligence or other brain functions.

Temporal lobe epilepsy (TLE), is the most common epilepsy syndrome with focal seizures. These seizures are often associated with auras. TLE often begins in childhood. Research has shown that repeated temporal lobe seizures can cause a brain structure called the hippocampus to shrink over time. The hippocampus is important for memory and learning. While it may take years of temporal lobe seizures for measurable hippocampal damage to occur, this finding underlines the need to treat TLE early and as effectively as possible.

Neocortical epilepsy is characterized by seizures that originate from the brain's cortex, or outer layer. The seizures can be either focal or generalized. They may include strange sensations, visual hallucinations, emotional changes, muscle spasms, convulsions, and a variety of other symptoms, depending on where in the brain the seizures originate.

There are many other types of epilepsy, each with its own characteristic set of symptoms. Many of these, including Lennox-Gastaut syndrome and Rasmussen encephalitis, begin in childhood. Children with Lennox-Gastaut syndrome have severe epilepsy with several different types of seizures, including atonic seizures, which cause sudden falls and are also called drop attacks. This severe form of epilepsy can be very difficult to treat effectively. Rasmussen encephalitis is a progressive type of epilepsy in which half of the brain shows continual inflammation. It sometimes is treated with a radical surgical procedure called hemispherectomy. Some childhood epilepsy syndromes, such as childhood absence epilepsy, tend to go into remission or stop entirely during adolescence, whereas other syndromes such as juvenile myoclonic epilepsy and Lennox-Gastaut syndrome are usually present for life once they develop. However, seizure syndromes do not always appear in childhood.

Epilepsy syndromes that are easily treated, do not seem to impair cognitive functions or development, and usually stop spontaneously, are often described as benign. Benign epilepsy syndromes include benign infantile encephalopathy and benign neonatal convulsions. Other syndromes, such as early myoclonic encephalopathy, include neurological and developmental problems. However, these problems may be caused by underlying neurodegenerative processes rather than by the seizures. Epilepsy syndromes in which the seizures or the person's cognitive abilities get worse over time are called progressive epilepsy.

Several types of epilepsy begin in infancy. The most common type of infantile epilepsy is infantile spasms, clusters of seizures that usually begin before the age of six months. During these seizures the infant may bend and cry out. Anticonvulsant drugs often do not work for infantile spasms, but the seizures can be treated with adrenocorticotropic hormone (ACTH) or prednisone.

How is epilepsy diagnosed?

Doctors have developed a number of different tests to determine whether a person has epilepsy and, if so, what kind of seizures the person has. In some cases, people may have symptoms that look very much like a seizure but in fact are nonepileptic events caused by other disorders. Even doctors may not be able to tell the difference between these disorders and epilepsy without close observation and intensive testing. Tests used include electroencephalogram (EEG) monitoring, brain scans, medical history, and blood tests.

Can epilepsy be prevented?

Many cases of epilepsy can be prevented by wearing seat belts and bicycle helmets, putting children in car seats, and other measures that prevent head injury and other trauma. Prescribing medication after first or second seizures or febrile seizures also may help prevent epilepsy in some cases. Good prenatal care, including treatment of high blood pressure and infections during pregnancy, can prevent brain damage in the developing baby that may lead to epilepsy and other neurological problems later. Treating cardiovascular disease, high blood pressure, infections, and other disorders that can affect the brain during adulthood and aging also may prevent many cases of epilepsy. Finally, identifying the genes for many neurological disorders can provide opportunities for genetic screening and prenatal diagnosis that may ultimately prevent many cases of epilepsy.

Chapter 51

Treating Epilepsy

Chapter Contents

Section 51.1

Medications and Surgery

Excerpted from "Seizures and Epilepsy: Hope through Research,"
National Institute of Neurological Disorders (NINDS), NIH Publication
No. 04–156, updated February 9, 2010.

Medications

By far the most common approach to treating epilepsy is to prescribe antiepileptic drugs. More than 20 different antiepileptic drugs are on the market, all with different benefits and side effects. The choice of which drug to prescribe, and at what dosage, depends on many different factors, including the type of seizures a person has, the person's lifestyle and age, how frequently the seizures occur, and, for a woman, the likelihood that she will become pregnant. People with epilepsy should follow their doctor's advice and share any concerns they may have regarding their medication.

Doctors seeing a patient with newly developed epilepsy often prescribe carbamazepine, valproate, lamotrigine, oxcarbazepine, or phenytoin first, unless the epilepsy is a type that is known to require a different kind of treatment. For absence seizures, ethosuximide is often the primary treatment. Other commonly prescribed drugs include clonazepam, phenobarbital, and primidone. Some relatively new epilepsy drugs include tiagabine, gabapentin, topiramate, levetiracetam, and felbamate. Other drugs are used in combination with one of the standard drugs or for intractable seizures that do not respond to other medications. A few drugs, such as fosphenytoin, are approved for use only in hospital settings to treat specific problems such as status epilepticus. For people with stereotyped recurrent severe seizures that can be easily recognized by the person's family, the drug diazepam is now available as a gel that can be administered rectally by a family member. This method of drug delivery may be able to stop prolonged or repeated seizures before they develop into status epilepticus.

For most people with epilepsy, seizures can be controlled with just one drug at the optimal dosage. Combining medications usually amplifies side effects such as fatigue and decreased appetite, so doctors usually prescribe monotherapy, or the use of just one drug, whenever possible. Combinations of drugs are sometimes prescribed if monotherapy fails to effectively control a patient's seizures.

Most side effects of antiepileptic drugs are relatively minor, such as fatigue, dizziness, or weight gain. However, severe and life-threatening side effects such as allergic reactions can occur. Epilepsy medication also may predispose people to developing depression or psychoses. People with epilepsy should consult a doctor immediately if they develop any kind of rash while on medication, or if they find themselves depressed or otherwise unable to think in a rational manner. Other danger signs that should be discussed with a doctor immediately are extreme fatigue, staggering or other movement problems, and slurring of words. People with epilepsy should be aware that their epilepsy medication can interact with many other drugs in potentially harmful ways. For this reason, people with epilepsy should always tell doctors who treat them which medications they are taking. Women also should know that some antiepileptic drugs can interfere with the effectiveness of oral contraceptives, and they should discuss this possibility with their doctors. People taking epilepsy medication should be sure to check with their doctor or seek a second medical opinion if their medication does not appear to be working or if it causes unexpected side effects.

Surgery

When seizures cannot be adequately controlled by medications, doctors may recommend that the person be evaluated for surgery. Surgery for epilepsy is performed by teams of doctors at medical centers. To decide if a person may benefit from surgery, doctors consider the type or types of seizures he or she has. They also take into account the brain region involved and how important that region is for everyday behavior. Surgeons usually avoid operating in areas of the brain that are necessary for speech, language, hearing, or other important abilities. Doctors may perform tests such as a Wada test (administration of the drug amobarbital into the carotid artery) to find areas of the brain that control speech and memory. They often monitor the patient intensively prior to surgery in order to pinpoint the exact location in the brain where seizures begin. They also may use implanted electrodes to record brain activity from the surface of the brain. This yields better information than an external electroencephalogram (EEG).

A 1990 National Institutes of Health (NIH) consensus conference on surgery for epilepsy concluded that there are three broad categories of epilepsy that can be treated successfully with surgery. These include focal seizures, seizures that begin as focal seizures before spreading to the rest of the brain, and unilateral multifocal epilepsy with infantile hemiplegia (such as Rasmussen encephalitis). Doctors generally recommend surgery only after patients have tried two or three different medications without success, or if there is an identifiable brain lesion—a damaged or dysfunctional area—believed to cause the seizures.

A study published in 2000 compared surgery to an additional year of treatment with antiepileptic drugs in people with longstanding temporal lobe epilepsy. The results showed that 64% of patients receiving surgery became seizure-free, compared to 8% of those who continued with medication only. Because of this study and other evidence, the American Academy of Neurology (AAN) now recommends surgery for temporal lobe epilepsy (TLE) when antiepileptic drugs are not effective. However, the study and the AAN guidelines do not provide guidance on how long seizures should occur, how severe they should be, or how many drugs should be tried before surgery is considered. A nationwide study is now underway to determine how soon surgery for TLE should be performed.

If a person is considered a good candidate for surgery and has seizures that cannot be controlled with available medication, experts generally agree that surgery should be performed as early as possible. Surgery should always be performed with support from rehabilitation specialists and counselors who can help the person deal with the many psychological, social, and employment issues he or she may face.

While surgery can significantly reduce or even halt seizures for some people, it is important to remember that any kind of surgery carries some amount of risk (usually small). Surgery for epilepsy does not always successfully reduce seizures, and it can result in cognitive or personality changes, even in people who are excellent candidates for surgery. Patients should ask their surgeon about his or her experience, success rates, and complication rates with the procedure they are considering.

Even when surgery completely ends a person's seizures, it is important to continue taking seizure medication for some time to give the brain time to re-adapt. Doctors generally recommend medication for two years after a successful operation to avoid new seizures.

Surgery to treat underlying conditions: In cases where seizures are caused by a brain tumor, hydrocephalus, or other conditions that can be treated with surgery, doctors may operate to treat these underlying conditions. In many cases, once the underlying condition is successfully treated, a person's seizures will disappear as well.

Surgery to remove a seizure focus: The most common type of surgery for epilepsy is removal of a seizure focus, or small area of the brain where seizures originate. This type of surgery, which doctors may refer to as a lobectomy or lesionectomy, is appropriate only for focal seizures that originate in just one area of the brain. In general, people have a better chance of becoming seizure-free after surgery if they have a small, well-defined seizure focus. Lobectomies have a 55–70% success rate when the type of epilepsy and the seizure focus is well-defined.

Multiple subpial transection: When seizures originate in part of the brain that cannot be removed, surgeons may perform a procedure called a multiple subpial transection. In this type of operation, which has been commonly performed since 1989, surgeons make a series of cuts that are designed to prevent seizures from spreading into other parts of the brain while leaving the person's normal abilities intact. About 70% of patients who undergo a multiple subpial transection have satisfactory improvement in seizure control.

Corpus callosotomy: Corpus callosotomy, or severing the network of neural connections between the right and left halves, or hemispheres, of the brain, is done primarily in children with severe seizures that start in one half of the brain and spread to the other side. Corpus callosotomy can end drop attacks and other generalized seizures. However, the procedure does not stop seizures in the side of the brain where they originate, and these focal seizures may even increase after surgery.

Hemispherectomy and hemispherotomy: These procedures remove half of the brain's cortex, or outer layer. They are used predominantly in children who have seizures that do not respond to medication because of damage that involves only half the brain, as occurs with conditions such as Rasmussen encephalitis and Sturge-Weber syndrome. While this type of surgery is very radical and is performed only as a last resort, children often recover very well from the procedure, and their seizures usually cease altogether. With intense rehabilitation, they often recover nearly normal abilities. Since the chance of a full recovery is best in young children, hemispherectomy should be performed as early in a child's life as possible. It is rarely performed in children older than 13 years.

Section 51.2

Vagus Nerve Stimulation

Vagus nerve stimulation (VNS) is designed to prevent seizures by sending regular, mild pulses of electrical energy to the brain via the vagus nerve. These pulses are supplied by a device something like a pacemaker. The VNS device is sometimes referred to as a pacemaker for the brain. It is placed under the skin on the chest wall and a wire runs from it to the vagus nerve in the neck.

The vagus nerve is part of the autonomic nervous system, which controls functions of the body that are not under voluntary control, such as the heart rate. The vagus nerve passes through the neck as it travels between the chest and abdomen and the lower part of the brain.

What is the surgery like?

The surgeon first makes an incision along the outer side of the chest on the left side, and the device is implanted under the skin. Then a second incision is made horizontally in the lower neck, along a crease of skin, and the wire from the stimulator is wound around the vagus nerve in the left side of the neck. The brain itself is not involved in the surgery.

The device (also called an implant) is a flat, round battery, about the size of a silver dollar—that is, about an inch and a half (four centimeters [cm]) across—and 10–13 millimeters thick, depending on the model used. Newer models may be somewhat smaller.

The procedure usually lasts about 50–90 minutes with the patient under general anesthesia. Sometimes a hospital stay of one night is required. Some surgeons have performed the procedure with local anesthesia and the patient has been discharged the same day.

How is VNS used?

The neurologist programs the strength and timing of the impulses according to each patient's individual needs. The settings can be programmed and changed without entering the body, just by using a programming wand connected to a laptop computer.

For all patients, the device is programmed to go on for a certain period (for example, seven seconds or thirty seconds) and then to go off for another period (for example, fourteen seconds or five minutes). The device runs continuously, usually with thirty seconds of stimulation alternating with five minutes of no stimulation. The patient is usually not aware that it's operating.

Holding a special magnet near the implanted device causes the device to become active outside of the programmed interval. For people with warnings (auras) before their seizures, activating the stimulator with the magnet when the warning occurs may help to stop the seizure. Many patients without auras also experience improved seizure control, however.

Settings (also called stimulation parameters) set by the neurologist typically include a stimulation amplitude of 1.0–3.0 mA (milliamperes), a stimulation frequency of 30 Hz (hertz), and a pulse width of 500 microseconds. By adjusting these settings, the doctor not only may be able to control more of the patient's seizures, but often can also relieve side effects. One study, for instance, found that changing the pulse width eliminated pain that some patients were experiencing. The battery for the stimulator lasts approximately 5–10 years.

Resources: The VNS implant devices are built by Cyberonics, Inc. Additional information for patients and physicians is available at their website (www.cyberonics.com).

Section 51.3

Ketogenic Diet

The ketogenic diet is a special high-fat, low-carbohydrate diet that helps to control seizures in some people with epilepsy. It is prescribed by a physician and carefully monitored by a dietitian. It is stricter, with calorie, fluid, and protein measurement and occasional restriction, than the modified Atkins diet, which is also used today.

The name ketogenic means that it produces ketones in the body (keto = ketone, genic = producing). Ketones are formed when the body uses fat for its source of energy. Usually the body usually uses carbohydrates (such as sugar, bread, pasta) for its fuel, but because the ketogenic diet is very low in carbohydrates, fats become the primary fuel instead. Ketones are not dangerous. They can be detected in the urine, blood, and breath. Ketones are one of the more likely mechanisms of action of the diet; with higher ketone levels often leading to improved seizure control. However, there are many other theories for why the diet will work.

Who will it help?

Doctors usually recommend the ketogenic diet for children whose seizures have not responded to several different seizure medicines. It is particularly recommended for children with the Lennox-Gastaut syndrome.

Doctors seldom recommend the ketogenic diet for adults. However, in the limited studies that have been done, the diet seems to work just as well, although it is very restrictive for most adults. Studies are underway to evaluate the modified Atkins diet in this population.

The ketogenic diet has been shown in case reports and case series to be particularly effective for some epilepsy conditions. These include infantile spasms, Rett syndrome, tuberous sclerosis complex, Dravet syndrome, Doose syndrome, and GLUT-1 deficiency. Using a formula-only ketogenic diet for infants and gastrostomy-tube fed children may lead to better compliance and possibly even improved efficacy. The diet works well for children with focal seizures, but may be less likely to lead to an immediate seizure-free result. In general, the diet can always be considered as long as there are no clear metabolic or mitochondrial reasons not to use it.

What is it like?

The typical ketogenic diet, called the long-chain triglyceride diet, provides 3–4 grams of fat for every one gram of carbohydrate and protein. The dietician recommends a daily diet that contains 75 to 100 calories for every kilogram (2.2 pounds) of body weight and 1–2 grams of protein for every kilogram of body weight. If this sounds complicated, it is. That's why parents need a dietitian's help.

A ketogenic diet ratio is the ratio of fat to carbohydrate and protein grams combined. A 4:1 ratio is stricter than a 3:1 ratio, and is typically used for most children. A 3:1 ratio is typically used for infants, adolescents, and children who require higher amounts of protein or carbohydrate for some other reason.

The kinds of foods that provide fat for the ketogenic diet are butter, heavy whipping cream, mayonnaise, and oils (canola or olive). Because the amount of carbohydrate and protein in the diet have to be restricted, it is very important that the meals be prepared carefully. No other sources of carbohydrates can be eaten. (Even toothpaste might have some sugar in it.). For this reason, the ketogenic diet is supervised by a dietician. The parents and the child become very familiar with what can and cannot be eaten.

What happens first?

Typically the diet is started in the hospital. The child usually begins by fasting (except for water) under close medical supervision for 24 hours. For instance, the child might go into the hospital on Monday, start fasting at 6:00 p.m. and continue to have only water until 6:00 a.m. on Tuesday. The diet is started at that point, either by slowly increasing the calories or the ratio. This is the typical Hopkins protocol. There is growing evidence that fasting is probably not necessary for long-term efficacy, although it does lead to quicker onset of ketosis. The primary reason for admission in most centers is to monitor for any increase in seizures on the diet, ensure all medications are carbohydrate-free, and educate the families.

Does it work?

Several studies have shown that the ketogenic diet does reduce or prevent seizures in many children whose seizures could not be controlled by medications. Over half of children who go on the diet have at least a 50% reduction in the number of their seizures. Some children, usually 10–15%, even become seizure-free.

Children who are on the ketogenic diet continue to take seizure medicines. Some are able to take smaller doses or fewer medicines than before they started the diet, however. The time when medications can be lowered depends on the child and the comfort level of the neurologist. Evidence suggests it can be done as early as the diet initiation period safely in many circumstances.

If the person goes off the diet for even one meal, it may lose its good effect. So it is very important to stick with the diet as prescribed. It can be especially hard to follow the diet 100% if there are other children at home who are on a normal diet. Small children who have free access to the refrigerator are tempted by forbidden foods. Parents need to work as closely as possible with a dietician.

Are there any side effects?

A person starting the ketogenic diet may feel sluggish for a few days after the diet is started. This can worsen if a child is sick at the same time as the diet is started. Make sure to encourage carbohydrate-free fluids during illnesses.

Other side effects that might occur if the person stays on the diet for a long time are:

- kidney stones,
- high cholesterol levels in the blood,
- dehydration,
- constipation,
- slowed growth or weight gain, and
- bone fractures.

Because the diet does not provide all the vitamins and minerals found in a balanced diet, the dietician will recommend vitamin and mineral supplements. The most important of these are calcium and vitamin D (to prevent thinning of the bones), iron, and folic acid.

There are no anticonvulsants that should be stopped while on the diet. Topamax (topiramate) and Zonegran (zonisamide) do not have a higher risk of acidosis or kidney stones while on the diet. Depakote (valproic acid) does not lead to carnitine deficiency or other difficulties while on the diet either. Medication levels do not change while on the diet according to recent studies.

How is the patient monitored over time?

Early on, the doctor will usually see the child every 1–3 months. Blood and urine tests are performed to make sure there are no medical problems. The height and weight are measured to see if growth has slowed down. As the child gains weight, the diet may need to be adjusted by the dietician.

Can the diet ever be stopped?

If seizures have been well controlled for some time, usually two years, the doctor might suggest going off the diet. Usually, the patient is gradually taken off the diet over several months or even longer. Just as happens if seizure medicines are stopped suddenly, seizures may become much worse if the ketogenic diet is stopped all at once. Children usually continue to take seizure medicines after they go off the diet. In many situations, the diet has led to significant, but not total, seizure control. Families may choose to remain on the ketogenic diet for many years in these situations.

Where can I find out more information about the diet?

Other than the internet, there are several books about the ketogenic diet available. One is *The Ketogenic Diet: A Treatment for Children and Others with Epilepsy*, by Drs. Freeman and Kossoff, which discusses the Johns Hopkins approach and experience. The Charlie Foundation at www.charliefoundation.org and Matthew's Friends at www.matthewsfriends.org are parent-run organizations for support.

Section 51.4

Research Progress in Epilepsy

Excerpted from "Curing Epilepsy: The Promise of Research," National Institute of Neurological Disorders and Stroke (NINDS), NIH Publication No. 07–6120, April 24, 2009.

While the ultimate goal of curing epilepsy has not yet been achieved, researchers have made a great deal of progress. For example, the number of studies aimed at understanding how and why epilepsy develops has increased substantially, and researchers are banding together in collaborative efforts to overcome the limitations of individual research. Researchers also have identified a number of genes associated with epilepsy. Many technical advances, from improved brain imaging to the widespread use of micro-arrays, are allowing new insights. Partly as a result of these advances, a variety of new antiepileptic drugs and other treatments are now being tested in clinical studies.

Here is a look at how progress being made in laboratories, clinical settings, and voluntary groups across the country.

Discovering what creates epileptic seizures: To understand how to prevent, treat, and cure epilepsy, researchers first must learn how it develops. Where, how, when, and why do neurons begin to display the abnormal firing patterns that cause epileptic seizures? This process, known as epileptogenesis, is at the core of our understanding of epilepsy. Investigators are using a number of strategies to learn about epileptogenesis.

- Many studies have shown that having one seizure increases the risk of others.

- Recent studies have shown that non-neuronal cells in the brain, called astrocytes, play a central role in brain function and even produce the nerve-signaling chemical glutamate. Research has shown that glutamate produced by astrocytes can trigger seizures. This suggests that factors which impair astrocyte function, ranging from genetic variations to brain damage from stroke or head injury, can cause epilepsy.

The search for genes that increase the risk: Current science suggests that a majority of epilepsy syndromes involve multiple genes and variable symptoms. Most common epilepsies are probably the result of environmental factors acting in combination with genes. This would explain why there are so many epilepsy syndromes and may also explain why epilepsy is often associated with other disorders, neurological or otherwise.

New ways to observe brain chemistry and function during seizures: Another challenge in epilepsy research is finding ways to identify when and where seizures begin in the brain. The search for epilepsy markers is complicated because there are multiple types of epilepsy. Also, investigators have a very limited knowledge of the processes that lead to chronic epilepsy. A number of laboratories are using transcranial magnetic stimulation (TMS) as a diagnostic and therapeutic tool for epilepsy. Many studies have shown that TMS can be used to measure excitability in this region.

Developing new treatments that eliminate seizures without side effects: Individuals with seizures that are not controlled by drugs or surgery make up approximately 25–30% of the epilepsy patient population. Even when seizures are controlled, the quality of life for some people with epilepsy is severely affected by the long- and short-term side effects of medication or surgery. Fortunately, the improved understanding of epilepsy resulting from research on epileptogenesis (how a normal brain develops epilepsy) has led to many potential new treatments. Some of these treatments are now in clinical trials, while others are still in early development. If these treatments work as anticipated, they should greatly improve the care of people with epilepsy.

Anticonvulsant Screening Program: Record numbers of researchers are continuing to search for new compounds that might be used to treat epilepsy. One of the largest drug screening programs is the National Institute of Neurological Disorders and Stroke (NINDS) Anticonvulsant Screening Program (ASP). The major goals of this program are to find safer, more effective antiepileptic compounds, to discover effective treatments for patients with drug-resistant epilepsy, and to one day develop ways of stopping disease progression. The ASP screens an average of 700 new chemicals each year, using both animal and laboratory tests.

Surgery: Researchers have greatly refined surgical treatment of epilepsy in the past decade. Many investigators now consider surgery the most suitable option for many people with epilepsy that is not well controlled by drug therapy. Surgery is currently the only treatment that can truly cure epilepsy, at least in some people. Technological improvements in imaging techniques are some of the most important factors for increasing the success of epilepsy surgery. Improvements in hardware, software, and data acquisition and storage have also increased the usefulness of surgery.

New developments in neuroimaging have made it possible to identify the brain regions where seizures begin in many people who were not formerly considered good candidates for surgery. One study showed that using magnetic resonance spectroscopy to identify specific chemical abnormalities in the brain can predict the success of surgery in temporal lobe epilepsy but not neocortical epilepsy. Another study found that single photon emission computed tomography (SPECT) was superior to photo emission tomography (PET) in the imaging of receptors for the neurotransmitter acetylcholine, which made it better for identifying where seizures begin. Several studies have now shown that focal surgery in properly selected patients with tuberous sclerosis can have excellent results if the seizure focus is carefully located by electrophysiology.

Brain stimulation: Many studies have shown that brain stimulation can reduce seizures in some people with epilepsy. Several types of brain stimulation other than (vagus nerve stimulation) are now being tested for epilepsy. These include chronic deep brain stimulation, trigeminal nerve stimulation, transcranial magnetic stimulation, and transcranial direct current stimulation.

Therapies to predict or interrupt seizures: A major new area in epilepsy investigation is developing systems that anticipate epileptic seizures and then deliver a therapy to stop them. For example, researchers might be able to use electrical stimulation, a local drug infusion, or cooling of one part of the brain to arrest seizures. This type of therapy could be very useful for people who don't respond well to standard epilepsy treatments and who are not good candidates for surgery. However, the success of seizure-interrupting treatment depends upon the development of methods to detect patterns of brain activity that predict seizures. One seizure-interrupting device, called a responsive neurostimulator system, is now being tested in a multi-center clinical trial of patients with temporal lobe epilepsy, bi-temporal epilepsy, and neocortical epilepsy. This therapy uses a pacemaker-like device implanted in the brain to deliver a small amount of electricity when it detects the onset of a seizure.

Chapter 52

Living with Epilepsy

Epilepsy affects an estimated 2.5 million people in the United States and each year accounts for $15.5 billion in direct costs (medical) and indirect costs (lost or reduced earnings and productivity). More than one-third of people with epilepsy continue to have seizures despite treatment. Each year, about 200,000 new cases of epilepsy are diagnosed in the United States with children younger than two years of age and adults older than 65 most likely to be affected. In addition, people of low socioeconomic status, those who live in urban areas, and members of some minority populations are at increased risk for epilepsy.

Delayed recognition of seizures and inadequate treatment, which may result from lack of specialty care, greatly increases a person's risk for subsequent seizures, brain damage, disability, and death from injuries incurred during a seizure. Epilepsy is a widely recognized health condition, but one that is poorly understood by the public, even among people who know someone with the disorder. Lack of knowledge about the causes of epilepsy has been associated with negative attitudes, beliefs, and stigma. Lack of understanding about epilepsy is a leading cause of discrimination in the workplace and in schools.

This chapter begins with excerpts from "At a Glance: Targeting Epilepsy," Centers for Disease Control and Prevention (CDC), 2009; and concludes with excerpts from "Seizures and Epilepsy: Hope through Research," National Institute of Neurological Disorders (NINDS), NIH Publication No. 04–156, updated February 9, 2010.

During the past 14 years, the Centers for Disease Control and Prevention (CDC) Epilepsy Program has steadily increased its ability to effectively address public health issues related to epilepsy. The program works to protect the health of people living with epilepsy, improve the quality of life of people living with this condition, and decrease the stigma associated with the disorder. To achieve these goals, the program has established national and local partnerships to increase public awareness and deliver targeted educational messages. The Epilepsy Program supports activities in several key areas, including communication, education, and self-management.

Communication and education: CDC has a long-standing partnership with the national Epilepsy Foundation to conduct multifaceted public education and awareness campaigns. These campaigns are designed to increase awareness about and acceptance of people with epilepsy and to counteract the social stigma associated with this disorder through education and community programs.

In 2000, CDC developed the tool kit *No Label Required* for teenagers with epilepsy to help them make informed decisions about issues of greatest concern in their lives. Building on the success of this tool kit, CDC worked with the Epilepsy Foundation to develop and test an award-winning tool kit for parents, *You Are Not Alone: Toolkit for Parents of Teens with Epilepsy*. Tool kit components are designed to empower and support parents while encouraging their teenagers toward self-management and are available at http://www.cdc.gov/epilepsy.

Self-management and mental health: Improving the ability of people with epilepsy to better manage the disorder is a priority for CDC's Epilepsy Program. In 2008, a computer-based, theory-driven epilepsy self-management program developed for adults with epilepsy was found to be an effective management tool.

How Does Epilepsy Affect Daily Life?

Most people with epilepsy lead outwardly normal lives. Approximately 80% can be significantly helped by modern therapies, and some may go months or years between seizures. However, the condition can and does affect daily life for people with epilepsy, their family, and their friends. People with severe seizures that resist treatment have, on average, a shorter life expectancy and an increased risk of cognitive impairment, particularly if the seizures developed in early childhood. These impairments may be related to the underlying conditions that cause epilepsy or to epilepsy treatment rather than the epilepsy itself.

Behavior and emotions: It is not uncommon for people with epilepsy, especially children, to develop behavioral and emotional problems. Families must learn to accept and live with the seizures without blaming or resenting the affected person. Counseling services can help families cope with epilepsy in a positive manner. Epilepsy support groups also can help by providing a way for people with epilepsy and their family members to share their experiences, frustrations, and tips for coping with the disorder.

People with epilepsy have an increased risk of poor self-esteem, depression, and suicide. These problems may be a reaction to a lack of understanding or discomfort about epilepsy that may result in cruelty or avoidance by other people. Many people with epilepsy also live with an ever-present fear that they will have another seizure.

Driving and recreation: For many people with epilepsy, the risk of seizures restricts their independence, in particular the ability to drive. Most states and the District of Columbia will not issue a driver's license to someone with epilepsy unless the person can document that they have gone a specific amount of time without a seizure (the waiting period varies from a few months to several years). The risk of seizures also restricts people's recreational choices. For instance, people with epilepsy should not participate in sports such as skydiving or motor racing where a moment's inattention could lead to injury. Other activities, such as swimming and sailing, should be done only with precautions and supervision. However, jogging, football, and many other sports are reasonably safe for a person with epilepsy. Studies to date have not shown any increase in seizures due to sports, although these studies have not focused on any activity in particular. There is some evidence that regular exercise may even improve seizure control in some people. Sports are often such a positive factor in life that it is best for the person to participate, although the person with epilepsy and the coach or other leader should take appropriate safety precautions. It is important to take steps to avoid potential sports-related problems such as dehydration, overexertion, and hypoglycemia, as these problems can increase the risk of seizures.

Education and employment: By law, people with epilepsy or other handicaps in the United States cannot be denied employment or access to any educational, recreational, or other activity because of their seizures. However, one survey showed that only about 56% of people with epilepsy finish high school and about 15% finish college—rates much lower than those for the general population. The same survey found that about 25% of working-age people with epilepsy are unemployed. These numbers indicate that significant barriers still exist for people with epilepsy in school and work. Restrictions on driving limit the employment opportunities for many people with epilepsy, and many find it difficult to face the misunderstandings and social pressures they encounter in public situations. Antiepileptic drugs also may cause side effects that interfere with concentration and memory. Children with epilepsy may need extra time to complete schoolwork, and they sometimes may need to have instructions or other information repeated for them. Teachers should be told what to do if a child in their classroom has a seizure, and parents should work with the school system to find reasonable ways to accommodate any special needs their child may have.

Pregnancy and motherhood: Women with epilepsy are often concerned about whether they can become pregnant and have a healthy child. This is usually possible. While some seizure medications and some types of epilepsy may reduce a person's interest in sexual activity, most people with epilepsy can become pregnant. Moreover, women with epilepsy have a 90% or better chance of having a normal, healthy baby, and the risk of birth defects is only about 4–6%. The risk that children of parents with epilepsy will develop epilepsy themselves is only about 5% unless the parent has a clearly hereditary form of the disorder.

There are several precautions women can take before and during pregnancy to reduce the risks associated with pregnancy and delivery. Women who are thinking about becoming pregnant should talk with their doctors to learn any special risks associated with their epilepsy and the medications they may be taking. Some seizure medications, particularly valproate, trimethadione, and phenytoin, are known to increase the risk of having a child with birth defects such as cleft palate, heart problems, or finger and toe defects. For this reason, a woman's doctor may advise switching to other medications during pregnancy. Whenever possible, a woman should allow her doctor enough time to properly change medications, including phasing in the new medications and checking to determine when blood levels are stabilized, before she tries to become pregnant. Women should also begin prenatal vitamin supplements—especially with folic acid, which may reduce the risk of some birth defects—well before pregnancy. Women who discover that they are pregnant but have not already spoken with their doctor about ways to reduce the risks should do so as soon as possible. However, they should continue taking seizure medication as prescribed until that time to avoid preventable seizures. Seizures during pregnancy can harm the developing baby or lead to miscarriage, particularly if the seizures are severe. Nevertheless, many women who have seizures during pregnancy have normal, healthy babies.

The frequency of seizures during pregnancy may be influenced by a variety of factors, including the woman's increased blood volume during pregnancy, which can dilute the effect of medication. Women should have their blood levels of seizure medications monitored closely during and after pregnancy, and the medication dosage should be adjusted accordingly.

Pregnant women with epilepsy should take prenatal vitamins and get plenty of sleep to avoid seizures caused by sleep deprivation. They also should take vitamin K supplements after 34 weeks of pregnancy to reduce the risk of a blood-clotting disorder in infants called neonatal coagulopathy that can result from fetal exposure to epilepsy medications. Finally, they should get good prenatal care; avoid tobacco, caffeine, alcohol, and illegal drugs; and try to avoid stress.

Labor and delivery usually proceed normally for women with epilepsy, although there is a slightly increased risk of hemorrhage, eclampsia, premature labor, and cesarean section. Doctors can administer antiepileptic drugs intravenously and monitor blood levels of anticonvulsant medication during labor to reduce the risk that the labor will trigger a seizure. Babies sometimes have symptoms of withdrawal from the mother's seizure medication after they are born, but these problems wear off in a few weeks or months and usually do not cause serious or long-term effects. A mother's blood levels of anticonvulsant medication should be checked frequently after delivery as medication often needs to be decreased.

Epilepsy medications need not influence a woman's decision about breastfeeding her baby. Only minor amounts of epilepsy medications are secreted in breast milk, usually not enough to harm the baby and much less than the baby was exposed to in the womb. On rare occasions, the baby may become excessively drowsy or feed poorly, and these problems should be closely monitored. However, experts believe the benefits of breastfeeding outweigh the risks except in rare circumstances.

To increase doctors' understanding of how different epilepsy medications affect pregnancy and the chances of having a healthy baby,

Massachusetts General Hospital has begun a nationwide registry for women who take antiepileptic drugs while pregnant. Women who enroll in this program are given educational materials on preconception planning and perinatal care and are asked to provide information about the health of their children (this information is kept confidential). Women and physicians can contact this registry by calling 888-233-2334 or 617-726-1742 (Fax: 617-724-8307).

Women with epilepsy should be aware that some epilepsy medications can interfere with the effectiveness of oral contraceptives. Women who wish to use oral contraceptives to prevent pregnancy should discuss this with their doctors, who may be able to prescribe a different kind of antiepileptic medication or suggest other ways of avoiding an unplanned pregnancy.

Chapter 53

Nonepileptic Seizures

Chapter Contents

Section 53.1

Physiologic and Psychogenic Nonepileptic Seizures

This section begins with "The Truth about Psychogenic NonEpileptic Seizures," © 2005 Epilepsy.com. All rights reserved. Reprinted with permission. Updated in January, 2010 by David A. Cooke, MD, FACP, Diplomate, American Board of Internal Medicine. Text continues with "Study Finds Cognitive Behavioral Therapy Can Alleviate Nonepileptic Seizures, April 15, 2009." © 2009 Lifespan (www.lifespan.org). All rights reserved. Reprinted with permission.

The Truth about Psychogenic Nonepileptic Seizures

Psychogenic nonepileptic seizures (PNES) are an uncomfortable topic, one which is difficult for both patients and health care professionals to discuss as well as treat, and yet it is estimated that PNES are diagnosed in 20–30% of patients seen at epilepsy centers for intractable seizures.[1] Moreover, in the general population the prevalence rate is 2–33 per 100,000, making PNES nearly as prevalent as multiple sclerosis or trigeminal neuralgia.[2] Despite these startling statistics, PNES has largely remained a conversation held behind closed doors and in hushed tones throughout the medical community—until now.

"In addition to being common, psychogenic symptoms pose an uncomfortable and often frustrating challenge, both in diagnosis and management," said Selim R. Benbadis, MD, Director of Comprehensive Epilepsy Program, Professor, Departments of Neurology and Neurosurgery, University of South Florida and Tampa General Hospital. Benbadis is a leading pioneer in the study of PNES and has openly encouraged both the psychiatric and neurological community to broaden their clinical knowledge base when diagnosing and treating patients with PNES. In an editorial published in *Epilepsy & Behavior*, Benbadis wrote, "The American Psychiatric Association has abundant written patient education material available on diverse topics, but none on somatoform disorders. Psychogenic symptoms are also not the subject of much clinical research. Thus, there seems to be a severe disconnect between the frequency of the problem and the amount of attention devoted to it."[3]

Misdiagnosis

Benbadis also contends that the misdiagnosis of epilepsy in patients with PNES is common. In fact, approximately 25% of patients who have a previous diagnosis of epilepsy and are not responding to drug therapy are found to be misdiagnosed. "Unfortunately, once the diagnosis of epilepsy is made, it is easily perpetuated without being questioned, which explains the usual diagnostic delay and cost associated with PNES." It is important to note that the diagnosis of PNES may be difficult initially for several reasons. First, physicians are taught almost exclusively to consider (and exclude) physical disorders as the cause of physical symptoms. Furthermore, physicians are more likely to treat for the more serious condition if they are in doubt of the diagnosis, which explains why many patients misdiagnosed with epilepsy are prescribed antiepileptic drugs. Second, the diagnosis of seizures depends largely on the observations of others who may not be trained to notice the subtle differences between an epileptic and nonepileptic seizure. Third, many physicians do not have access to electroencephalogram (EEG)-video monitoring, which has to be performed by an epileptologist (a neurologist that specializes in epilepsy).

Editor's note: Dr. David A. Cooke notes that the situation is complicated by the fact that up to 50% of patients with PNES also, in fact, do have epilepsy as well, and they may be having both epileptic and nonepileptic spells. (David A. Cooke, MD, FACP, Diplomate, American Board of Internal Medicine, January, 2010.)

What Exactly Are PNES?

PNES are attacks that may look like epileptic seizures, but are not caused by abnormal brain electrical discharges. They are a manifestation of psychological distress. Frequently, patients with PNES may look like they are experiencing generalized convulsions similar to tonic clonic seizures with falling and shaking. Less frequently, PNES may mimic absence seizures or complex partial seizures with temporary loss of attention or staring. A physician may suspect PNES when the seizures have unusual features such as type of movements, duration, triggers, and frequency.[4]

What Causes PNES?

A specific traumatic event, such as physical or sexual abuse, incest, divorce, death of a loved one, or other great loss or sudden change, can be identified in many patients with PNES. By definition, PNES are a physical manifestation of a psychological disturbance and are a type of somatoform disorder called a conversion disorder.[1] Somatoform disorders are those conditions that are suggestive of a physical disorder, but upon examination cannot be accounted for by an underlying physical condition. Conversion disorder is a somatoform disorder that is defined as physical symptoms caused by psychologic conflict, unconsciously converted to resemble those of a neurologic disorder. Conversion disorder tends to develop during adolescence or early adulthood but may occur at any age. It appears to be somewhat more common among women.[5]

How Are PNES Diagnosed?

According to Benbadis, while EEGs are helpful in the diagnosis of epilepsy, they are often normal in patients with proven epilepsy and should not be used alone as a diagnostic tool for epilepsy. The most reliable test to make the diagnosis of PNES is EEG-video monitoring. During a video-EEG, the patient is monitored (over a time-period spanning anywhere from several hours to several days) with both a video camera and an EEG until a seizure occurs. Through analysis of the video and EEG recordings, the diagnosis of PNES can be made with near certainty. Upon diagnosis, the patient will usually be referred to a psychiatrist for further care.

Treatment Issues

"Somatoform disorders are very difficult to treat because as soon as you extinguish one symptom another one pops up. These disorders consume a lot of time and money and tend to invoke a tremendous amount of frustration on the part of the health care professionals working with this population," said Susan Kelley, PhD, Professor of Behavioral Health at the University of South Florida, Tampa, and psychotherapist in private practice. Kelley has been able to circumvent this frustration as she has adopted a trauma-focused clinical approach, which not only serves her well as a clinician, but also helps her patients with PNES to overcome their seizures. "For some patients with psychogenic non-epileptic seizures, the seizures are a manifestation of trauma, which is also known as post-traumatic stress disorder (PTSD). In order to treat patients with PTSD, the clinician has to take the seizure apart to see what the seizure represents in terms of emotions and memory as well as where this trauma is stored in the body." She postulates that when a person experiences trauma such as physical abuse, sexual abuse, witnessing violence, his or her body can absorb this trauma. Therefore, a seizure is the body's way of expressing what the mind and mouth cannot. What Kelley has found to be the most effective treatment for PNES is a therapeutic technique called eye movement desensitization and reprocessing (EMDR).

EMDR integrates elements of many psychotherapies including: psychodynamic, cognitive behavioral, interpersonal, experiential, and body-centered therapies. During EMDR the client attends to past and present experiences in brief sequential doses while simultaneously focusing on an external stimulus. Then the client is instructed to let new material become the focus of the next set of dual attention. This sequence of dual attention and personal association is repeated many times in the session.[6]

Dealing with the Stigma Associated with Psychiatric Disorders

Understandably, many patients' first reactions upon hearing they have PNES, and not epilepsy, is one of disbelief, denial, and confusion. That is because mental health issues come with highly stigmatized labels such as crazy, insane, and so forth. These stigmas are embedded in our language and even more deeply in our unconscious belief system. However, people with PNES are not crazy or insane. Some of them are victims of trauma and their recovery from the trauma as well as the seizures depends largely on their ability to overcome the stigma and follow-up with a mental health professional. "PNES is a real condition that arises in response to real stressors. These seizures are not consciously produced and are not the patient's fault," said Benbadis. Kelley agreed and said, "We need to take the shame and stigma away associated with psychiatric illnesses and instead focus on the fact that many people with PNES have a trauma history. It is so vital for people suffering with PNES to know that there is hope and that PNES is treatable through such techniques as EMDR." While EMDR works for patients with PNES who have experienced trauma it does not work with patients who have not. Kelley emphasizes the need for "greater cooperation and collaboration among the neurology, psychiatry, and psychology disciplines, so that we can find more treatments that will bring relief to these patients."

Research

In his latest study, Benbadis and colleagues examined the relationship between chronic pain or fibromyalgia and psychogenic seizures.

They designated two groups: (1) patients who had been diagnosed with fibromyalgia or chronic pain, and (2) patients who had a seizure during their visit, either in the waiting room or in the examining room. Benbadis et al. derived their data from the records of all patients evaluated over five years in a single epilepsy clinic for refractory seizures as well as through EEG-video monitoring. In the first group, they identified 28 patients with a diagnosis of fibromyalgia and eight with a diagnosis of chronic pain. After EEG-video monitoring, 27 were diagnosed with PNES. In the second group, they identified 13 patients who had a seizure during their clinic visit. After EEG-video monitoring, ten were diagnosed with PNES. "These findings suggest that a history of fibromyalgia or chronic pain and the occurrence of an episode during the visit both have a high predictive value (75% each) and a very high specificity (99%) for an eventual diagnosis of PNES," said Benbadis. He speculates that the association between chronic pain and PNES may be "because chronic discomfort can cause psychological distress, which may result in PNES." He also points out that another possibility is that "fibromyalgia and chronic pain are loosely made diagnoses that are largely psychogenic in themselves."

Whether fibromyalgia and chronic pain are largely psychogenic in nature remains a highly controversial subject. Some researchers believe fibromyalgia is a disorder of central processing with neuroendocrine/neurotransmitter dysregulation. While others in the medical community strongly believe fibromyalgia and chronic pain are psychogenic in their etiology since there is no clear underlying medical cause. Currently, the rift between these two schools of thought still remains.

If you would like more information regarding PNES you may go to: http://hsc.usf.edu/COM/epilepsy/PNESbrochure.pdf.

References

1. Benbadis SR, A spell in the epilepsy clinic and a history of "chronic pain" or "fibromyalgia" independently predict a diagnosis of psychogenic seizures. *Epilepsy Behav* 2005(6):264–265.

2. Benbadis SR, *Psychogenic Seizures*. http://www.emedicine.com/NEURO/topic403.htm.

3. Benbadis SR, The problem of psychogenic symptoms: is the psychiatric community in denial? *Epilepsy Behav* 2005(6): 9–14.

4. Benbadis SR, Heriaud L., Psychogenic (Non-Epileptic) *Seizures, a Guide for Families and Patients*. http://hsc.usf.edu/COM/epilepsy/PNESbrochure.pdf.

5. *The Merck Manual of Therapy and Diagnosis*, Section 15, Chapter 186, Conversion Disorder. www.merck.com.

6. EMDR Institute Inc., *A Brief Description of EMDR*. http:// www.emdr.com/briefdes.htm.

Study Finds Cognitive Behavioral Therapy Can Alleviate Nonepileptic Seizures

Researchers at Rhode Island Hospital have found that cognitive behavioral therapy (CBT) can reduce the frequency of seizures in patients with psychogenic nonepileptic seizures (PNES), along with improving their overall quality of life. The study was published in *Epilepsy & Behavior*.

Key findings of Rhode Island Hospital study:

* Cognitive behavioral therapy can reduce the number of PNES seizures

* Quality of life scores improve

* Depression, anxiety, and somatic symptoms associated with PNES improve

PNES is a condition that is marked by seizures resembling epileptic seizures. Unlike epilepsy, however, seizures in patients with PNES are not caused by the same brain cell firing that occurs with epilepsy. Estimates indicate that approximately 20–30% of patients who are seen in epilepsy centers actually suffer from PNES as opposed to epilepsy. Patients who suffer from PNES often exhibit a higher incidence of symptoms such as anxiety and depression than patients with epilepsy, along with a reduced quality of life due to the effect of the seizures themselves. It is recognized, however, that conditions such as anxiety and depression often respond well to CBT. To date, treatment trials for PNES are few, despite the disabling nature of the disorder.

With this in mind, senior author W. Curt LaFrance, Jr., MD, MPH, director of the division of neuropsychiatry and behavioral neurology at Rhode Island Hospital, developed a CBT for PNES treatment manual. Modified from a CBT for patients with epilepsy workbook, the treatment manual has been developed over the past five years to address core issues in patients with PNES. LaFrance, who is also an assistant professor of psychiatry and neurology (research) at the Warren Alpert Medical School of Brown University, worked with colleagues at Rhode Island Hospital's comprehensive epilepsy center to conduct an open, prospective clinical trial assessing the outcomes of outpatients with video-electroencephalogram (EEG)-confirmed PNES who were treated using the CBT for PNES manual.

LaFrance and the researchers have outlined a clinical model for management of PNES, where a key component is to identify precursors, precipitants, and perpetuating factors of the seizures. LaFrance says, "Based on the tendency of patients with PNES to somatize (to manifest mental pain as pain in one's body), we hypothesized that identifying and modifying cognitive distortions and environmental triggers for PNES would reduce PNES."

The researchers then identified patients who were referred to the Rhode Island Hospital neuropsychiatry/behavioral neurology clinic after being diagnosed with PNES and at least one typical PNES was captured on video EEG. Of the 101 patients who were assessed for eligibility, 21 patients met the criteria or agreed to participate. Of those 21, 17 completed the 12-week session of CBT intervention and were included in the analysis.

LaFrance notes that the results of the clinical trial showed the CBT to be effective in terms of reducing the frequency of PNES. He notes, "Upon completion of the CBT, 16 of the 21 participants reported a 50%reduction in seizure frequency, and 11 of the 17 who completed the CBT reported no seizures per week by their final CBT session." He also points out, "treating the seizure is not the sum total of treating the patient with a seizure disorder, so we assessed other important measures, as well." The evaluation of quality of life scores, as well as assessments of depression, anxiety, somatic symptoms, and psychosocial functioning also showed statistically significant improvement from baseline to final session.

The doctor concludes, "In this small clinical trial, treatment with the CBT for PNES program appears to be a beneficial approach in helping patients with PNES reduce their seizure frequency and significantly improve quality of life. We have also seen patients referred with other somatoform disorders, such as psychogenic movement disorders, respond to the treatment." The results of this trial will be used for an upcoming National Institutes of Health proposal for a multi-center randomized controlled trial for PNES.

Section 53.2

Febrile Seizures

Excerpted from "Febrile Seizures Fact Sheet,"
National Institute of Neurological Disorders and Stroke (NINDS),
NIH Publication No. 06–3930, updated February 9, 2010.

Febrile seizures are convulsions brought on by a fever in infants or small children. During a febrile seizure, a child often loses consciousness and shakes, moving limbs on both sides of the body. Less commonly, the child becomes rigid or has twitches in only a portion of the body, such as an arm or a leg, or on the right or the left side only. Most febrile seizures last a minute or two, although some can be as brief as a few seconds while others last for more than 15 minutes.

The majority of children with febrile seizures have rectal temperatures greater than 102 degrees Fahrenheit (F). Most febrile seizures occur during the first day of a child's fever. Children prone to febrile seizures are not considered to have epilepsy, since epilepsy is characterized by recurrent seizures that are not triggered by fever.

Approximately one in every 25 children will have at least one febrile seizure, and more than one-third of these children will have additional febrile seizures before they outgrow the tendency to have them. Febrile seizures usually occur in children between the ages of six months and five years and are particularly common in toddlers.

A few factors appear to boost a child's risk of having recurrent febrile seizures, including young age (less than 15 months) during the first seizure, frequent fevers, and having immediate family members with a history of febrile seizures. If the seizure occurs soon after a fever has begun or when the temperature is relatively low, the risk of recurrence is higher. A long initial febrile seizure does not substantially boost the risk of recurrent febrile seizures, either brief or long.

Although they can be frightening to parents, the vast majority of febrile seizures are harmless. There is no evidence that febrile seizures cause brain damage. Even in the rare instances of very prolonged seizures (more than one hour), most children recover completely. Between 95%–98% of children who have experienced febrile seizures do not go on to develop epilepsy.

Diagnosis: Before diagnosing febrile seizures in infants and children, doctors sometimes perform tests to be sure that seizures are not caused by something other than simply the fever itself. For example, if a doctor suspects the child has meningitis, a spinal tap may be needed. If there has been severe diarrhea or vomiting, dehydration could be responsible for seizures.

Prevention: If a child has a fever most parents will use fever-lowering drugs such as acetaminophen or ibuprofen to make the child more comfortable, although there are no studies that prove that this will reduce the risk of a seizure.

Children especially prone to febrile seizures may be treated with the drug diazepam orally or rectally, whenever they have a fever. The majority of children with febrile seizures do not need to be treated with medication, but in some cases a doctor may decide that medicine given only while the child has a fever may be the best alternative. This medication may lower the risk of having another febrile seizure.

Chapter 54

Myoclonus: Involuntary Muscle Jerking

Myoclonus describes a symptom and generally is not a diagnosis of a disease. It refers to sudden, involuntary jerking of a muscle or group of muscles. Myoclonic twitches or jerks usually are caused by sudden muscle contractions, called positive myoclonus, or by muscle relaxation, called negative myoclonus. Myoclonic jerks may occur alone or in sequence, in a pattern or without pattern. They may occur infrequently or many times each minute. Myoclonus sometimes occurs in response to an external event or when a person attempts to make a movement. The twitching cannot be controlled by the person experiencing it.

In its simplest form, myoclonus consists of a muscle twitch followed by relaxation. A hiccup is an example of this type of myoclonus. Other familiar examples of myoclonus are the jerks or sleep starts that some people experience while drifting off to sleep. These simple forms of myoclonus occur in normal, healthy persons and cause no difficulties. When more widespread, myoclonus may involve persistent, shock-like contractions in a group of muscles. In some cases, myoclonus begins in one region of the body and spreads to muscles in other areas. More severe cases of myoclonus can distort movement and severely limit a person's ability to eat, talk, or walk. These types of myoclonus may indicate an underlying disorder in the brain or nerves.

Excerpted from "Myoclonus Fact Sheet," National Institute of Neurological Disorders and Stroke (NINDS), NIH Publication No. 00–4793, December 18, 2009.

What are the causes of myoclonus?

Myoclonus may develop in response to infection, head or spinal cord injury, stroke, brain tumors, kidney or liver failure, lipid storage disease, chemical or drug poisoning, or other disorders. Prolonged oxygen deprivation to the brain, called hypoxia, may result in post-hypoxic myoclonus. Myoclonus can occur by itself, but most often it is one of several symptoms associated with a wide variety of nervous system disorders. For example, myoclonic jerking may develop in patients with multiple sclerosis, Parkinson disease, Alzheimer disease, or Creutzfeldt-Jakob disease. Myoclonic jerks commonly occur in persons with epilepsy, a disorder in which the electrical activity in the brain becomes disordered leading to seizures.

What are the types of myoclonus?

Classifying the many different forms of myoclonus is difficult because the causes, effects, and responses to therapy vary widely. Following are the types most commonly described.

Action myoclonus is characterized by muscular jerking triggered or intensified by voluntary movement or even the intention to move. It may be made worse by attempts at precise, coordinated movements. Action myoclonus is the most disabling form of myoclonus and can affect the arms, legs, face, and even the voice. This type of myoclonus often is caused by brain damage that results from a lack of oxygen and blood flow to the brain when breathing or heartbeat is temporarily stopped.

Cortical reflex myoclonus is thought to be a type of epilepsy that originates in the cerebral cortex—the outer layer, or gray matter, of the brain, responsible for much of the information processing that takes place in the brain. In this type of myoclonus, jerks usually involve only a few muscles in one part of the body, but jerks involving many muscles also may occur. Cortical reflex myoclonus can be intensified when individuals attempt to move in a certain way or perceive a particular sensation.

Essential myoclonus occurs in the absence of epilepsy or other apparent abnormalities in the brain or nerves. It can occur randomly in people with no family history, but it also can appear among members of the same family, indicating that it sometimes may be an inherited disorder. Essential myoclonus tends to be stable without increasing in severity over time. In some families, there is an association of essential myoclonus, essential tremor, and even a form of dystonia, called myoclonus dystonia. Other forms of essential myoclonus may be a type of epilepsy with no known cause.

Palatal myoclonus is a regular, rhythmic contraction of one or both sides of the rear of the roof of the mouth, called the soft palate. These contractions may be accompanied by myoclonus in other muscles, including those in the face, tongue, throat, and diaphragm. The contractions are very rapid, occurring as often as 150 times a minute, and may persist during sleep. The condition usually appears in adults and can last indefinitely. People with palatal myoclonus usually regard it as a minor problem, although some occasionally complain of a clicking sound in the ear, a noise made as the muscles in the soft palate contract.

Progressive myoclonus epilepsy (PME) is a group of diseases characterized by myoclonus, epileptic seizures, and other serious symptoms such as trouble walking or speaking. These rare disorders often get worse over time and sometimes are fatal. Studies have identified many forms of PME. Lafora body disease is inherited as an autosomal recessive disorder, meaning that the disease occurs only when a child inherits two copies of a defective gene, one from each parent. Lafora body disease is characterized by myoclonus, epileptic seizures, and dementia (progressive loss of memory and other intellectual functions). A second group of PME diseases belonging to the class of cerebral storage diseases usually involves myoclonus, visual problems, dementia, and dystonia (sustained muscle contractions that cause twisting movements or abnormal postures). Another group of PME disorders in the class of system degenerations often is accompanied by action myoclonus, seizures, and problems with balance and walking. Many of these PME diseases begin in childhood or adolescence.

Reticular reflex myoclonus is thought to be a type of generalized epilepsy that originates in the brain stem, the part of the brain that connects to the spinal cord and controls vital functions such as breathing and heartbeat. Myoclonic jerks usually affect the whole body, with muscles on both sides of the body affected simultaneously. In some people, myoclonic jerks occur in only a part of the body, such as the legs, with all the muscles in that part being involved in each jerk. Reticular reflex myoclonus can be triggered by either a voluntary movement or an external stimulus.

559

Stimulus-sensitive myoclonus is triggered by a variety of external events, including noise, movement, and light. Surprise may increase the sensitivity of the individual.

Sleep myoclonus occurs during the initial phases of sleep, especially at the moment of dropping off to sleep. Some forms appear to be stimulus-sensitive. Some persons with sleep myoclonus are rarely troubled by, or need treatment for, the condition. However, myoclonus may be a symptom in more complex and disturbing sleep disorders, such as restless legs syndrome, and may require treatment by a doctor.

What do scientists know about myoclonus?

Although rare cases of myoclonus are caused by an injury to the peripheral nerves (defined as the nerves outside the brain and spinal cord, or the central nervous system), most myoclonus is caused by a disturbance of the central nervous system. Studies suggest that several locations in the brain are involved in myoclonus. One such location, for example, is in the brain stem close to structures that are responsible for the startle response, an automatic reaction to an unexpected stimulus involving rapid muscle contraction.

How is myoclonus treated?

Treatment of myoclonus focuses on medications that may help reduce symptoms. The drug of first choice to treat myoclonus, especially certain types of action myoclonus, is clonazepam, a type of tranquilizer. Dosages of clonazepam usually are increased gradually until the individual improves or side effects become harmful. Drowsiness and loss of coordination are common side effects. The beneficial effects of clonazepam may diminish over time if the individual develops a tolerance for the drug.

Many of the drugs used for myoclonus, such as barbiturates, levetiracetam, phenytoin, and primidone, are also used to treat epilepsy. Barbiturates slow down the central nervous system and cause tranquilizing or antiseizure effects. Phenytoin, levetiracetam, and primidone are effective antiepileptic drugs, although phenytoin can cause liver failure or have other harmful long-term effects in individuals with PME. Sodium valproate is an alternative therapy for myoclonus and can be used either alone or in combination with clonazepam. Although clonazepam and sodium valproate are effective in the majority

560

of people with myoclonus, some people have adverse reactions to these drugs.

The complex origins of myoclonus may require the use of multiple drugs for effective treatment. Although some drugs have a limited effect when used individually, they may have a greater effect when used with drugs that act on different pathways or mechanisms in the brain. By combining several of these drugs, scientists hope to achieve greater control of myoclonic symptoms. Some drugs currently being studied in different combinations include clonazepam, sodium valproate, levetiracetam, and primidone. Hormonal therapy also may improve responses to anti-myoclonic drugs in some people.

Chapter 55

Restless Legs Syndrome

Restless legs syndrome (RLS) is a neurological disorder characterized by unpleasant sensations in the legs and an uncontrollable urge to move when at rest in an effort to relieve these feelings. RLS sensations are often described by people as burning, creeping, tugging, or like insects crawling inside the legs. Also called paresthesias (abnormal sensations), or dysesthesias (unpleasant abnormal sensations), the sensations range in severity from uncomfortable to irritating to painful.

The most distinctive or unusual aspect of the condition is that lying down and trying to relax activates the symptoms. As a result, most people with RLS have difficulty falling asleep and staying asleep. Left untreated, the condition causes exhaustion and daytime fatigue. Many people with RLS report that their job, personal relations, and activities of daily living are strongly affected as a result of their exhaustion. They are often unable to concentrate, have impaired memory, or fail to accomplish daily tasks.

Some researchers estimate that RLS affects as many as 12 million Americans. However, others estimate a much higher occurrence because RLS is thought to be underdiagnosed and, in some cases, misdiagnosed. Some people with RLS will not seek medical attention, believing that they will not be taken seriously, that their symptoms are too mild, or that their condition is not treatable. Some physicians

Text in this chapter is excerpted from "Restless Legs Syndrome Fact Sheet," National Institute of Neurological Disorders and Stroke (NINDS), NIH Publication No. 01–4847, December 18, 2009.

wrongly attribute the symptoms to nervousness, insomnia, stress, arthritis, muscle cramps, or aging.

RLS occurs in both genders, although the incidence may be slightly higher in women. Although the syndrome may begin at any age, even as early as infancy, most patients who are severely affected are middle-aged or older. In addition, the severity of the disorder appears to increase with age. Older patients experience symptoms more frequently and for longer periods of time.

More than 80% of people with RLS also experience a more common condition known as periodic limb movement disorder (PLMD). PLMD is characterized by involuntary leg twitching or jerking movements during sleep that typically occur every 10–60 seconds, sometimes throughout the night. The symptoms cause repeated awakening and severely disrupted sleep. Unlike RLS, the movements caused by PLMD are involuntary—people have no control over them. Although many patients with RLS also develop PLMD, most people with PLMD do not experience RLS. Like RLS, the cause of PLMD is unknown.

What are common signs and symptoms of restless legs?

As described, people with RLS feel uncomfortable sensations in their legs, especially when sitting or lying down, accompanied by an irresistible urge to move about. These sensations usually occur deep inside the leg, between the knee and ankle; more rarely, they occur in the feet, thighs, arms, and hands. Although the sensations can occur on just one side of the body, they most often affect both sides.

Because moving the legs (or other affected parts of the body) relieves the discomfort, people with RLS often keep their legs in motion to minimize or prevent the sensations. They may pace the floor, constantly move their legs while sitting, and toss and turn in bed.

Most people find the symptoms to be less noticeable during the day and more pronounced in the evening or at night, especially during the onset of sleep. For many people, the symptoms disappear by early morning, allowing for more refreshing sleep at that time. Other triggering situations are periods of inactivity such as long car trips, sitting in a movie theater, long-distance flights, immobilization in a cast, or relaxation exercises.

The symptoms of RLS vary in severity and duration from person to person. Mild RLS occurs episodically, with only mild disruption of sleep onset, and causes little distress. In moderately severe cases, symptoms occur only once or twice a week but result in significant delay of sleep onset, with some disruption of daytime function. In severe cases of RLS, the symptoms occur more than twice a week and result in burdensome interruption of sleep and impairment of daytime function. Symptoms may begin at any stage of life, although the disorder is more common with increasing age. Sometimes people will experience spontaneous improvement over a period of weeks or months. Although rare, spontaneous improvement over a period of years also can occur. If these improvements occur, it is usually during the early stages of the disorder. In general, however, symptoms become more severe over time.

People who have both RLS and an associated condition tend to develop more severe symptoms rapidly. In contrast, those whose RLS is not related to any other medical condition and whose onset is at an early age show a very slow progression of the disorder and many years may pass before symptoms occur regularly.

What causes restless legs syndrome?

In most cases, the cause of RLS is unknown (referred to as idiopathic). A family history of the condition is seen in approximately 50% of such cases, suggesting a genetic form of the disorder. People with familial RLS tend to be younger when symptoms start and have a slower progression of the condition. In other cases, RLS appears to be related to the following factors or conditions, although researchers do not yet know if these factors actually cause RLS.

* People with low iron levels or anemia may be prone to developing RLS. Once iron levels or anemia is corrected, patients may see a reduction in symptoms.

* Chronic diseases such as kidney failure, diabetes, Parkinson disease, and peripheral neuropathy are associated with RLS. Treating the underlying condition often provides relief from RLS symptoms.

* Some pregnant women experience RLS, especially in their last trimester. For most of these women, symptoms usually disappear within four weeks after delivery.

* Certain medications—such as antinausea drugs (prochlorperazine or metoclopramide), antiseizure drugs (phenytoin or droperidol), antipsychotic drugs (haloperidol or phenothiazine derivatives), and some cold and allergy medications—may aggravate symptoms. Patients can talk with their physicians about the possibility of changing medications.

Researchers also have found that caffeine, alcohol, and tobacco may aggravate or trigger symptoms in patients who are predisposed to develop RLS. Some studies have shown that a reduction or complete elimination of such substances may relieve symptoms, although it remains unclear whether elimination of such substances can prevent RLS symptoms from occurring at all.

How is restless legs syndrome diagnosed?

Currently, there is no single diagnostic test for RLS. The disorder is diagnosed clinically by evaluating the patient's history and symptoms. Despite a clear description of clinical features, the condition is often misdiagnosed or underdiagnosed. In 1995, the International Restless Legs Syndrome Study Group identified four basic criteria for diagnosing RLS: (1) a desire to move the limbs, often associated with paresthesias or dysesthesias; (2) symptoms that are worse or present only during rest and are partially or temporarily relieved by activity; (3) motor restlessness; and (4) nocturnal worsening of symptoms. Although about 80% of those with RLS also experience PLMD, it is not necessary for a diagnosis of RLS. In more severe cases, patients may experience dyskinesia (uncontrolled, often continuous movements) while awake, and some experience symptoms in one or both of their arms as well as their legs. Most people with RLS have sleep disturbances, largely because of the limb discomfort and jerking. The result is excessive daytime sleepiness and fatigue.

If a patient's history is suggestive of RLS, laboratory tests may be performed to rule out other conditions and support the diagnosis of RLS. Blood tests to exclude anemia, decreased iron stores, diabetes, and renal dysfunction should be performed. Electromyography and nerve conduction studies may also be recommended to measure electrical activity in muscles and nerves, and Doppler sonography may be used to evaluate muscle activity in the legs. Such tests can document any accompanying damage or disease in nerves and nerve roots (such as peripheral neuropathy and radiculopathy) or other leg-related movement disorders. Negative results from tests may indicate that the diagnosis is RLS. In some cases, sleep studies such as polysomnography (a test that records the patient's brain waves, heartbeat, and breathing during an entire night) are undertaken to identify the presence of PLMD.

How is restless legs syndrome treated?

Although movement brings relief to those with RLS, it is generally only temporary. However, RLS can be controlled by finding any possible underlying disorder. Often, treating the associated medical condition, such as peripheral neuropathy or diabetes, will alleviate many symptoms. For patients with idiopathic RLS, treatment is directed toward relieving symptoms.

For those with mild to moderate symptoms, prevention is key, and many physicians suggest certain lifestyle changes and activities to reduce or eliminate symptoms. Decreased use of caffeine, alcohol, and tobacco may provide some relief. Physicians may suggest that certain individuals take supplements to correct deficiencies in iron, folate, and magnesium. Studies also have shown that maintaining a regular sleep pattern can reduce symptoms. Some individuals, finding that RLS symptoms are minimized in the early morning, change their sleep patterns. Others have found that a program of regular moderate exercise helps them sleep better; on the other hand, excessive exercise has been reported by some patients to aggravate RLS symptoms. Taking a hot bath, massaging the legs, or using a heating pad or ice pack can help relieve symptoms in some patients. Although many patients find some relief with such measures, rarely do these efforts completely eliminate symptoms.

Physicians also may suggest a variety of medications to treat RLS. Generally, physicians choose from dopaminergics, benzodiazepines (central nervous system depressants), opioids, and anticonvulsants. Dopaminergic agents, largely used to treat Parkinson disease, have been shown to reduce RLS symptoms and PLMD and are considered the initial treatment of choice. In 2005, ropinirole became the only drug approved by the U.S. Food and Drug Administration (FDA) specifically for the treatment of moderate to severe RLS. The drug was first approved in 1997 for patients with Parkinson disease.

Benzodiazepines (such as clonazepam and diazepam) may be prescribed for patients who have mild or intermittent symptoms. These drugs help patients obtain a more restful sleep but they do not fully alleviate RLS symptoms and can cause daytime sleepiness. Because these depressants also may induce or aggravate sleep apnea in some cases, they should not be used in people with this condition.

For more severe symptoms, opioids such as codeine, propoxyphene, or oxycodone may be prescribed for their ability to induce relaxation and diminish pain. Side effects include dizziness, nausea, vomiting, and the risk of addiction.

Anticonvulsants such as carbamazepine and gabapentin are also useful for some patients, as they decrease the sensory disturbances (creeping and crawling sensations). Dizziness, fatigue, and sleepiness are among the possible side effects.

Unfortunately, no one drug is effective for everyone with RLS. What may be helpful to one individual may actually worsen symptoms for another. In addition, medications taken regularly may lose their effect, making it necessary to change medications periodically.

What is the prognosis of people with restless legs?

RLS is generally a lifelong condition for which there is no cure. Symptoms may gradually worsen with age, though more slowly for those with the idiopathic form of RLS than for patients who also suffer from an associated medical condition. Nevertheless, current therapies can control the disorder, minimizing symptoms and increasing periods of restful sleep. In addition, some patients have remissions, periods in which symptoms decrease or disappear for days, weeks, or months, although symptoms usually eventually reappear. A diagnosis of RLS does not indicate the onset of another neurological disease.

Chapter 56

Narcolepsy

Narcolepsy is a chronic neurological disorder caused by the brain's inability to regulate sleep-wake cycles normally. At various times throughout the day, people with narcolepsy experience fleeting urges to sleep. If the urge becomes overwhelming, patients fall asleep for periods lasting from a few seconds to several minutes. In rare cases, some people may remain asleep for an hour or longer.

Narcoleptic sleep episodes can occur at any time, and thus frequently prove profoundly disabling. People may involuntarily fall asleep while at work or at school, when having a conversation, playing a game, eating a meal, or most dangerously, when driving an automobile or operating other types of potentially hazardous machinery. In addition to daytime sleepiness, three other major symptoms frequently characterize narcolepsy: cataplexy or the sudden loss of voluntary muscle tone; vivid hallucinations during sleep onset or upon awakening; and brief episodes of total paralysis at the beginning or end of sleep.

Contrary to common beliefs, people with narcolepsy do not spend a substantially greater proportion of their time asleep during a 24-hour period than do normal sleepers. In addition to daytime drowsiness and involuntary sleep episodes, most patients also experience frequent awakenings during nighttime sleep. For these reasons, narcolepsy is considered to be a disorder of the normal boundaries between the sleeping and waking states.

This chapter is excerpted from "Narcolepsy Fact Sheet," National Institute of Neurological Disorders and Stroke (NINDS), NIH Publication No. 03–1637, October 2, 2009.

For most adults, a normal night's sleep lasts about eight hours and is composed of four to six separate sleep cycles. A sleep cycle is defined by a segment of non-rapid eye movement (NREM) sleep followed by a period of rapid eye movement (REM) sleep. The NREM segment can be further divided into stages according to the size and frequency of brain waves. REM sleep, in contrast, is accompanied by bursts of rapid eye movement (hence the acronym REM sleep) along with sharply heightened brain activity and temporary paralysis of the muscles that control posture and body movement. When subjects are awakened from sleep, they report that they were "having a dream" more often if they had been in REM sleep than if they had been in NREM sleep. Transitions from NREM to REM sleep are governed by interactions among groups of neurons (nerve cells) in certain parts of the brain.

Scientists now believe that narcolepsy results from disease processes affecting brain mechanisms that regulate REM sleep. For normal sleepers a typical sleep cycle is about 100–110 minutes long, beginning with NREM sleep and transitioning to REM sleep after 80–100 minutes. But, people with narcolepsy frequently enter REM sleep within a few minutes of falling asleep.

Who gets narcolepsy?

Narcolepsy is not rare, but it is an under-recognized and underdiagnosed condition. The disorder is estimated to affect about one in every 2,000 Americans. But the exact prevalence rate remains uncertain, and the disorder may affect a larger segment of the population.

Narcolepsy appears throughout the world in every racial and ethnic group, affecting males and females equally. But prevalence rates vary among populations. Compared to the United States (U.S.) population, for example, the prevalence rate is substantially lower in Israel (about one per 500,000) and considerably higher in Japan (about one per 600).

Most cases of narcolepsy are sporadic—that is, the disorder occurs independently in individuals without strong evidence of being inherited. But familial clusters are known to occur. Up to 10% of patients diagnosed with narcolepsy with cataplexy report having a close relative with the same symptoms. Genetic factors alone are not sufficient to cause narcolepsy. Other factors—such as infection, immune-system dysfunction, trauma, hormonal changes, and stress—may also be present before the disease develops. Thus, while close relatives of people with narcolepsy have a statistically higher risk of developing the disorder than do members of the general population, that risk remains low in comparison to diseases that are purely genetic in origin.

What are the symptoms?

People with narcolepsy experience highly individualized patterns of REM sleep disturbances that tend to begin subtly and may change dramatically over time. The most common major symptom, other than excessive daytime sleepiness (EDS), is cataplexy, which occurs in about 70% of all patients. Sleep paralysis and hallucinations are somewhat less common. Only 10–25% of patients, however, display all four of these major symptoms during the course of their illness.

What causes narcolepsy?

The cause of narcolepsy remains unknown but during the past decade, scientists have made considerable progress in understanding its pathogenesis and in identifying genes strongly associated with the disorder. Researchers have also discovered abnormalities in various parts of the brain involved in regulating REM sleep that appear to contribute to symptom development. Experts now believe it is likely that—similar to many other complex, chronic neurological diseases—narcolepsy involves multiple factors interacting to cause neurological dysfunction and REM sleep disturbances.

Other factors appear to play important roles in the development of narcolepsy. Some rare cases are known to result from traumatic injuries to parts of the brain involved in REM sleep or from tumor growth and other disease processes in the same regions. Infections, exposure to toxins, dietary factors, stress, hormonal changes such as those occurring during puberty or menopause, and alterations in a person's sleep schedule are just a few of the many factors that may exert direct or indirect effects on the brain, thereby possibly contributing to disease development.

How is narcolepsy diagnosed?

Narcolepsy is not definitively diagnosed in most patients until 10–15 years after the first symptoms appear. This unusually long lag-time is due to several factors, including the disorder's subtle onset and the variability of symptoms. As important, however, is the fact that the public is largely unfamiliar with the disorder, as are many health professionals. When symptoms initially develop, people often do not recognize that they are experiencing the onset of a distinct neurological disorder and thus fail to seek medical treatment.

Two tests in particular are considered essential in confirming a diagnosis of narcolepsy: the polysomnogram (PSG) and the multiple sleep latency test (MSLT). The PSG is an overnight test that takes continuous multiple measurements while a patient is asleep to document abnormalities in the sleep cycle. It records heart and respiratory rates, electrical activity in the brain through electroencephalography (EEG), and nerve activity in muscles through electromyography (EMG). A PSG can help reveal whether REM sleep occurs at abnormal times in the sleep cycle and can eliminate the possibility that an individual's symptoms result from another condition.

The MSLT is performed during the day to measure a person's tendency to fall asleep and to determine whether isolated elements of REM sleep intrude at inappropriate times during the waking hours. As part of the test, an individual is asked to take four or five short naps usually scheduled two hours apart over the course of a day. As the name suggests, the sleep latency test measures the amount of time it takes for a person to fall asleep. Because sleep latency periods are normally ten minutes or longer, a latency period of five minutes or less is considered suggestive of narcolepsy. The MSLT also measures heart and respiratory rates, records nerve activity in muscles, and pinpoints the occurrence of abnormally timed REM episodes through EEG recordings. If a person enters REM sleep either at the beginning or within a few minutes of sleep onset during at least two of the scheduled naps, this is also considered a positive indication of narcolepsy.

What treatments are available?

Narcolepsy cannot yet be cured. But EDS and cataplexy, the most disabling symptoms of the disorder, can be controlled in most patients with drug treatment. Often the treatment regimen is modified as symptoms change.

For decades, doctors have used central nervous system stimulants—amphetamines such as methylphenidate, dextroamphetamine, methamphetamine, and pemoline—to alleviate EDS and reduce the incidence of sleep attacks. For most patients these medications are generally quite effective at reducing daytime drowsiness and improving levels of alertness. However, they are associated with a wide array of undesirable side effects so their use must be carefully monitored. Common side effects include irritability and nervousness, shakiness, disturbances in heart rhythm, stomach upset, nighttime sleep disruption, and anorexia. Patients may also develop tolerance with long-term use, leading to the need for increased dosages to maintain effectiveness. In addition, doctors should be careful when prescribing these drugs and patients should be careful using them because the potential for abuse is high with any amphetamine.

In 1999, the U.S. Food and Drug Administration (FDA) approved a new non-amphetamine wake-promoting drug called modafinil for the treatment of EDS. In clinical trials, modafinil proved to be effective in alleviating EDS while producing fewer, less serious side effects than do amphetamines. Headache is the most commonly reported adverse effect. Long-term use of modafinil does not appear to lead to tolerance.

Two classes of antidepressant drugs have proved effective in controlling cataplexy in many patients: tricyclics (including imipramine, desipramine, clomipramine, and protriptyline) and selective serotonin reuptake inhibitors (including fluoxetine and sertraline). In general, antidepressants produce fewer adverse effects than do amphetamines. But troublesome side effects still occur in some patients, including impotence, high blood pressure, and heart rhythm irregularities.

On July 17, 2002, the FDA approved Xyrem (sodium oxybate or gamma hydroxybutyrate, also known as GHB) for treating people with narcolepsy who experience episodes of cataplexy. Due to safety concerns associated with the use of this drug, the distribution of Xyrem is tightly restricted.

What behavioral strategies help people cope with symptoms?

None of the currently available medications enables people with narcolepsy to consistently maintain a fully normal state of alertness. Thus, drug therapy should be supplemented by various behavioral strategies according to the needs of the individual patient.

To gain greater control over their symptoms, many patients take short, regularly scheduled naps at times when they tend to feel sleepiest. Adults can often negotiate with employers to modify their work schedules so they can take naps when necessary and perform their most demanding tasks when they are most alert.

Improving the quality of nighttime sleep can combat EDS and help relieve persistent feelings of fatigue. Exercising for at least 20 minutes per day at least 4–5 hours before bedtime also improves sleep quality and can help people with narcolepsy avoid gaining excess weight.

Safety precautions, particularly when driving, are of paramount importance for all persons with narcolepsy. Although the disorder, in itself, is not fatal, EDS and cataplexy can lead to serious injury or death if left uncontrolled. Suddenly falling asleep or losing muscle control can transform actions that are ordinarily safe, such as walking down a long flight of stairs, into hazards. People with untreated narcoleptic symptoms are involved in automobile accidents roughly ten times more frequently than the general population. However, accident rates are normal among patients who have received appropriate medication.

Part Nine

Additional Help and Information

Chapter 57

Glossary of Terms Related to Brain Disorders

aneurysm: A blood-filled sac formed by disease related stretching of an artery or blood vessel.

angiogram: An x-ray of blood vessels. The person receives an injection of dye to outline the vessels on the x-ray.[1]

anoxia: An absence of oxygen supply to an organ's tissues leading to cell death.

aphasia: Difficulty understanding and/or producing spoken and written language.

apoptosis: Cell death that occurs naturally as part of normal development, maintenance, and renewal of tissues within an organism.

arachnoid membrane: One of the three membranes that cover the brain; it is between the pia mater and the dura. Collectively, these three membranes form the meninges.

Terms in this chapter are excerpted from "Traumatic Brain Injury: Hope through Research," National Institute of Neurological Disorders and Stroke (NINDS), NIH Publication No. 02–2478, updated February 9, 2010. Terms marked with a [1] are from "Childhood Brain and Spinal Cord Tumors Treatment Overview (PDQ®): Patient Version." PDQ® Cancer Information Summary. National Cancer Institute; Bethesda, MD. Updated October 15, 2009. Available at: http://www. cancer.gov. Accessed January 7, 2010. Terms marked with a [2] are from "Dementia: Hope through Research," NINDS, updated February 12, 2010. Terms marked with a [3] are from "Seizures and Epilepsy: Hope through Research," NINDS, NIH Publication 04–156, February 9, 2010.

benign: Not cancerous. Benign tumors may grow larger but do not spread to other parts of the body.[1]

biopsy: The removal of cells or tissues for examination by a pathologist. The pathologist may study the tissue under a microscope or perform other tests on the cells or tissue.[1]

brain death: An irreversible cessation of measurable brain function.

Broca aphasia: See non-fluent aphasia.

cancer: A term for diseases in which abnormal cells divide without control. Cancer cells can invade nearby tissues and can spread to other parts of the body through the blood and lymph systems.[1]

cerebellum: The portion of the brain in the back of the head between the cerebrum and the brain stem. The cerebellum controls balance for walking and standing, and other complex motor functions.[1]

cerebral hemisphere: One half of the cerebrum, the part of the brain that controls muscle functions and also controls speech, thought, emotions, reading, writing, and learning. The right hemisphere controls the muscles on the left side of the body, and the left hemisphere controls the muscles on the right side of the body.[1]

cerebrospinal fluid (CSF): The fluid that bathes and protects the brain and spinal cord.

cerebrum: The largest part of the brain. It is divided into two hemispheres, or halves, called the cerebral hemispheres. Areas within the cerebrum control muscle functions and also control speech, thought, emotions, reading, writing, and learning.[1]

chemotherapy: Treatment with drugs that kill cancer cells.[1]

clinical trial: A type of research study that tests how well new medical approaches work in people. These studies test new methods of screening, prevention, diagnosis, or treatment of a disease.[1]

closed head injury: An injury that occurs when the head suddenly and violently hits an object but the object does not break through the skull.

cognitive training: Patients practice tasks designed to improve mental performance.[2]

coma: A state of profound unconsciousness caused by disease, injury, or poison.

compressive cranial neuropathies: Degeneration of nerves in the brain caused by pressure on those nerves.

computed tomography (CT): A scan that creates a series of cross-sectional x-rays of the head and brain; also called computerized axial tomography or CAT scan.

concussion: Injury to the brain caused by a hard blow or violent shaking, causing a sudden and temporary impairment of brain function, such as a short loss of consciousness or disturbance of vision and equilibrium.

contrecoup: A contusion caused by the shaking of the brain back and forth within the confines of the skull.

contusion: Distinct area of swollen brain tissue mixed with blood released from broken blood vessels.

cortical atrophy: Degeneration of the brain's cortex (outer layer), common in many forms of dementia.[2]

deep vein thrombosis: Formation of a blood clot deep within a vein.

dementia: A term for a collection of symptoms that significantly impair thinking and normal activities and relationships.[2]

dementia pugilistica: Brain damage caused by cumulative and repetitive head trauma; common in career boxers.

depressed skull fracture: A fracture occurring when pieces of broken skull press into the tissues of the brain.

diffuse axonal injury: See shearing.

dura: A tough, fibrous membrane lining the brain; the outermost of the three membranes collectively called the meninges.

dysarthria: Inability or difficulty articulating words due to emotional stress, brain injury, paralysis, or spasticity of the muscles needed for speech.

early seizures: Seizures that occur within one week after a traumatic brain injury.

epidural hematoma: Bleeding into the area between the skull and the dura.

fluent aphasia: A condition in which patients display little meaning in their speech even though they speak in complete sentences. Also called Wernicke or motor aphasia.

Glasgow Coma Scale: A clinical tool used to assess the degree of consciousness and neurological functioning: and therefore severity of brain injury: by testing motor responsiveness, verbal acuity, and eye opening.

global aphasia: A condition in which patients suffer severe communication disabilities as a result of extensive damage to portions of the brain responsible for language.

grade: The grade of a tumor depends on how abnormal the cancer cells look under a microscope and how quickly the tumor is likely to grow and spread. Grading systems are different for each type of cancer.[1]

hematoma: Heavy bleeding into or around the brain caused by damage to a major blood vessel in the head.

hemorrhagic stroke: Stroke caused by bleeding out of one of the major arteries leading to the brain.

hypermetabolism: A condition in which the body produces too much heat energy.

hypothyroidism: Decreased production of thyroid hormone leading to low metabolic rate, weight gain, chronic drowsiness, dry skin and hair, and fluid accumulation and retention in connective tissues.

hypoxia: Decreased oxygen levels in an organ, such as the brain; less severe than anoxia.

immediate seizures: Seizures that occur within 24 hours of a traumatic brain injury.

intracerebral hematoma: Bleeding within the brain caused by damage to a major blood vessel.

intracranial pressure: Buildup of pressure in the brain as a result of injury.

ischemic stroke: Stroke caused by the formation of a clot that blocks blood flow through an artery to the brain.

ketogenic diet: A strict diet rich in fats and low in carbohydrates that causes the body to break down fats instead of carbohydrates to survive.[3]

lesion: Damaged or dysfunctional part of the brain or other parts of the body mutation an abnormality in a gene.[3]

locked-in syndrome: A condition in which a patient is aware and awake, but cannot move or communicate due to complete paralysis of the body.

lumbar puncture: See spinal tap.

magnetic resonance imaging (MRI): A noninvasive diagnostic technique that uses magnetic fields to detect subtle changes in brain tissue.

malignant: Cancerous. Malignant tumors can invade and destroy nearby tissue and spread to other parts of the body.[1]

meningitis: Inflammation of the three membranes that envelop the brain and spinal cord, collectively known as the meninges; the meninges include the dura, pia mater, and arachnoid.

metastatic: Having to do with metastasis, which is the spread of cancer from one part of the body to another.[1]

mild cognitive impairment: A condition associated with impairments in understanding and memory not severe enough to be diagnosed as dementia, but more pronounced than those associated with normal aging.[2]

Mini-Mental Status Examination: A test used to assess cognitive skills in people with suspected dementia. The test examines orientation, memory, and attention, as well as the ability to name objects, follow verbal and written commands, write a sentence spontaneously, and copy a complex shape.[2]

motor aphasia: See non-fluent aphasia.

multi-infarct dementia: A type of vascular dementia caused by numerous small strokes in the brain.[2]

myelin: A fatty substance that coats and insulates nerve cells.[2]

myoclonic seizures: Seizures that cause sudden jerks or twitches, especially in the upper body, arms, or legs.[3]

neural stem cells: Cells found only in adult neural tissue that can develop into several different cell types in the central nervous system.

neuro-excitation: The electrical activation of cells in the brain; neuro-excitation is part of the normal functioning of the brain or can also be the result of abnormal activity related to an injury.

neuron: A nerve cell that is one of the main functional cells of the brain and nervous system.

neurotransmitters: Chemicals that transmit nerve signals from one neuron to another.

non-fluent aphasia: A condition in which patients have trouble recalling words and speaking in complete sentences, also called Broca or motor aphasia.

penetrating head injury: A brain injury in which an object pierces the skull and enters the brain tissue.

penetrating skull fracture: A brain injury in which an object pierces the skull and injures brain tissue.

persistent vegetative state: An ongoing state of severely impaired consciousness, in which the patient is incapable of voluntary motion.

plaques: Unusual clumps of material found between tissues of the brain in Alzheimer disease.[2]

plasticity: Ability of the brain to adapt to deficits and injury.

post-concussion syndrome (PCS): A complex, poorly understood problem that may cause headache after head injury; in most cases, patients cannot remember the event that caused the concussion and a variable period of time prior to the injury.

post-traumatic amnesia (PTA): A state of acute confusion due to a traumatic brain injury, marked by difficulty with perception, thinking, remembering, and concentration; during this acute stage, patients often cannot form new memories.

post-traumatic dementia: A condition marked by mental deterioration and emotional apathy following trauma.

post-traumatic epilepsy: Recurrent seizures occurring more than one week after a traumatic brain injury.

pruning: Process whereby an injury destroys an important neural network in children, and another less useful neural network that would have eventually died takes over the responsibilities of the damaged network.

seizure focus: An area of the brain where seizures originate.[3]

seizures: Abnormal activity of nerve cells in the brain causing strange sensations, emotions, and behavior, or sometimes convulsions, muscle spasms, and loss of consciousness.

sensory aphasia: See fluent aphasia.

shaken baby syndrome: A severe form of head injury that occurs when an infant or small child is shaken forcibly enough to cause the brain to bounce against the skull; the degree of brain damage depends on the extent and duration of the shaking.

shearing (or diffuse axonal injury): Damage to individual neurons resulting in disruption of neural networks and the breakdown of overall communication among neurons in the brain.

shunt: In medicine, a passage that is made to allow blood or other fluid to move from one part of the body to another.[1]

spinal tap: A procedure in which a thin needle called a spinal needle is put into the lower part of the spinal column to collect cerebrospinal fluid or to give drugs. Also called lumbar puncture.[1]

stereotactic biopsy: A biopsy procedure that uses a computer and a three-dimensional (3D) scanning device to find a tumor site and guide the removal of tissue for examination under a microscope.[1]

stupor: A state of impaired consciousness in which the patient is unresponsive but can be aroused briefly by a strong stimulus.

subdural hematoma: Bleeding confined to the area between the dura and the arachnoid membranes.

thrombosis or thrombus: The formation of a blood clot at the site of an injury.

tumor: An abnormal mass of tissue that results when cells divide more than they should or do not die when they should, also called neoplasm. Tumors may be benign (not cancerous), or malignant (cancerous).[1]

vasospasm: Exaggerated, persistent contraction of the walls of a blood vessel.

vegetative state: A condition in which patients are unconscious and unaware of their surroundings, but continue to have a sleep/wake cycle and can have periods of alertness.

Wernicke aphasia: See fluent aphasia.

Chapter 58

Directory of Organizations with Information about Brain Disorders

Government Organizations

Agency for Healthcare Research and Quality (AHRQ)
540 Gaither Rd.
Rockville, MD 20850
Toll-Free: 800-358-9295
Phone: 301-427-1364
Website: http://www.ahrq.gov

Agency for Toxic Substances and Disease Registry
4770 Buford Hwy. NE
Atlanta, GA 30341
Toll-Free: 800-232-4636
TTY: 888-232-6348
Website: http://www.atsdr.cdc
.gov
E-mail: cdcinfo@cdc.gov

Alzheimer's Disease Education and Referral Center (ADEAR)
P.O. Box 8250
Silver Spring, MD 20907
Toll-Free: 800-438-4380
Fax: 301-495-3334
Website: http://www.alzheimers
.nia.nih.gov
E-mail: adear@nia.nih.gov

Brain Attack Coalition
Building 31, Rm. 8A-16
31 Center Dr., MSC 2540
Bethesda, MD 20892
Phone: 301-496-5751
Fax: 301-402-2186
Website: http://www.stroke-site
.org

Resources in this chapter were compiled from several sources deemed reliable; all contact information was verified and updated in February, 2010. Inclusion does not imply endorsement. This list is not comprehensive, it is intended as a starting point for gathering of information.

Centers for Disease Control and Prevention (CDC)
1600 Clifton Rd.
Atlanta, GA 30333
Toll-Free: 800-232-4636
Toll-Free TTY: 888-232-6348
Website: http://www.cdc.gov
E-mail: cdcinfo@cdc.gov

Eldercare Locator
Toll-Free: 800-677-1116
Website: http://www.eldercare
.gov

National Cancer Institute (NCI)
NCI Public Inquiries Office
6116 Executive Blvd.
Room 3036A
Bethesda, MD 20892
Toll-Free: 800-4-CANCER
(800-422-6237)
Website: http://www.cancer.gov

National Heart, Lung, and Blood Institute (NHBLI)
Building 31, Room 5A52
31 Center Dr., MSC 2486
Bethesda, MD 20892
Phone: 301-592-8573
TTY: 240-629-3255
Fax: 240-629-3246
Website: http://www.nhlbi.nih
.gov

National Institute of Mental Health (NIMH)
6001 Executive Blvd.
Rm. 8184, MSC 9663
Bethesda, MD 20892
Toll-Free: 866-615-6464
Phone: 301-443-4513
TTY: 301-443-8431
Fax: 301-443-4279
Website: http://www.nimh.nih.gov
E-mail: nimhinfo@nih.gov

National Institute on Aging (NIA)
Building 31, Rm. 5C27
31 Center Dr., MSC 2292
Bethesda, MD 20892
Phone: 301-496-1752
Toll-Free TTY: 800-222-4225
Fax: 301-496-1072
Website: http://www.nia.nih.gov

National Institute on Disability and Rehabilitation Research (NIDRR)
U.S. Department of Education
400 Maryland Ave. SW
Mailstop PCP-6038
Washington, DC 20202
Phone/TTY: 202-245-7460
Fax: 202-245-7323
Website: http://www.ed.gov/
about/offices/list/osers/nidrr

National Rehabilitation Information Center (NARIC)
8201 Corporate Dr., Ste. 600
Landover, MD 20785
Toll-Free: 800-346-2742
Phone: 301-459-5900
TTY: 301-459-5984
Fax: 301-562-2401
Website: http://www.naric.com
E-mail:
naricinfo@heitechservices.com

National Institute of Neurological Disorders and Stroke (NINDS)
P.O. Box 5801
Bethesda, MD 20824
Toll-Free: 800-352-9424
Phone: 301-496-5751
TTY: 301-468-5981
Website: http://www.ninds.nih
.gov

Patient Recruitment and Public Liaison Office
Clinical Center
National Institutes of Health
10 Cloister Ct., Bldg. 61
Bethesda, MD 20892
Toll-Free: 800-411-1222
Toll-Free TTY: 866-411-1010
Fax: 301-480-9793
Website: http://www.cc.nih.gov/
participate.shtml

Private Organizations

Acoustic Neuroma Association
600 Peachtree Pkwy., Ste. 108
Cumming, GA 30041
Toll-Free: 877-200-8211
Toll-Free Fax: 877-202-0239
Phone: 770-205-8211
Fax: 770-205-0239
Website: http://www.anausa.org
E-mail: info@anausa.org

ALS Association
27001 Agoura Rd., Ste. 250
Calabasas Hills, CA 91301
Toll-Free: 800-782-4747
Phone: 818-880-9007
Fax: 818-880-9006
Website: http://www.alsa.org

Alzheimer's Association
225 N. Michigan Ave., 17th Fl.
Chicago, IL 60601-7633
Toll-Free Helpline:
800-272-3900 (24-hr.)
Toll-Free TDD Helpline:
866-403-3073 (24-hr.)
Phone: 312-335-8700
TDD: 312-335-5886
Fax: 866-699-1246
Website: http://www.alz.org
E-mail: info@alz.org

Alzheimer's Foundation of America
322 8th Ave., 7th Fl.
New York, NY 10001
Toll-Free: 866-AFA-8484
(232-8484)
Fax: 646-638-1546
Website: http://www.alzfdn.org
E-mail: info@alzfdn.org

American Brain Tumor Association
2720 River Road
Des Plaines, IL 60018
Toll-Free: 800-866-2282
Phone: 847-827-9910
Fax: 847-827-9918
Website: http://www.abta.org
E-mail: info@abta.org

American Pain Foundation
201 N. Charles St., Ste. 710
Baltimore, MD 21201
Toll-Free: 888-615-PAIN (7246)
Website: http://www.
painfoundation.org
E-mail: info@painfoundation.org

American Stroke Association
Division of American Heart
Association
7272 Greenville Ave.
Dallas, TX 75231
Toll-Free: 888-4STROKE
(478-7653)
Website: http://www.
strokeassociation.org
E-mail: strokeassociation@heart
.org

Angioma Alliance
520 W. 21st St.
Suite G2-411
Norfolk, VA 23517
Website: http://www.
angiomaalliance.org

Association for Frontotemporal Dementias (AFTD)
Radnor Station, Bldg. #2, Ste. 200
290 King of Prussia Road
Radnor, PA 19087
Toll-Free: 866-507-7222
Phone: 267-514-7221
Website: http://www.ftd-picks.org
E-mail: info@ftd-picks.org

Batten Disease Support and Research Association
166 Humphries Dr.
Reynoldsburg, OH 43068
Toll-Free: 800-448-4570
Phone: 740-927-4298
Fax: 740-927-7683
Website: http://www.bdsra.org
E-mail: bdsra1@bdsra.org

Brain Aneurysm Foundation
269 Hanover St., Bldg. 3
Hanover, MA 02339
Toll-Free: 888-272-4602
Phone: 781-826-5556
Website: http://www.bafound.org
E-mail: office@bafound.org

Brain Injury Association of America
1608 Spring Hill Rd., Ste. 110
Vienna, VA 22182
Toll-Free: 800-444-6443
Phone: 703-761-0750
Fax: 703-761-0755
Website: http://www.biausa.org
E-mail: braininjuryinfo@biausa.org

Brain Injury Resource Center
Phone: 206-621-8558
Website: http://www.headinjury.com

Children's Hemiplegia and Stroke Assoc. (CHASA)
4101 W. Green Oaks Blvd.
Ste. 305, #149
Arlington, TX 76016
Phone: 817-492-4325
Website: http://www.chasa.org

CJD Aware!
2527 S. Carrollton Ave.
New Orleans, LA 70118
Phone: 504-861-4627
Website: http://www.cjdaware.com
E-mail: info@cjdaware.com

Creutzfeldt-Jakob Disease (CJD) Foundation Inc.
P.O. Box 5312
Akron, OH 44334
Toll-Free: 800-659-1991
Phone: 330-665-5590
Fax: 330-668-2474
Website: http://www.cjdfoundation.org
E-mail: help@cjdfoundation.org

CUREPSP (Foundation for PSP | CBD and Related Brain Diseases)
Executive Plaza III
11350 McCormick Rd., Ste. 906
Hunt Valley, MD 21031
Toll-Free: 800-457-4777
Phone: 410-785-7004
Fax: 410-785-7009
Website: http://www.curepsp.org
E-mail: info@curepsp.org

Family Caregiver Alliance/ National Center on Caregiving
180 Montgomery St., Ste. 1100
San Francisco, CA 94104
Toll-Free: 800-445-8106
Phone: 415-434-3388
Fax: 415-434-3508
Website: http://www.caregiver.org
E-mail: info@caregiver.org

Family Center on Technology and Disability
Academy for Educational Development
1825 Connecticut Ave., NW 7th FL
Washington DC 20009
Phone: 202-884-8068
Fax: 202-884-8441
Website: http://www.fctd.info
E-mail: fctd@aed.org

Hydrocephalus Association
870 Market St., Ste. 705
San Francisco, CA 94102
Toll-Free: 888-598-3789
Phone: 415-732-7040
Fax: 415-732-7044
Website:
http://www.hydroassoc.org
E-mail: info@hydroassoc.org

Les Turner ALS Foundation
5550 W. Touhy Ave., Ste 302
Skokie, IL 60077-3254
Toll-Free: 888-ALS-1107
(257-1107)
Phone: 847-679-3311
Fax: 847-679-9109
Website:
http://www.lesturnerals.org
E-mail: info@lesturnerals.org

Lewy Body Dementia Association
912 Killian Hill Rd. SW
Suite 202C
Atlanta, GA 30047
Toll-Free: 800-539-9767
Phone: 404-935-6444
Fax: 480-422-5434
Website: http://www.
lewybodydementia.org
E-mail: lbda@lbda.org

Multiple Sclerosis Association of America
706 Haddonfield Rd.
Cherry Hill, NJ 08002
Toll-Free: 800-532-7667
Phone: 856-488-4500
Fax: 856-661-9797
Website:
http://www.msassociation.org
E-mail: webmaster@msaa.com

Multiple Sclerosis Foundation
6350 N. Andrews Ave.
Ft. Lauderdale, FL 33309
Toll-Free: 888-MSFOCUS
(673-6287)
Phone: 954-776-6805
Fax: 954-351-0630
Website: http://www.msfocus.org
E-mail: support@msfocus.org

Narcolepsy Network
P.O. Box 294
Pleasantville, NY 10570
Toll-Free: 888-292-6522
Phone: 401-667-2523
Fax: 401-633-6567
Website: http://www.
narcolepsynetwork.org
E-mail:
narnet@narcolepsynetwork.org

National Aphasia Association
350 7th Ave., Ste. 902
New York, NY 10001
Toll-Free: 800-922-4622
Website: http://www.aphasia.org
E-mail: naa@aphasia.org

National Ataxia Foundation (NAF)
2600 Fernbrook Ln., Ste. 119
Minneapolis, MN 55447
Phone: 763-553-0020
Fax: 763-553-0167
Website: http://www.ataxia.org
E-mail: naf@ataxia.org

National Easter Seal Society
233 S. Wacker Dr.
Suite 2400
Chicago, IL 60606
Toll-Free: 800-221-6827
Phone: 312-726-6200
TTY: 312-726-4258
Fax: 312-726-1494
Website: http://www.easter-seals.org

National Family Caregivers Association
10400 Connecticut Ave.
Suite 500
Kensington, MD 20895
Toll-Free: 800-896-3650
Phone: 301-942-6430
Fax: 301-942-2302
Website: http://www.thefamilycaregiver.org
E-mail: info@thefamilycaregiver.org

National Headache Foundation
820 N. Orleans, Ste. 217
Chicago, IL 60610
Toll-Free: 888-NHF-5552 (643-5552)
Phone: 312-274-2650
Fax: 312-640-9049
Website: http://www.headaches.org
E-mail: info@headaches.org

National Hospice and Palliative Care Organization
1731 King St., Ste. 100
Alexandria, VA 22314
Toll-Free: 800-658-8898
Phone: 703-837-1500
Fax: 703-837-1233
Website: http://www.nhpco.org
E-mail: nhpco_info@nhpco.org

National Hydrocephalus Foundation
12413 Centralia Rd.
Lakewood, CA 90715
Toll-Free: 888-857-3434
Phone: 562-924-6666
Website: http://nhfonline.org
E-mail: nhf@earthlink.net

National Multiple Sclerosis Society
733 Third Ave., 3rd Fl.
New York, NY 10017
Toll-Free: 800-344-4867 (FIGHTMS)
Website: http://www.nationalmssociety.org
E-mail: nat@nmss.org

National Organization for Rare Disorders (NORD)
55 Kenosia Ave.
P.O. Box 1968
Danbury, CT 06813
Toll-Free Voice Mail:
800-999-6673
TDD: 203-797-9590
Fax: 203-798-2291
Website:
http://www.rarediseases.org
E-mail:
orphan@rarediseases.org

National Rehabilitation Information Center (NARIC)
8201 Corporate Dr.
Suite 600
Landover, MD 20785
Toll-Free: 800-346-2742
Phone: 301-459-5900
TTY: 301-459-5984
Fax: 301-562-2401
Website: http://www.naric.com
E-mail:
naricinfo@heitechservices.com

National Respite Network and Resource Center
800 Eastowne Dr.
Suite 105
Chapel Hill, NC 27514
Phone: 919-490-5577 x222
Fax: 919-490-4905
Website: http://www.archrespite
.org

National Sleep Foundation
1522 K St. NW, Ste. 500
Washington, DC 20005
Phone: 202-347-3471
Fax: 202-347-3472
Website:
http://www.sleepfoundation.org
E-mail: nsf@sleepfoundation.org

National Stroke Association
9707 E. Easter Ln., Bldg. B
Centennial, CO 80112
Toll-Free: 800-STROKES
(787-6537)
Fax: 303-649-1328
Website: http://www.stroke.org
E-mail: info@stroke.org

Paralyzed Veterans of America (PVA)
801 18th St., NW
Washington, DC 20006
Health Care Hotline:
800-232-1782
Toll-Free TTY: 800-795-4327
Website: http://www.pva.org
E-mail: info@pva.org

Project ALS
3960 Broadway, Ste. 420
New York, NY 10032
Toll-Free: 800-603-0270
Phone: 212-420-7382
Fax: 212-420-7387
Website: http://www.projectals
.org
E-mail: info@projectals.org

Restless Legs Syndrome Foundation
1610 14th St. NW
Suite 300
Rochester, MN 55901
Phone: 507-287-6465
Fax: 507-287-6312
Website: http://www.rls.org
E-mail: rlsfoundation@rls.org

United Leukodystrophy Foundation
2304 Highland Dr.
Sycamore, IL 60178
Toll-Free: 800-728-5483
Fax: 815-895-2432
Website: http://www.ulf.org
E-mail: office@ulf.org

WE MOVE (Worldwide Education and Awareness for Movement Disorders)
204 W. 84th St.
New York, NY 10024
Phone: 212-875-8312
Fax: 212-875-8389
Website: http://www.wemove.org
E-mail: wemove@wemove.org

World Health Organization (WHO)
Avenue Appia 20
1211 Geneva 27
Switzerland
Phone: + 41 22 791 21 11
Fax: + 41 22 791 3111
Website: http://www.who.int
E-mail: info@who.int

Index

Index

Health Reference Series
Complete Catalog
List price $93 per volume. School and library price $84 per volume.

Adolescent Health Sourcebook, 3rd Edition

Basic Consumer Health Information about Adolescent Growth and Development, Puberty, Sexuality, Reproductive Health, and Physical, Emotional, Social, and Mental Health Concerns of Teens and Their Parents, Including Facts about Nutrition, Physical Activity, Weight Management, Acne, Allergies, Cancer, Diabetes, Growth Disorders, Juvenile Arthritis, Infections, Substance Abuse, and More

Along with Information about Adolescent Safety Concerns, Youth Violence, a Glossary of Related Terms, and a Directory of Resources

Edited by Amy L. Sutton. 600 pages. 2010. 978-0-7808-1140-9.

Adult Health Concerns Sourcebook

Basic Consumer Health Information about Medical and Mental Concerns of Adults, Including Facts about Choosing Healthcare Providers, Navigating Insurance Options, Maintaining Wellness, Preventing Cancer, Heart Disease, Stroke, Diabetes, and Osteoporosis, and Understanding Aging-Related Health Concerns, Including Menopause, Cognitive Changes, and Changes in the Coronary and Vascular Systems

Along with Tips on Caring for Aging Parents and Dealing with Health-Related Work and Travel Issues, a Glossary, and a Directory of Resources for Additional Help and Information

Edited by Sandra J. Judd. 648 pages. 2008. 978-0-7808-0999-4.

"Provides a thorough list of topics that are important to adult health and for caregivers."
—*CHOICE, Nov '08*

"Written in easy-to-understand language... the content is well-organized and is intended to aid adults in making health care-related decisions."
—*AORN Journal, Dec '08*

AIDS Sourcebook, 4th Edition

Basic Consumer Health Information about Human Immunodeficiency Virus (HIV) and Acquired Immunodeficiency Syndrome (AIDS), Featuring Updated Statistics and Facts about Risks, Prevention, Screening, Diagnosis, Treatments, Side Effects, and Complications, and Including a Section about the Impact of HIV/AIDS on the Health of Women, Children, and Adolescents

Along with Tips on Managing Life with AIDS, Reports on Current Research Initiatives and Clinical Trials, a Glossary of Related Terms, and Resource Directories for Further Help and Information

Edited by Ivy L. Alexander. 680 pages. 2008. 978-0-7808-0997-0.

SEE ALSO *Contagious Diseases Sourcebook, 2nd Edition*

Alcoholism Sourcebook, 3rd Edition

Basic Consumer Health Information about Alcohol Use, Abuse, and Dependence, Featuring Facts about the Physical, Mental, and Social Health Effects of Alcohol Addiction, Including Alcoholic Liver Disease, Pancreatic Disease, Cardiovascular Disease, Neurological Disorders, and the Effects of Drinking during Pregnancy

Along with Information about Alcohol Treatment, Medications, and Recovery Programs, in Addition to Tips for Reducing the Prevalence of Underage Drinking, Statistics about Alcohol Use, a Glossary of Related Terms, and Directories of Resources for More Help and Information

Edited by Joyce Brennfleck Shannon. 600 pages. 2010. 978-0-7808-1141-6.

SEE ALSO *Drug Abuse Sourcebook, 3rd Edition*

Allergies Sourcebook, 3rd Edition

Basic Consumer Health Information about Allergic Disorders, Such as Anaphylaxis, Hives,

Eczema, Rhinitis, Sinusitis, and Conjunctivitis, and Their Triggers, Including Pollen, Mold, Dust Mites, Animal Dander, Insects, Chemicals, Food, Food Additives, and Medications

Along with Advice about the Diagnosis and Treatment of Allergy Symptoms, a Glossary of Related Terms, a Directory of Resources for Help and Information, and Suggestions for Additional Reading

Edited by Amy L. Sutton. 588 pages. 2007. 978-0-7808-0950-5.

SEE ALSO Asthma Sourcebook, 2nd Edition

Alzheimer Disease Sourcebook, 4th Edition

Basic Consumer Health Information about Alzheimer Disease, Other Dementias, and Related Disorders, Including Multi-Infarct Dementia, Dementia with Lewy Bodies, Frontotemporal Dementia (Pick Disease), Wernicke-Korsakoff Syndrome (Alcohol-Related Dementia), AIDS Dementia Complex, Huntington Disease, Creutzfeldt-Jacob Disease, and Delirium

Along with Information about Coping with Memory Loss and Forgetfulness, Maintaining Skills, and Long-Term Planning for People with Dementia, and Suggestions Addressing Common Caregiver Concerns, Updated Information about Current Research Efforts, a Glossary of Related Terms, and Directories of Sources for Additional Help and Information

Edited by Karen Bellenir. 603 pages. 2008. 978-0-7808-1001-3.

"An invaluable resource for persons who have received a diagnosis, for caregivers, and for family members dealing with this insidious disease. It is recommended for public, community college, and ready-reference sections in academic libraries."
—American Reference Books Annual, 2009

SEE ALSO Brain Disorders Sourcebook, 3rd Edition

Arthritis Sourcebook, 3rd Edition

Basic Consumer Health Information about the Risk Factors, Symptoms, Diagnosis, and

Treatment of Osteoarthritis, Rheumatoid Arthritis, Juvenile Arthritis, Gout, Infectious Arthritis, and Autoimmune Disorders Associated with Arthritis

Along with Facts about Medications, Surgeries, and Self-Care Techniques to Manage Pain and Disability, Tips on Living with Arthritis, a Glossary of Related Terms, and Resources for Additional Help and Information

Edited by Amy L. Sutton. 600 pages. 2010. 978-0-7808-1077-8.

Asthma Sourcebook, 2nd Edition

Basic Consumer Health Information about the Causes, Symptoms, Diagnosis, and Treatment of Asthma in Infants, Children, Teenagers, and Adults, Including Facts about Different Types of Asthma, Common Co-Occurring Conditions, Asthma Management Plans, Triggers, Medications, and Medication Delivery Devices

Along with Asthma Statistics, Research Updates, a Glossary, a Directory of Asthma-Related Resources, and More

Edited by Karen Bellenir. 581 pages. 2006. 978-0-7808-0866-9.

SEE ALSO Lung Disorders Sourcebook; Respiratory Disorders Sourcebook, 2nd Edition

Attention Deficit Disorder Sourcebook

Basic Consumer Health Information about Attention Deficit/Hyperactivity Disorder in Children and Adults, Including Facts about Causes, Symptoms, Diagnostic Criteria, and Treatment Options Such as Medications, Behavior Therapy, Coaching, and Homeopathy

Along with Reports on Current Research Initiatives, Legal Issues, and Government Regulations, and Featuring a Glossary of Related Terms, Internet Resources, and a List of Additional Reading Material

Edited by Dawn D. Matthews. 447 pages. 2002. 978-0-7808-0624-5.

"Recommended reference source."
—Booklist, Jan '03

SEE ALSO Learning Disabilities Sourcebook, 3rd Edition

Autism and Pervasive Developmental Disorders Sourcebook

Basic Consumer Health Information about Autism Spectrum and Pervasive Developmental Disorders, Such as Classical Autism, Asperger Syndrome, Rett Syndrome, and Childhood Disintegrative Disorder, Including Information about Related Genetic Disorders and Medical Problems and Facts about Causes, Screening Methods, Diagnostic Criteria, Treatments and Interventions, and Family and Education Issues

Along with a Glossary of Related Terms, Tips for Evaluating the Validity of Health Claims, and a Directory of Resources for Additional Help and Information

Edited by Sandra J. Judd. 603 pages. 2007. 978-0-7808-0953-6.

"This book provides a current overview of disorders on the autism spectrum and information about various therapies, educational resources, and help for families with practical issues such as workplace adjustments, living arrangements, and estate planning. It is a useful resource for public and consumer health libraries."
—American Reference Books Annual, 2009

SEE ALSO Learning Disabilities Sourcebook, 3rd Edition

Back and Neck Disorders Sourcebook, 2nd Edition

Basic Consumer Health Information about Spinal Pain, Spinal Cord Injuries, and Related Disorders, Such as Degenerative Disk Disease, Osteoarthritis, Scoliosis, Sciatica, Spina Bifida, and Spinal Stenosis, and Featuring Facts about Maintaining Spinal Health, Self-Care, Pain Management, Rehabilitative Care, Chiropractic Care, Spinal Surgeries, and Complementary Therapies

Along with Suggestions for Preventing Back and Neck Pain, a Glossary of Related Terms, and a Directory of Resources

Edited by Amy L. Sutton. 607 pages. 2004. 978-0-7808-0738-9.

"Recommended... An easy to use, comprehensive medical reference book."
—E-Streams, Sep '05

"For anyone who has back or neck problems, this book is ideal. Its easy-to-understand language and variety of topics makes this sourcebook a worthwhile read. The price... is reasonable for the amount of information contained in the book"
—Occupational Therapy in Health Care, 2007

Blood & Circulatory Disorders Sourcebook, 3rd Edition

Basic Consumer Health Information about Blood and Circulatory System Disorders, Such as Anemia, Leukemia, Lymphoma, Rh Disease, Hemophilia, Thrombophilia, Other Bleeding and Clotting Deficiencies, and Artery, Vascular, and Venous Diseases, Including Facts about Blood Types, Blood Donation, Bone Marrow and Stem Cell Transplants, Tests and Medications, and Tips for Maintaining Circulatory Health

Along with a Glossary of Related Terms and a List of Resources for Additional Help and Information

Edited by Sandra J. Judd. 600 pages. 2010. 978-0-7808-1081-5.

SEE ALSO Leukemia Sourcebook

Brain Disorders Sourcebook, 3rd Edition

Basic Consumer Health Information about Acquired and Traumatic Brain Injuries, Brain Tumors, Cerebral Palsy and Other Genetic and Congenital Brain Disorders, Infections of the Brain, Epilepsy, and Degenerative Neurological Disorders Such as Dementia, Huntington Disease, and Amyotrophic Lateral Sclerosis (ALS)

Along with Information on Brain Structure and Function, Treatment and Rehabilitation Options, a Glossary of Terms Related to Brain Disorders, and a Directory of Resources for More Information

Edited by Joyce Brennfleck Shannon. 600 pages. 2010. 978-0-7808-1083-9.

SEE ALSO Alzheimer Disease Sourcebook, 4th Edition

Breast Cancer Sourcebook, 3rd Edition

Basic Consumer Health Information about Breast Health and Breast Cancer, Including Facts about Environmental, Genetic, and Other Risk Factors, Prevention Efforts, Screening and Diagnostic Methods, Surgical Treatment Options and Other Care Choices, Complementary and Alternative Therapies, and Post-Treatment Concerns

Along with Statistical Data, News about Research Advances, a Glossary of Related Terms, and Directories of Resources for Additional Information and Support

Edited by Karen Bellenir. 606 pages. 2009. 978-0-7808-1030-3.

"A very useful reference for people wanting to learn more about breast cancer and how to negotiate their care or the care of a loved one. The third edition is necessary as information/treatment options continue to evolve."
—*Doody's Review Service, 2009*

SEE ALSO Cancer Sourcebook for Women, 3rd Edition, Women's Health Concerns Sourcebook, 3rd Edition

---

Breastfeeding Sourcebook

Basic Consumer Health Information about the Benefits of Breastmilk, Preparing to Breastfeed, Breastfeeding as a Baby Grows, Nutrition, and More, Including Information on Special Situations and Concerns Such as Mastitis, Illness, Medications, Allergies, Multiple Births, Prematurity, Special Needs, and Adoption

Along with a Glossary and Resources for Additional Help and Information

Edited by Jenni Lynn Colson. 367 pages. 2002. 978-0-7808-0332-9.

SEE ALSO Pregnancy and Birth Sourcebook, 3rd Edition

Burns Sourcebook

Basic Consumer Health Information about Various Types of Burns and Scalds, Including Flame, Heat, Cold, Electrical, Chemical, and Sun Burns

Along with Information on Short-Term and Long-Term Treatments, Tissue Reconstruction, Plastic Surgery, Prevention Suggestions, and First Aid

Edited by Allan R. Cook. 604 pages. 1999. 978-0-7808-0204-9.

"This is an exceptional addition to the series and is highly recommended for all consumer health collections, hospital libraries, and academic medical centers."
—*E-Streams, Mar '00*

"This key reference guide is an invaluable addition to all health care and public libraries in confronting this ongoing health issue."
—*American Reference Books Annual, 2000*

SEE ALSO Dermatological Disorders Sourcebook, 2nd Edition

Cancer Sourcebook, 5th Edition

Basic Consumer Health Information about Major Forms and Stages of Cancer, Featuring Facts about Head and Neck Cancers, Lung Cancers, Gastrointestinal Cancers, Genitourinary Cancers, Lymphomas, Blood Cell Cancers, Endocrine Cancers, Skin Cancers, Bone Cancers, Metastatic Cancers, and More

Along with Facts about Cancer Treatments, Cancer Risks and Prevention, a Glossary of Related Terms, Statistical Data, and a Directory of Resources for Additional Information

Edited by Karen Bellenir. 1105 pages. 2007. 978-0-7808-0947-5.

"The 5th, updated edition of Cancer Sourcebook should be in every public and health lending library collection... An unparalleled discussion essential for any health collections considering an all-in-one basic general reference."
—*California Bookwatch, Aug '07*

SEE ALSO Breast Cancer Sourcebook, 3rd Edition, Cancer Survivorship Sourcebook, Leukemia Sourcebook

---

Cancer Sourcebook for Women, 4th Edition

Basic Consumer Health Information about Gynecologic Cancers and Other Cancers of Special Concern to Women, Including Cancers of the Breast, Cervix, Colon, Lung, Ovaries, Thyroid, and Uterus

Along with Facts about Benign Conditions of the Female Reproductive System, Cancer Risk

630

Factors, Diagnostic and Treatment Procedures, Side Effects of Cancer and Cancer Treatments, Women's Issues in Cancer Survivorship, a Glossary of Related Terms, and a Directory of Resources for Additional Help and Information

Edited by Karen Bellenir. 600 pages. 2010. 978-0-7808-1139-3.

SEE ALSO Breast Cancer Sourcebook, 3rd Edition, Women's Health Concerns Sourcebook, 3rd Edition

Cancer Survivorship Sourcebook

Basic Consumer Health Information about the Physical, Educational, Emotional, Social, and Financial Needs of Cancer Patients from Diagnosis, through Cancer Treatment, and Beyond, Including Facts about Researching Specific Types of Cancer and Learning about Clinical Trials and Treatment Options, and Featuring Tips for Coping with the Side Effects of Cancer Treatments and Adjusting to Life after Cancer Treatment Concludes

Along with Suggestions for Caregivers, Friends, and Family Members of Cancer Patients, a Glossary of Cancer Care Terms, and Directories of Related Resources

Edited by Karen Bellenir. 633 pages. 2007. 978-0-7808-0985-7.

"Well organized and comprehensive in coverage, the book speaks to issues encountered both during and after cancer treatment. Recommended for consumer health and public libraries."
—Library Journal, Aug 1 '07

"Cancer Survivorship Sourcebook will be useful to anyone who has a friend or loved one with a cancer diagnosis."
—American Reference Books Annual, 2008

SEE ALSO Cancer Sourcebook, 5th Edition, Disease Management Sourcebook

Cardiovascular Disorders Sourcebook, 4th Edition

Basic Consumer Health Information about Heart and Blood Vessel Diseases and Disorders, Such as Angina, Heart Attack, Heart Failure, Cardiomyopathy, Arrhythmias, Valve Disease, Atherosclerosis, Aneurysms, and

Congenital Heart Defects, Including Information about Cardiovascular Disease in Women, Men, Children, Adolescents, and Minorities

Along with Facts about Diagnosing, Managing, and Preventing Cardiovascular Disease, a Glossary of Related Medical Terms, and a Directory of Resources for Additional Information

Edited by Amy L. Sutton. 600 pages. 2010. 978-0-7808-1080-8.

Caregiving Sourcebook

Basic Consumer Health Information for Caregivers, Including a Profile of Caregivers, Caregiving Responsibilities and Concerns, Tips for Specific Conditions, Care Environments, and the Effects of Caregiving

Along with Facts about Legal Issues, Financial Information, and Future Planning, a Glossary, and a Listing of Additional Resources

Edited by Joyce Brennfleck Shannon. 583 pages. 2001. 978-0-7808-0331-2.

"Essential for most collections."
—Library Journal, Apr 1 '02

"An ideal addition to the reference collection of any public library. Health sciences information professionals may also want to acquire the Caregiving Sourcebook for their hospital or academic library for use as a ready reference tool by health care workers interested in aging and caregiving."
—E-Streams, Jan '02

Child Abuse Sourcebook, 2nd Edition

Basic Consumer Health Information about the Physical, Sexual, and Emotional Abuse of Children, Neglect, Münchhausen Syndrome by Proxy (MSBP), and Shaken Baby Syndrome, and Featuring Facts about Withholding Medical Care, Corporal Punishment, Child Maltreatment in Youth Sports, and Parental Substance Abuse

Along with Information about Child Protective Services, Foster Care, Adoption, Parenting Challenges, Abuse Prevention Programs, and Intervention, Treatment, and Recovery Guidelines, a Glossary of Related Terms, and Resources for Additional Help and Information

Edited by Joyce Brennfleck Shannon. 600 pages. 2009. 978-0-7808-1037-2.

SEE ALSO Domestic Violence Sourcebook, 3rd Edition

Childhood Diseases and Disorders Sourcebook, 2nd Edition

Basic Consumer Health Information about the Physical, Mental, and Developmental Health of Pre-Adolescent Children, Including Facts about Infectious Diseases, Asthma, Allergies, Diabetes, and Other Acute and Chronic Conditions Affecting the Gastrointestinal Tract, Ears, Nose, Throat, Liver, Kidneys, Heart, Blood, Brain, Muscles, Bones, and Skin

Along with Reports on Recommended Childhood Vaccinations, Wellness Guidelines, a Glossary of Related Medical Terms, and a List of Resources for Parents

Edited by Sandra J. Judd. 694 pages. 2009. 978-0-7808-1031-0.

"The strength of this source is the wide range of information given about childhood health issues... It is most appropriate for public libraries and academic libraries that field medical questions."
—*American Reference Books Annual, 2009*

SEE ALSO Healthy Children Sourcebook

Colds, Flu and Other Common Ailments Sourcebook

Basic Consumer Health Information about Common Ailments and Injuries, Including Colds, Coughs, the Flu, Sinus Problems, Headaches, Fever, Nausea and Vomiting, Menstrual Cramps, Diarrhea, Constipation, Hemorrhoids, Back Pain, Dandruff, Dry and Itchy Skin, Cuts, Scrapes, Sprains, Bruises, and More

Along with Information about Prevention, Self-Care, Choosing a Doctor, Over-the-Counter Medications, Folk Remedies, and Alternative Therapies, and Including a Glossary of Important Terms and a Directory of Resources for Further Help and Information

Edited by Chad T. Kimball. 622 pages. 2001. 978-0-7808-0435-7.

"A good starting point for research on common illnesses. It will be a useful addition to

public and consumer health library collections."
—*American Reference Books Annual, 2002*

"Will prove valuable to any library seeking to maintain a current, comprehensive reference collection of health resources... Excellent reference."
—*The Bookwatch, Aug '01*

SEE ALSO Contagious Diseases Sourcebook, 2nd Edition

Communication Disorders Sourcebook

Basic Information about Deafness and Hearing Loss, Speech and Language Disorders, Voice Disorders, Balance and Vestibular Disorders, and Disorders of Smell, Taste, and Touch

Edited by Linda M. Ross. 533 pages. 1996. 978-0-7808-0077-9.

"This is skillfully edited and is a welcome resource for the layperson. It should be found in every public and medical library."
—*Booklist Health Sciences Supplement,*
Oct '97

Complementary & Alternative Medicine Sourcebook, 4th Edition

Basic Consumer Health Information about Ayurveda, Acupuncture, Aromatherapy, Chiropractic Care, Diet-Based Therapies, Guided Imagery, Herbal and Vitamin Supplements, Homeopathy, Hypnosis, Massage, Meditation, Naturopathy, Pilates, Reflexology, Reiki, Shiatsu, Tai Chi, Traditional Chinese Medicine, Yoga, and Other Complementary and Alternative Medical Therapies

Along with Statistics, Tips for Selecting a Practitioner, Treatments for Specific Health Conditions, a Glossary of Related Terms, and a Directory of Resources for Additional Help and Information

Edited by Amy L. Sutton. 600 pages. 2010. 978-0-7808-1082-2.

Congenital Disorders Sourcebook, 2nd Edition

Basic Consumer Health Information about Nonhereditary Birth Defects and Disorders

Related to Prematurity, Gestational Injuries, Congenital Infections, and Birth Complications, Including Heart Defects, Hydrocephalus, Spina Bifida, Cleft Lip and Palate, Cerebral Palsy, and More

Along with Facts about the Prevention of Birth Defects, Fetal Surgery and Other Treatment Options, Research Initiatives, a Glossary of Related Terms, and Resources for Additional Information and Support

Edited by Sandra J. Judd. 619 pages. 2007. 978-0-7808-0945-1.

"Congenital Disorders Sourcebook provides an excellent, non-technical overview of many aspects of pregnancy with the focus on congenital disorders."

—American Reference Books Annual, 2008

"An excellent readable reference aimed at the lay public for difficult to understand medical problems. An excellent starting point for the interested parent or family member who may then be motivated to seek more information."

—Doody's Review Service, 2007

SEE ALSO Pregnancy and Birth Sourcebook, 3rd Edition

Contagious Diseases Sourcebook, 2nd Edition

Basic Consumer Health Information about Diseases Spread from Person to Person through Direct Physical Contact, Airborne Transmissions, Sexual Contact, or Contact with Blood or Other Body Fluids, Including Pneumococcal, Staphylococcal, and Streptococcal Diseases, Colds, Influenza, Lice, Measles, Mumps, Tuberculosis, and Others

Along with Facts about Self-Care and Over-the-Counter Medications, Antibiotics and Drug Resistance, Disease Prevention, Vaccines, and Bioterrorism, a Glossary, and a Directory of Resources for More Information

Edited by Joyce Brennfleck Shannon. 600 pages. 2010. 978-0-7808-1075-4.

SEE ALSO AIDS Sourcebook, 4th Edition, Hepatitis Sourcebook

Cosmetic and Reconstructive Surgery Sourcebook, 2nd Edition

Basic Consumer Information about Plastic Surgery and Non-Surgical Appearance-Enhancing Procedures, Including Facts about Botulinum Toxin, Collagen Replacement, Dermabrasion, Chemical Peels, Eyelid Surgery, Nose Reshaping, Lip Augmentation, Liposuction, Breast Enlargement and Reduction, Tummy Tucking, and Other Skin, Hair, Facial, and Body Shaping Procedures

Along with Information about Reconstructive Procedures for Congenital Disorders, Disfiguring Diseases, Burns, and Traumatic Injuries, a Glossary of Related Terms, and a Directory of Additional Resources

Edited by Karen Bellenir. 483 pages. 2007. 978-0-7808-0951-2.

"A comprehensive source for people considering cosmetic surgery... also recommended for medical students who will perform these procedures later in their careers; and public librarians and academic medical librarians who may assist patrons interested in this information."

—Medical Reference Services Quarterly, Fall '08

"A practical guide for health care consumers and health care workers... This easy-to-read reference guide would be useful for novice and veteran health care consumers, surgical technology students, nursing students, and perioperative nurses new to plastic and reconstructive surgery. It also may be helpful for medical-surgical nurses as a guide for patient teaching in their practices."

—AORN Journal, Aug '08

SEE ALSO Surgery Sourcebook, 2nd Edition

Death and Dying Sourcebook, 2nd Edition

Basic Consumer Health Information about End-of-Life Care and Related Perspectives and Ethical Issues, Including End-of-Life Symptoms and Treatments, Pain Management, Quality-of-Life Concerns, the Use of Life Support, Patients' Rights and Privacy Issues, Advance Directives, Physician-Assisted Suicide, Caregiving, Organ and Tissue Donation, Autopsies, Funeral Arrangements, and Grief

Along with Statistical Data, Information about the Leading Causes of Death, a Glossary, and Directories of Support Groups and Other Resources

Edited by Joyce Brennfleck Shannon. 626 pages. 2006. 978-0-7808-0871-3.

Dental Care and Oral Health Sourcebook, 3rd Edition

Basic Consumer Health Information about Dental Care and Oral Health Throughout the Lifespan, Including Facts about Cavities, Bad Breath, Cold and Canker Sores, Dry Mouth, Toothaches, Gum Disease, Malocclusion, Temporomandibular Joint and Muscle Disorders, Oral Cancers, and Dental Emergencies

Along with Information about Mouth Hygiene, Crowns, Bridges, Implants, and Fillings, Surgical, Orthodontic, and Cosmetic Dental Procedures, Pain Management, Health Conditions that Impact Oral Care, a Glossary of Related Terms, and a Directory of Additional Resources

Edited by Amy L. Sutton. 619 pages. 2008. 978-0-7808-1032-7.

"Could serve as turning point in the battle to educate consumers in issues concerning oral health. Tightly written in terms the average person can understand, yet comprehensive in scope and authoritative in tone, it is another excellent sourcebook in the Health Reference Series... Should be in the reference department of all public libraries, and in academic libraries that have a public constituency."
—American Reference Books Annual, 2009

Depression Sourcebook, 2nd Edition

Basic Consumer Health Information about Unipolar Depression, Bipolar Disorder, Dysthymia, Seasonal Affective Disorder, Postpartum Depression, and Other Depressive Disorders, Including Facts about Populations at Special Risk, Coexisting Medical Conditions, Symptoms, Treatment Options, and Suicide Prevention

Along with Statistical Data, a Glossary of Related Terms, and a Directory of Resources for Additional Help and Information

Edited by Sandra J. Judd. 646 pages. 2008. 978-0-7808-1003-7.

"Recommended for public libraries."
—American Reference Books Annual, 2009

SEE ALSO Mental Health Disorders Sourcebook, 4th Edition

Dermatological Disorders Sourcebook, 2nd Edition

Basic Consumer Health Information about Conditions and Disorders Affecting the Skin, Hair, and Nails, Such as Acne, Rosacea, Rashes, Dermatitis, Pigmentation Disorders, Birthmarks, Skin Cancer, Skin Injuries, Psoriasis, Scleroderma, and Hair Loss, Including Facts about Medications and Treatments for Dermatological Disorders and Tips for Maintaining Healthy Skin, Hair, and Nails

Along with Information about How Aging Affects the Skin, a Glossary of Related Terms, and a Directory of Resources for Additional Help and Information

Edited by Amy L. Sutton. 617 pages. 2006. 978-0-7808-0795-2.

"Well organized... presents a plethora of information in a manner that is appropriate in style and readability for the intended audience."
—Physical Therapy, Nov '06

"Helpfully brings together... sources in one convenient place, saving the user hours of research time."
—American Reference Books Annual, 2006

SEE ALSO Burns Sourcebook

Diabetes Sourcebook, 4th Edition

Basic Consumer Health Information about Type 1 and Type 2 Diabetes Mellitus, Gestational Diabetes, Monogenic Forms of Diabetes, and Insulin Resistance, with Guidelines for Lifestyle Modifications and the Medical Management of Diabetes, Including Facts about Insulin, Insulin Delivery Devices, Oral Diabetes Medications, Self-Monitoring of Blood Glucose, Meal Planning, Physical Activity Recommendations, Foot Care, and Treatment Options for People with Kidney Failure

Along with a Section about Diabetes Complications and Co-Occurring Conditions, a Glossary of Related Terms, and Directories of Resources for Additional Help and Information

Edited by Karen Bellenir. 627 pages. 2008. 978-0-7808-1005-1.

"Completely and comprehensively covering almost everything a student or physician would need to know... well worth the investment."

—*Internet Bookwatch, Dec '08*

SEE ALSO *Endocrine and Metabolic Disorders Sourcebook, 2nd Edition*

Diet and Nutrition Sourcebook, 3rd Edition

Basic Consumer Health Information about Dietary Guidelines and the Food Guidance System, Recommended Daily Nutrient Intakes, Serving Proportions, Weight Control, Vitamins and Supplements, Nutrition Issues for Different Life Stages and Lifestyles, and the Needs of People with Specific Medical Concerns, Including Cancer, Celiac Disease, Diabetes, Eating Disorders, Food Allergies, and Cardiovascular Disease

Along with Facts about Federal Nutrition Support Programs, a Glossary of Nutrition and Dietary Terms, and Directories of Additional Resources for More Information about Nutrition

Edited by Joyce Brennfleck Shannon. 605 pages. 2006. 978-0-7808-0800-3.

"A valuable resource tool for any individual."

—*Journal of Dental Hygiene, Apr '07*

"From different recommended eating habits to reduce disease and common ailments to nutrition advice for those with specific conditions, Diet and Nutrition Sourcebook is especially important because so much is changing in this area, and so rapidly."

—*California Bookwatch, Jun '06*

SEE ALSO *Eating Disorders Sourcebook, 2nd Edition, Vegetarian Sourcebook*

Digestive Diseases and Disorders Sourcebook

Basic Consumer Health Information about Diseases and Disorders that Impact the Upper and Lower Digestive System, Including Celiac Disease, Constipation, Crohn's Disease, Cyclic Vomiting Syndrome, Diarrhea, Diverticulosis and Diverticulitis, Gallstones, Heartburn, Hemorrhoids, Hernias, Indigestion (Dyspepsia), Irritable Bowel Syndrome, Lactose Intolerance, Ulcers, and More

Along with Information about Medications and Other Treatments, Tips for Maintaining a Healthy Digestive Tract, a Glossary, and Directory of Digestive Diseases Organizations

Edited by Karen Bellenir. 323 pages. 2000. 978-0-7808-0327-5.

"An excellent addition to all public or patient-research libraries."

—*American Reference Books Annual, 2001*

"Recommended reference source."

—*Booklist, May '00*

SEE ALSO *Gastrointestinal Diseases and Disorders Sourcebook, 2nd Edition*

Disabilities Sourcebook

Basic Consumer Health Information about Physical and Psychiatric Disabilities, Including Descriptions of Major Causes of Disability, Assistive and Adaptive Aids, Workplace Issues, and Accessibility Concerns

Along with Information about the Americans with Disabilities Act, a Glossary, and Resources for Additional Help and Information

Edited by Dawn D. Matthews. 602 pages. 2000. 978-0-7808-0389-3.

"A must for libraries with a consumer health section."

—*American Reference Books Annual, 2002*

"A much needed addition to the Omnigraphics Health Reference Series. A current reference work to provide people with disabilities, their families, caregivers or those who work with them, a broad range of information in one volume, has not been available until now... It is recommended for all public and academic library reference collections."

—*E-Streams, May '01*

"An excellent source book in easy-to-read format covering many current topics; highly recommended for all libraries."

—*CHOICE, Jan '01*

Disease Management Sourcebook

Basic Consumer Health Information about Coping with Chronic and Serious Illnesses, Navigating the Health Care System, Communicating with Health Care Providers, Assessing Health Care Quality, and Making Informed Health Care Decisions, Including Facts about Second Opinions, Hospitalization, Surgery, and Medications

Along with a Section about Children with Chronic Conditions, Information about Legal, Financial, and Insurance Issues, a Glossary of Related Terms, and Directories of Additional Resources

Edited by Joyce Brennfleck Shannon. 621 pages. 2008. 978-0-7808-1002-0.

"Consumers need to know how to manage their health care the same way they manage anything else in their lives. The text is very readable and is written for the layperson and consumer. The cost is not prohibitive. This book should be in all collections of health care libraries and public libraries."
— *American Reference Books Annual, 2009*

"The information is very current, and the selection of font and layout make the book easy to read. A hardback that will stand up to much usage, this is an excellent resource for consumers... Recommended. General readers."
—*CHOICE, Nov '08*

"Intended for lay readers, this resource clarifies the many confusing and overwhelming details associated with chronic disease care. Meticulous and clearly explained, the book even includes diagrams intended to ease comprehension of over-the-counter medication labels. An essential guide to navigating the health-care rapids."
—*Library Journal, Aug '08*

Domestic Violence Sourcebook, 3rd Edition

Basic Consumer Health Information about Warning Signs, Risk Factors, and Health Consequences of Intimate Partner Violence, Sexual Violence and Rape, Stalking, Human Trafficking, Child Maltreatment, Teen Dating Violence, and Elder Abuse

Along with Facts about Victims and Perpetrators, Strategies for Violence Prevention, and Emergency Interventions, Safety Plans, and Financial and Legal Tips for Victims, a Glossary of Related Terms, and Directories of Resources for Additional Information and Support

Edited by Joyce Brennfleck Shannon. 634 pages. 2009. 978-0-7808-1038-9.

"A recommended pick for any library interested in consumer health and social issues... A 'must' for any serious health collection."
—*California Bookwatch, Jul '09*

SEE ALSO *Child Abuse Sourcebook, 2nd Edition*

Drug Abuse Sourcebook, 3rd Edition

Basic Consumer Health Information about the Abuse of Cocaine, Club Drugs, Hallucinogens, Heroin, Inhalants, Marijuana, and Other Illicit Substances, Prescription Medications, and Over-the-Counter Medicines

Along with Facts about Addiction and Related Health Effects, Drug Abuse Treatment and Recovery, Drug Testing, Prevention Programs, Glossaries of Drug-Related Terms, and Directories of Resources for More Information

Edited by Joyce Brennfleck Shannon. 600 pages. 2010. 978-0-7808-1079-2.

SEE ALSO *Alcoholism Sourcebook, 3rd Edition*

Ear, Nose, and Throat Disorders Sourcebook, 2nd Edition

Basic Consumer Health Information about Disorders of the Ears, Hearing Loss, Vestibular Disorders, Nasal and Sinus Problems, Throat and Vocal Cord Disorders, and Otolaryngologic Cancers, Including Facts about Ear Infections and Injuries, Genetic and Congenital Deafness, Sensorineural Hearing Disorders, Tinnitus, Vertigo, Ménière Disease, Rhinitis, Sinusitis, Snoring, Sore Throats, Hoarseness, and More

Along with Reports on Current Research Initiatives, a Glossary of Related Medical Terms, and a Directory of Sources for Further Help and Information

Edited by Sandra J. Judd. 631 pages. 2007. 978-0-7808-0872-0.

636

"A resource book for the general public that provides comprehensive coverage of basic up-to-date medical information about the causes, symptoms, diagnosis, and treatment of diseases and disorders that affect the ears, nose, sinuses, throat, and voice... The majority of information is presented in question and answer format, much like questions a patient might ask of a health care provider. An extensive index facilitates the reader's ability to easily access information on any specific topic."
—*Journal of Dental Hygiene, Oct '07*

"A handy compilation of information on common and some not so common ailments of the ears, nose, and throat."
—*Doody's Review Service, 2007*

Eating Disorders Sourcebook, 2nd Edition

Basic Consumer Health Information about Anorexia Nervosa, Bulimia, Binge Eating, Compulsive Exercise, Female Athlete Triad, and Other Eating Disorders, Including Facts about Body Image and Other Cultural and Age-Related Risk Factors, Prevention Efforts, Adverse Health Effects, Treatment Options, and the Recovery Process

Along with Guidelines for Healthy Weight Control, a Glossary, and Directories of Additional Resources

Edited by Joyce Brennfleck Shannon. 557 pages. 2007. 978-0-7808-0948-2.

"Recommended for the reference collection of large public libraries."
—*American Reference Books Annual, 2008*

"A basic health reference any health or general library needs."
—*Internet Bookwatch, Jun '07*

SEE ALSO *Diet and Nutrition Sourcebook, 3rd Edition, Mental Health Disorders Sourcebook, 4th Edition*

Emergency Medical Services Sourcebook

Basic Consumer Health Information about Preventing, Preparing for, and Managing Emergency Situations, When and Who to Call for Help, What to Expect in the Emergency Room, the Emergency Medical Team,

Patient Issues, and Current Topics in Emergency Medicine

Along with Statistical Data, a Glossary, and Sources of Additional Help and Information

Edited by Jenni Lynn Colson. 472 pages. 2002. 978-0-7808-0420-3.

"Handy and convenient for home, public, school, and college libraries. Recommended."
—*CHOICE, Apr '03*

"This reference can provide the consumer with answers to most questions about emergency care in the United States, or it will direct them to a resource where the answer can be found."
—*American Reference Books Annual, 2003*

SEE ALSO *Injury and Trauma Sourcebook*

Endocrine and Metabolic Disorders Sourcebook, 2nd Edition

Basic Consumer Health Information about Hormonal and Metabolic Disorders that Affect the Body's Growth, Development, and Functioning, Including Disorders of the Pancreas, Ovaries and Testes, and Pituitary, Thyroid, Parathyroid, and Adrenal Glands, with Facts about Growth Disorders, Addison Disease, Cushing Syndrome, Conn Syndrome, Diabetic Disorders, Multiple Endocrine Neoplasia, Inborn Errors of Metabolism, and More

Along with Information about Endocrine Functioning, Diagnostic and Screening Tests, a Glossary of Related Terms, and Directories of Additional Resources

Edited by Joyce Brennfleck Shannon. 597 pages. 2007. 978-0-7808-0952-9.

SEE ALSO *Diabetes Sourcebook, 4th Edition*

Environmental Health Sourcebook, 3rd Edition

Basic Consumer Health Information about the Environment and Its Effects on Human Health, Including Facts about Air, Water, and Soil Contamination, Hazardous Chemicals, Foodborne Hazards and Illnesses, Household Hazards Such as Radon, Mold, and Carbon Monoxide, Consumer Hazards from Toxic Products and Imported Goods, and Disorders

Linked to Environmental Causes, Including Chemical Sensitivity, Cancer, Allergies, and Asthma

Along with Information about the Impact of Environmental Hazards on Specific Populations, a Glossary of Related Terms, and Resources for Additional Help and Information.

Edited by Laura Larsen. 600 pages. 2010. 978-0-7808-1078-5

Ethnic Diseases Sourcebook

Basic Consumer Health Information for Ethnic and Racial Minority Groups in the United States, Including General Health Indicators and Behaviors, Ethnic Diseases, Genetic Testing, the Impact of Chronic Diseases, Women's Health, Mental Health Issues, and Preventive Health Care Services

Along with a Glossary and a Listing of Additional Resources

Edited by Joyce Brennfleck Shannon. 648 pages. 2001. 978-0-7808-0336-7.

"Not many books have been written on this topic to date, and the Ethnic Diseases Sourcebook is a strong addition to the list. It will be an important introductory resource for health consumers, students, health care personnel, and social scientists. It is recommended for public, academic, and large hospital libraries."
— American Reference Books Annual, 2002

"Will prove valuable to any library seeking to maintain a current, comprehensive reference collection of health resources... An excellent source of health information about genetic disorders which affect particular ethnic and racial minorities in the U.S."
—The Bookwatch, Aug '01

Eye Care Sourcebook, 3rd Edition

Basic Consumer Health Information about Eye Care and Eye Disorders, Including Facts about the Diagnosis, Prevention, and Treatment of Refractive Disorders, Cataracts, Glaucoma, Macular Degeneration, and Problems Affecting the Cornea, Retina, and Lacrimal Glands

Along with Advice about Preventing Eye Injuries and Tips for Living with Low Vision or Blindness, a Glossary of Related Terms, and Directories of Resources for More Help and Information

Edited by Amy L. Sutton. 646 pages. 2008. 978-0-7808-1000-6.

"A solid reference tool for eye care and a valuable addition to a collection."
—American Reference Books Annual, 2009

Family Planning Sourcebook

Basic Consumer Health Information about Planning for Pregnancy and Contraception, Including Traditional Methods, Barrier Methods, Hormonal Methods, Permanent Methods, Future Methods, Emergency Contraception, and Birth Control Choices for Women at Each Stage of Life

Along with Statistics, a Glossary, and Sources of Additional Information

Edited by Amy Marcaccio Keyzer. 503 pages. 2001. 978-0-7808-0379-4.

"Recommended for public, health, and undergraduate libraries as part of the circulating collection."
—E-Streams, Mar '02

"Will prove valuable to any library seeking to maintain a current, comprehensive reference collection of health resources... Excellent reference."
—The Bookwatch, Aug '01

SEE ALSO Pregnancy and Birth Sourcebook, 3rd Edition

Fitness and Exercise Sourcebook, 3rd Edition

Basic Consumer Health Information about the Physical and Mental Benefits of Fitness, Including Cardiorespiratory Endurance, Muscular Strength, Muscular Endurance, and Flexibility, with Facts about Sports Nutrition and Exercise-Related Injuries and Tips about Physical Activity and Exercises for People of All Ages and for People with Health Concerns

Along with Advice on Selecting and Using Exercise Equipment, Maintaining Exercise Motivation, a Glossary of Related Terms, and a Directory of Resources for More Help and Information

Edited by Amy L. Sutton. 635 pages. 2007. 978-0-7808-0946-8.

"Updates the consumer information on the physical and mental benefits of physical activity throughout the lifespan offered in earlier editions... Recommended. All readers; all levels."
—CHOICE, Oct '07

"An exceptionally well-rounded coverage perfect for any concerned about developing and understanding a fitness program."
—California Bookwatch, Jun '07

SEE ALSO Sports Injuries Sourcebook, 3rd Edition

Food Safety Sourcebook

Basic Consumer Health Information about the Safe Handling of Meat, Poultry, Seafood, Eggs, Fruit Juices, and Other Food Items, and Facts about Pesticides, Drinking Water, Food Safety Overseas, and the Onset, Duration, and Symptoms of Foodborne Illnesses, Including Types of Pathogenic Bacteria, Parasitic Protozoa, Worms, Viruses, and Natural Toxins

Along with the Role of the Consumer, the Food Handler, and the Government in Food Safety, a Glossary, and Resources for Additional Help and Information

Edited by Dawn D. Matthews. 327 pages. 1999. 978-0-7808-0326-8.

"Recommended reference source."
—Booklist, May '00

"This book takes the complex issues of food safety and foodborne pathogens and presents them in an easily understood manner. [It does] an excellent job of covering a large and often confusing topic."
— American Reference Books Annual, 2000

Forensic Medicine Sourcebook

Basic Consumer Information for the Layperson about Forensic Medicine, Including Crime Scene Investigation, Evidence Collection and Analysis, Expert Testimony, Computer-Aided Criminal Identification, Digital Imaging in the Courtroom, DNA Profiling, Accident Reconstruction, Autopsies, Ballistics, Drugs and Explosives Detection, Latent Fingerprints,

Product Tampering, and Questioned Document Examination

Along with Statistical Data, a Glossary of Forensics Terminology, and Listings of Sources for Further Help and Information

Edited by Annemarie S. Muth. 574 pages. 1999. 978-0-7808-0232-2.

"Given the expected widespread interest in its content and its easy to read style, this book is recommended for most public and all college and university libraries."
—E-Streams, Feb '01

"A wealth of information, useful statistics, references are up-to-date and extremely complete. This wonderful collection of data will help students who are interested in a career in any type of forensic field. It is a great resource for attorneys who need information about types of expert witnesses needed in a particular case. It also offers useful information for fiction and nonfiction writers whose work involves a crime. A fascinating compilation. All levels."
—CHOICE, Jan '00

"There are several items that make this book attractive to consumers who are seeking certain forensic data... This is a useful current source for those seeking general forensic medical answers."
—American Reference Books Annual, 2000

Gastrointestinal Diseases and Disorders Sourcebook, 2nd Edition

Basic Consumer Health Information about the Upper and Lower Gastrointestinal (GI) Tract, Including the Esophagus, Stomach, Intestines, Rectum, Liver, and Pancreas, with Facts about Gastroesophageal Reflux Disease, Gastritis, Hernias, Ulcers, Celiac Disease, Diverticulitis, Irritable Bowel Syndrome, Hemorrhoids, Gastrointestinal Cancers, and Other Diseases and Disorders Related to the Digestive Process

Along with Information about Commonly Used Diagnostic and Surgical Procedures, Statistics, Reports on Current Research Initiatives and Clinical Trials, a Glossary, and Resources for Additional Help and Information

Edited by Sandra J. Judd. 654 pages. 2006. 978-0-7808-0798-3.

the *Cause and Prevention of Headaches, the Effects of Stress and the Environment, Headaches during Pregnancy and Menopause, and Childhood Headaches*

Along with a Glossary and Other Resources for Additional Help and Information

Edited by Dawn D. Matthews. 342 pages. 2002. 978-0-7808-0337-4.

SEE ALSO *Pain Sourcebook, 3rd Edition*

Genetic Disorders Sourcebook, 4th Edition

Basic Consumer Health Information about Hereditary Diseases and Disorders, Including Facts about the Human Genome, Genetic Inheritance Patterns, Disorders Associated with Specific Genes, Such as Sickle Cell Disease, Hemophilia, and Cystic Fibrosis, Chromosome Disorders, Such as Down Syndrome, Fragile X Syndrome, and Turner Syndrome, and Complex Diseases and Disorders Resulting from the Interaction of Environmental and Genetic Factors, Such as Allergies, Cancer, and Obesity

Along with Facts about Genetic Testing, Suggestions for Parents of Children with Special Needs, Reports on Current Research Initiatives, a Glossary of Genetic Terminology, and Resources for Additional Help and Information

Edited by Sandra J. Judd. 600 pages. 2010. 978-0-7808-1076-1.

Head Trauma Sourcebook

Basic Information for the Layperson about Open-Head and Closed-Head Injuries, Treatment Advances, Recovery, and Rehabilitation

Along with Reports on Current Research Initiatives

Edited by Karen Bellenir. 414 pages. 1997. 978-0-7808-0208-7.

Headache Sourcebook

Basic Consumer Health Information about Migraine, Tension, Cluster, Rebound and Other Types of Headaches, with Facts about

Healthy Aging Sourcebook

Basic Consumer Health Information about Maintaining Health through the Aging Process, Including Advice on Nutrition, Exercise, and Sleep, Help in Making Decisions about Midlife Issues and Retirement, and Guidance Concerning Practical and Informed Choices in Health Consumerism

Along with Data Concerning the Theories of Aging, Different Experiences in Aging by Minority Groups, and Facts about Aging Now and Aging in the Future; and Featuring a Glossary, a Guide to Consumer Help, Additional Suggested Reading, and Practical Resource Directory

Edited by Jenifer Swanson. 537 pages. 1999. 978-0-7808-0390-9.

SEE ALSO *Adult Health Sourcebook, Physical and Mental Issues in Aging Sourcebook*

Healthy Children Sourcebook

Basic Consumer Health Information about the Physical and Mental Development of Children between the Ages of 3 and 12, Including Routine Health Care, Preventative Health Services, Safety and First Aid, Healthy Sleep, Dental Care, Nutrition, and Fitness, and Featuring Parenting Tips on Such Topics as Bedwetting, Choosing Day Care, Monitoring TV and Other Media, and Establishing a Foundation for Substance Abuse Prevention

Along with a Glossary of Commonly Used Pediatric Terms and Resources for Additional Help and Information.

Edited by Chad T. Kimball. 624 pages. 2003. 978-0-7808-0247-6.

"Should be required reading for parents and teachers."
—*E-Streams, Jun '04*

"It is hard to imagine that any other single resource exists that would provide such a comprehensive guide of timely information on health promotion and disease prevention for children aged 3 to 12."
—*American Reference Books Annual, 2004*

"This easy-to-read volume is a tremendous resource."
—*AORN Journal, May '05*

SEE ALSO *Childhood Diseases and Disorders Sourcebook, 2nd Edition*

Healthy Heart Sourcebook for Women

Basic Consumer Health Information about Cardiac Issues Specific to Women, Including Facts about Major Risk Factors and Prevention, Treatment and Control Strategies, and Important Dietary Issues

Along with a Special Section Regarding the Pros and Cons of Hormone Replacement Therapy and Its Impact on Heart Health, and Additional Help, Including Recipes, a Glossary, and a Directory of Resources

Edited by Dawn D. Matthews. 321 pages. 2000. 978-0-7808-0329-9.

"A good reference source and recommended for all public, academic, medical, and hospital libraries."
—*Medical Reference Services Quarterly, Summer '01*

"Contains very important information about coronary artery disease that all women should know. The information is current and presented in an easy-to-read format. The book will make a good addition to any library."
—*American Medical Writers Association Journal, Summer '00*

SEE ALSO *Cardiovascular Diseases and Disorders Sourcebook, 4th Edition, Women's Health Concerns Sourcebook, 3rd Edition*

Hepatitis Sourcebook

Basic Consumer Health Information about Hepatitis A, Hepatitis B, Hepatitis C, and Other Forms of Hepatitis, Including Autoimmune Hepatitis, Alcoholic Hepatitis, Nonalcoholic Steatohepatitis, and Toxic Hepatitis, with Facts about Risk Factors, Screening Methods, Diagnostic Tests, and Treatment Options

Along with Information on Liver Health, Tips for People Living with Chronic Hepatitis, Reports on Current Research Initiatives, a Glossary of Terms Related to Hepatitis, and a Directory of Sources for Further Help and Information

Edited by Sandra J. Judd. 570 pages. 2006. 978-0-7808-0749-5.

"The breadth of information found in this one book would not be readily found in another source. Highly recommended."
—*American Reference Books Annual, 2006*

SEE ALSO *Contagious Diseases Sourcebook, 2nd Edition*

Household Safety Sourcebook

Basic Consumer Health Information about Household Safety, Including Information about Poisons, Chemicals, Fire, and Water Hazards in the Home

Along with Advice about the Safe Use of Home Maintenance Equipment, Choosing Toys and Nursery Furniture, Holiday and Recreation Safety, a Glossary, and Resources for Further Help and Information

Edited by Dawn D. Matthews. 587 pages. 2002. 978-0-7808-0338-1.

"As a sourcebook on household safety this book meets its mark. It is encyclopedic in scope and covers a wide range of safety issues that are commonly seen in the home."
—*E-Streams, Jul '02*

Hypertension Sourcebook

Basic Consumer Health Information about the Causes, Diagnosis, and Treatment of High Blood Pressure, with Facts about Consequences, Complications, and Co-Occurring Disorders, Such as Coronary Heart Disease, Diabetes, Stroke, Kidney Disease, and Hypertensive Retinopathy, and Issues in Blood Pressure

Control, Including Dietary Choices, Stress Management, and Medications

Along with Reports on Current Research Initiatives and Clinical Trials, a Glossary, and Resources for Additional Help and Information

Edited by Dawn D. Matthews and Karen Bellenir. 588 pages. 2004. 978-0-7808-0674-0.

"Academic, public, and medical libraries will want to add the Hypertension Sourcebook to their collections."
—E-Streams, Aug '05

"The strength of this source is the wide range of information given about hypertension."
—American Reference Books Annual, 2005

SEE ALSO Stroke Sourcebook, 2nd Edition

Immune System Disorders Sourcebook, 2nd Edition

Basic Consumer Health Information about Disorders of the Immune System, Including Immune System Function and Response, Diagnosis of Immune Disorders, Information about Inherited Immune Disease, Acquired Immune Disease, and Autoimmune Diseases, Including Primary Immune Deficiency, Acquired Immunodeficiency Syndrome (AIDS), Lupus, Multiple Sclerosis, Type 1 Diabetes, Rheumatoid Arthritis, and Graves' Disease

Along with Treatments, Tips for Coping with Immune Disorders, a Glossary, and a Directory of Additional Resources

Edited by Joyce Brennfleck Shannon. 643 pages. 2005. 978-0-7808-0748-8.

"Highly recommended for academic and public libraries."
—American Reference Books Annual, 2006

"The updated second edition is a 'must' for any consumer health library seeking a solid resource covering the treatments, symptoms, and options for immune disorder sufferers... An excellent guide."
—MBR Bookwatch, Jan '06

SEE ALSO AIDS Sourcebook, 4th Edition, Arthritis Sourcebook, 3rd Edition

Infant and Toddler Health Sourcebook

Basic Consumer Health Information about the Physical and Mental Development of Newborns, Infants, and Toddlers, Including Neonatal Concerns, Nutrition Recommendations, Immunization Schedules, Common Pediatric Disorders, Assessments and Milestones, Safety Tips, and Advice for Parents and Other Caregivers

Along with a Glossary of Terms and Resource Listings for Additional Help

Edited by Jenifer Swanson. 570 pages. 2000. 978-0-7808-0246-9.

"As a reference for the general public, this would be useful in any library."
—E-Streams, May '01

"Recommended reference source."
—Booklist, Feb '01

Infectious Diseases Sourcebook

Basic Consumer Health Information about Non-Contagious Bacterial, Viral, Prion, Fungal, and Parasitic Diseases Spread by Food and Water, Insects and Animals, or Environmental Contact, Including Botulism, E. Coli, Encephalitis, Legionnaires' Disease, Lyme Disease, Malaria, Plague, Rabies, Salmonella, Tetanus, and Others, and Facts about Newly Emerging Diseases, Such as Hantavirus, Mad Cow Disease, Monkeypox, and West Nile Virus

Along with Information about Preventing Disease Transmission, the Threat of Bioterrorism, and Current Research Initiatives, with a Glossary and Directory of Resources for More Information

Edited by Karen Bellenir. 610 pages. 2004. 978-0-7808-0675-7.

"This reference continues the excellent tradition of the Health Reference Series in consolidating a wealth of information on a selected topic into a format that is easy to use and accessible to the general public."
—American Reference Books Annual, 2005

"Recommended for public and academic libraries."
—E-Streams, Jan '05

SEE ALSO Environmental Health Sourcebook, 3rd Edition

Injury and Trauma Sourcebook

Basic Consumer Health Information about the Impact of Injury, the Diagnosis and Treatment of Common and Traumatic Injuries, Emergency Care, and Specific Injuries Related to Home, Community, Workplace, Transportation, and Recreation

Along with Guidelines for Injury Prevention, a Glossary, and a Directory of Additional Resources

Edited by Joyce Brennfleck Shannon. 675 pages. 2002. 978-0-7808-0421-0.

"Practitioners should be aware of guides such as this in order to facilitate their use by patients and their families."
—Doody's Health Sciences Book Review Journal, Sep-Oct '02

"Recommended reference source."
—Booklist, Sep '02

"Highly recommended for academic and medical reference collections."
—Library Bookwatch, Sep '02

SEE ALSO Emergency Medical Services Sourcebook, Sports Injuries Sourcebook, 3rd Edition

Learning Disabilities Sourcebook, 3rd Edition

Basic Consumer Health Information about Dyslexia, Auditory and Visual Processing Disorders, Communication Disorders, Dyscalculia, Dysgraphia, and Other Conditions That Impede Learning, Including Attention Deficit/Hyperactivity Disorder, Autism Spectrum Disorders, Hearing and Visual Impairments, Chromosome-Based Disorders, and Brain Injury

Along with Facts about Brain Function, Assessment, Therapy and Remediation, Accommodations, Assistive Technology, Legal Protections, and Tips about Family Life, School Transitions, and Employment Strategies, a Glossary of Related Terms, and Directories of Additional Resources

Edited by Joyce Brennfleck Shannon. 613 pages. 2009. 978-0-7808-1039-6.

"Intended to be a starting point for people who need to know about learning disabilities. Each chapter on a specific disability includes readable,

well-organized descriptions... The book is well indexed and a glossary is included. Chapters on organizations and helpful websites will aid the reader who needs more information."
—American Reference Books Annual, 2009

"This book provides the necessary information to better understand learning disabilities and work with children who have them... It would be difficult to find another book that so comprehensively explains learning disabilities without becoming incomprehensible to the average parent who needs this information."
—Doody's Review Service, 2009

SEE ALSO Attention Deficit Disorder Sourcebook, Autism and Pervasive Developmental Disorders Sourcebook

Leukemia Sourcebook

Basic Consumer Health Information about Adult and Childhood Leukemias, Including Acute Lymphocytic Leukemia (ALL), Chronic Lymphocytic Leukemia (CLL), Acute Myelogenous Leukemia (AML), Chronic Myelogenous Leukemia (CML), and Hairy Cell Leukemia, and Treatments Such as Chemotherapy, Radiation Therapy, Peripheral Blood Stem Cell and Marrow Transplantation, and Immunotherapy

Along with Tips for Life During and After Treatment, a Glossary, and Directories of Additional Resources

Edited by Joyce Brennfleck Shannon. 564 pages. 2003. 978-0-7808-0627-6.

"Unlike other medical books for the layperson... the language does not talk down to the reader... This volume is highly recommended for all libraries."
—American Reference Books Annual, 2004

"A fine title which ranges from diagnosis to alternative treatments, staging, and tips for life during and after diagnosis."
—The Bookwatch, Dec '03

SEE ALSO Blood & Circulatory Disorders Sourcebook, 3rd Edition, Cancer Sourcebook, 5th Edition

Liver Disorders Sourcebook

Basic Consumer Health Information about the Liver and How It Works; Liver Diseases, Including Cancer, Cirrhosis, Hepatitis, and

Toxic and Drug Related Diseases; Tips for Maintaining a Healthy Liver; Laboratory Tests, Radiology Tests, and Facts about Liver Transplantation

Along with a Section on Support Groups, a Glossary, and Resource Listings

Edited by Joyce Brennfleck Shannon. 580 pages. 2000. 978-0-7808-0383-1.

"This title is recommended for health sciences and public libraries with consumer health collections."
—E-Streams, Oct '00

"Recommended reference source."
—Booklist, Jun '00

SEE ALSO Gastrointestinal Diseases and Disorders Sourcebook, 2nd Edition, Hepatitis Sourcebook

Lung Disorders Sourcebook

Basic Consumer Health Information about Emphysema, Pneumonia, Tuberculosis, Asthma, Cystic Fibrosis, and Other Lung Disorders, Including Facts about Diagnostic Procedures, Treatment Strategies, Disease Prevention Efforts, and Such Risk Factors as Smoking, Air Pollution, and Exposure to Asbestos, Radon, and Other Agents

Along with a Glossary and Resources for Additional Help and Information

Edited by Dawn D. Matthews. 657 pages. 2002. 978-0-7808-0339-8.

"Highly recommended for academic and medical reference collections."
—Library Bookwatch, Sep '02

SEE ALSO Asthma Sourcebook, 2nd Edition, Respiratory Disorders Sourcebook, 2nd Edition

Medical Tests Sourcebook, 3rd Edition

Basic Consumer Health Information about X-Rays, Blood Tests, Stool and Urine Tests, Biopsies, Mammography, Endoscopic Procedures, Ultrasound Exams, Computed Tomography, Magnetic Resonance Imaging (MRI), Nuclear Medicine, Genetic Testing, Home-Use Tests, and More

Along with Facts about Preventive Care and Screening Test Guidelines, Screening and

Assessment Tests Associated with Such Specific Concerns as Cancer, Heart Disease, Allergies, Diabetes, Thyroid Disfunction, and Infertility, a Glossary of Related Terms, and a Directory of Resources for Additional Help and Information

Edited by Karen Bellenir. 627 pages. 2008. 978-0-7808-1040-2

"This volume has a wide scope that makes it useful... Can be a valuable reference guide."
—American Reference Books Annual, 2009

"Would be a valuable contribution to any consumer health or public library."
—Doody's Book Review Service, 2009

Men's Health Concerns Sourcebook, 3rd Edition

Basic Consumer Health Information about Wellness in Men and Gender-Related Differences in Health, With Facts about Heart Disease, Cancer, Traumatic Injury, and Other Leading Causes of Death in Men, Reproductive Concerns, Sexual Dysfunction, Disorders of the Prostate, Penis, and Testes, Sex-Linked Genetic Disorders, and Other Medical and Mental Concerns of Men

Along with Statistical Data, a Glossary of Related Terms, and a Directory of Resources for Additional Information

Edited by Sandra J. Judd. 632 pages. 2009. 978-0-7808-1033-4.

"A good addition to any reference shelf in academic, consumer health, or hospital libraries."
—ARBAOnline, Oct '09

SEE ALSO Prostate and Urological Disorders Sourcebook

Mental Health Disorders Sourcebook, 4th Edition

Basic Consumer Health Information about the Causes and Symptoms of Mental Health Problems, Including Depression, Bipolar Disorder, Anxiety Disorders, Posttraumatic Stress Disorder, Obsessive-Compulsive Disorder, Eating Disorders, Addictions, and Personality and Psychotic Disorders

Along with Information about Medications and Treatments, Mental Health Concerns in

Children, Adolescents, and Adults, Tips on Living with Mental Health Disorders, a Glossary of Related Terms, and a Directory of Resources for Additional Help and Information

Edited by Amy L. Sutton. 680 pages. 2009. 978-0-7808-1041-9.

"Mental health concerns are presented in everyday language and intended for patients and their families as well as the general public... This resource is comprehensive and up to date... The easy-to-understand writing style helps to facilitate assimilation of needed facts and specifics on often challenging topics."
—*ARBA Online, Oct '09*

"No health collection should be without this resource, which will reach into many a general lending library as well."
—*Internet Bookwatch, Oct '09*

SEE ALSO Depression Sourcebook, 2nd Edition, Stress-Related Disorders Sourcebook, 2nd Edition

Mental Retardation Sourcebook

Basic Consumer Health Information about Mental Retardation and Its Causes, Including Down Syndrome, Fetal Alcohol Syndrome, Fragile X Syndrome, Genetic Conditions, Injury, and Environmental Sources

Along with Preventive Strategies, Parenting Issues, Educational Implications, Health Care Needs, Employment and Economic Matters, Legal Issues, a Glossary, and a Resource Listing for Additional Help and Information

Edited by Joyce Brennfleck Shannon. 627 pages. 2000. 978-0-7808-0377-0.

"Public libraries will find the book useful for reference and as a beginning research point for students, parents, and caregivers."
—*American Reference Books Annual, 2001*

"The strength of this work is that it compiles many basic fact sheets and addresses for further information in one volume. It is intended and suitable for the general public."
—*E-Streams, Nov '00*

"An invaluable overview."
—*Reviewer's Bookwatch, Jul '00*

Movement Disorders Sourcebook, 2nd Edition

Basic Consumer Health Information about the Symptoms and Causes of Movement Disorders, Including Parkinson Disease, Amyotrophic Lateral Sclerosis, Cerebral Palsy, Muscular Dystrophy, Multiple Sclerosis, Myasthenia, Myoclonus, Spina Bifida, Dystonia, Essential Tremor, Choreatic Disorders, Huntington Disease, Tourette Syndrome, and Other Disorders That Cause Slowed, Absent, or Excessive Movements

Along with Information about Surgical and Nonsurgical Interventions, Physical Therapies, Strategies for Independent Living, a Glossary of Related Terms, and a Directory of Resources for Additional Help and Information

Edited by Amy L. Sutton. 618 pages. 2009. 978-0-7808-1034-1.

"The second updated edition of Movement Disorders Sourcebook is a winner, providing the latest research and health findings on all kinds of movement disorders in children and adults... a top pick for any health or general lending library's health reference collection."
—*California Bookwatch, Aug '09*

SEE ALSO Muscular Dystrophy Sourcebook

Multiple Sclerosis Sourcebook

Basic Consumer Health Information about Multiple Sclerosis (MS) and Its Effects on Mobility, Vision, Bladder Function, Speech, Swallowing, and Cognition, Including Facts about Risk Factors, Causes, Diagnostic Procedures, Pain Management, Drug Treatments, and Physical and Occupational Therapies

Along with Guidelines for Nutrition and Exercise, Tips on Choosing Assistive Equipment, Information about Disability, Work, Financial, and Legal Issues, a Glossary of Related Terms, and a Directory of Additional Resources

Edited by Joyce Brennfleck Shannon. 553 pages. 2007. 978-0-7808-0998-7.

Muscular Dystrophy Sourcebook

Basic Consumer Health Information about Congenital, Childhood-Onset, and Adult-Onset

645

Forms of Muscular Dystrophy, Such as Duchenne, Becker, Emery-Dreifuss, Distal, Limb-Girdle, Facioscapulohumeral (FSHD), Myotonic, and Ophthalmoplegic Muscular Dystrophies, Including Facts about Diagnostic Tests, Medical and Physical Therapies, Management of Co-Occurring Conditions, and Parenting Guidelines

Along with Practical Tips for Home Care, a Glossary, and Directories of Additional Resources

Edited by Joyce Brennfleck Shannon. 552 pages. 2004. 978-0-7808-0676-4.

"This book is highly recommended for public and academic libraries as well as health care offices that support the information needs of patients and their families."
—E-Streams, Apr '05

"Excellent reference."
—The Bookwatch, Jan '05

SEE ALSO Movement Disorders Sourcebook, 2nd Edition

Obesity Sourcebook

Basic Consumer Health Information about Diseases and Other Problems Associated with Obesity, and Including Facts about Risk Factors, Prevention Issues, and Management Approaches

Along with Statistical and Demographic Data, Information about Special Populations, Research Updates, a Glossary, and Source Listings for Further Help and Information

Edited by Wilma Caldwell and Chad T. Kimball. 360 pages. 2001. 978-0-7808-0333-6.

"The book synthesizes the reliable medical literature on obesity into one easy-to-read and useful resource for the general public."
—American Reference Books Annual, 2002

"Well suited for the health reference collection of a public library or an academic health science library that serves the general population."
—E-Streams, Sep '01

Osteoporosis Sourcebook

Basic Consumer Health Information about Primary and Secondary Osteoporosis and Juvenile Osteoporosis and Related Conditions, Including Fibrous Dysplasia, Gaucher Disease, Hyperthyroidism, Hypophosphatasia,

Myeloma, Osteopetrosis, Osteogenesis Imperfecta, and Paget's Disease

Along with Information about Risk Factors, Treatments, Traditional and Non-Traditional Pain Management, a Glossary of Related Terms, and a Directory of Resources

Edited by Allan R. Cook. 568 pages. 2001. 978-0-7808-0239-1.

"This resource is recommended as a great reference source for public, health, and academic libraries, and is another triumph for the editors of Omnigraphics."
—American Reference Books Annual, 2002

"Will prove valuable to any library seeking to maintain a current, comprehensive reference collection of health resources... From prevention to treatment and associated conditions, this provides an excellent survey."
—The Bookwatch, Aug '01

SEE ALSO Healthy Aging Sourcebook, Women's Health Concerns Sourcebook, 3rd Edition

---

Pain Sourcebook, 3rd Edition

Basic Consumer Health Information about Acute and Chronic Pain, Including Nerve Pain, Bone Pain, Muscle Pain, Cancer Pain, and Disorders Characterized by Pain, Such as Arthritis, Temporomandibular Muscle and Joint (TMJ) Disorder, Carpal Tunnel Syndrome, Headaches, Heartburn, Sciatica, and Shingles, and Facts about Diagnostic Tests and Treatment Options for Pain, Including Over-the-Counter and Prescription Drugs, Physical Rehabilitation, Injection and Infusion Therapies, Implantable Technologies, and Complementary Medicine

Along with Tips for Living with Pain, a Glossary of Related Terms, and a Directory of Additional Resources

Edited by Joyce Brennfleck Shannon. 644 pages. 2008. 978-0-7808-1006-8.

"Excellent for ready-reference users and can be used for beginning students in health fields... appropriate for the consumer health collection in both public and academic libraries."
—American Reference Books Annual, 2009

SEE ALSO Arthritis Sourcebook, 3rd Edition; Back and Neck Sourcebook, 2nd Edition;

Headache Sourcebook; Sports Injuries Sourcebook, 3rd Edition

SEE ALSO *Healthy Aging Sourcebook*

Pediatric Cancer Sourcebook

Basic Consumer Health Information about Leukemias, Brain Tumors, Sarcomas, Lymphomas, and Other Cancers in Infants, Children, and Adolescents, Including Descriptions of Cancers, Treatments, and Coping Strategies

Along with Suggestions for Parents, Caregivers, and Concerned Relatives, a Glossary of Cancer Terms, and Resource Listings

Edited by Edward J. Prucha. 575 pages. 1999. 978-0-7808-0245-2.

"An excellent source of information. Recommended for public, hospital, and health science libraries with consumer health collections."
—*E-Streams, Jun '00*

"A valuable addition to all libraries specializing in health services and many public libraries."
—*American Reference Books Annual, 2000*

SEE ALSO *Childhood Diseases and Disorders Sourcebook, 2nd Edition, Healthy Children Sourcebook*

Physical and Mental Issues in Aging Sourcebook

Basic Consumer Health Information on Physical and Mental Disorders Associated with the Aging Process, Including Concerns about Cardiovascular Disease, Pulmonary Disease, Oral Health, Digestive Disorders, Musculoskeletal and Skin Disorders, Metabolic Changes, Sexual and Reproductive Issues, and Changes in Vision, Hearing, and Other Senses

Along with Data about Longevity and Causes of Death, Information on Acute and Chronic Pain, Descriptions of Mental Concerns, a Glossary of Terms, and Resource Listings for Additional Help

Edited by Jenifer Swanson. 660 pages. 1999. 978-0-7808-0233-9.

"This is a treasure of health information for the layperson."
—*CHOICE Health Sciences Supplement, May '00*

Podiatry Sourcebook, 2nd Edition

Basic Consumer Health Information about Disorders, Diseases, and Deformities that Affect the Foot and Ankle, Including Sprains, Corns, Calluses, Bunions, Plantar Warts, Plantar Fasciitis, Neuromas, Clubfoot, Flat Feet, Achilles Tendonitis, and Much More

Along with Information about Selecting a Foot Care Specialist, Foot Fitness, Shoes and Socks, Diagnostic Tests and Corrective Procedures, Financial Assistance for Corrective Devices, a Glossary of Related Terms, and a Directory of Resources for Additional Help and Information

Edited by Ivy L. Alexander. 516 pages. 2007. 978-0-7808-0944-4.

"An excellent resource... Although there have been various types of 'foot books' published in the past, none are as comprehensive as this one. 5 Stars (out of 5)!"
—*Doody's Review Service, 2007*

"Perfect for both health libraries and general-interest lending collections."
—*Internet Bookwatch, Jul '07*

Pregnancy and Birth Sourcebook, 3rd Edition

Basic Consumer Health Information about Pregnancy and Fetal Development, Including Facts about Fertility and Conception, Physical and Emotional Changes during Pregnancy, Prenatal Care and Diagnostic Tests, High-Risk Pregnancies and Complications, Labor, Delivery, and the Postpartum Period

Along with Tips on Maintaining Health and Wellness during Pregnancy and Caring for Newborn Infants, a Glossary of Related Terms, and Directories of Resources for Additional Help and Information

Edited by Amy L. Sutton. 645 pages. 2009. 978-0-7808-1074-7.

SEE ALSO *Breastfeeding Sourcebook, Congenital Disorders Sourcebook, 2nd Edition, Family Planning Sourcebook, Women's Health Concerns Sourcebook, 3rd Edition*

Prostate and Urological Disorders Sourcebook

Basic Consumer Health Information about Urogenital and Sexual Disorders in Men, Including Prostate and Other Andrological Cancers, Prostatitis, Benign Prostatic Hyperplasia, Testicular and Penile Trauma, Cryptorchidism, Peyronie Disease, Erectile Dysfunction, and Male Factor Infertility, and Facts about Commonly Used Tests and Procedures, Such as Prostatectomy, Vasectomy, Vasectomy Reversal, Penile Implants, and Semen Analysis

Along with a Glossary of Andrological Terms and a Directory of Resources for Additional Information

Edited by Karen Bellenir. 604 pages. 2006. 978-0-7808-0797-6.

"Certain to be a popular pick among library reference holdings... No prior knowledge is assumed for any of the conditions or terms herein, making it a most accessible general-interest reference."
—California Bookwatch, Apr '06

SEE ALSO Men's Health Concerns Sourcebook, 3rd Edition, Urinary Tract and Kidney Diseases and Disorders Sourcebook, 2nd Edition

Prostate Cancer Sourcebook

Basic Consumer Health Information about Prostate Cancer, Including Information about the Associated Risk Factors, Detection, Diagnosis, and Treatment of Prostate Cancer

Along with Information on Non-Malignant Prostate Conditions, and Featuring a Section Listing Support and Treatment Centers and a Glossary of Related Terms

Edited by Dawn D. Matthews. 340 pages. 2001. 978-0-7808-0324-4.

"Recommended reference source."
—Booklist, Jan '02

"A valuable resource for health care consumers seeking information on the subject... All text is written in a clear, easy-to-understand language that avoids technical jargon. Any library that collects consumer health resources would strengthen their collection with the addition of the Prostate Cancer Sourcebook."
—American Reference Books Annual, 2002

SEE ALSO Cancer Sourcebook, 5th Edition, Men's Health Concerns Sourcebook, 3rd Edition

Rehabilitation Sourcebook

Basic Consumer Health Information about Rehabilitation for People Recovering from Heart Surgery, Spinal Cord Injury, Stroke, Orthopedic Impairments, Amputation, Pulmonary Impairments, Traumatic Injury, and More, Including Physical Therapy, Occupational Therapy, Speech/Language Therapy, Massage Therapy, Dance Therapy, Art Therapy, and Recreational Therapy

Along with Information on Assistive and Adaptive Devices, a Glossary, and Resources for Additional Help and Information

Edited by Dawn D. Matthews. 519 pages. 2000. 978-0-7808-0236-0.

"This is an excellent resource for public library reference and health collections."
—American Reference Books Annual, 2001

"Recommended reference source."
—Booklist, May '00

Respiratory Disorders Sourcebook, 2nd Edition

Basic Consumer Health Information about Infectious, Inflammatory, and Chronic Conditions Affecting the Lungs and Respiratory System, Including Pneumonia, Bronchitis, Influenza, Tuberculosis, Sarcoidosis, Asthma, Cystic Fibrosis, Chronic Obstructive Pulmonary Disease, Lung Abscesses, Pulmonary Embolism, Occupational Lung Diseases, and Other Bacterial, Viral, and Fungal Infections

Along with Facts about the Structure and Function of the Lungs and Airways, Methods of Diagnosing Respiratory Disorders, and Treatment and Rehabilitation Options, a Glossary of Related Terms, and a Directory of Resources for Additional Help and Information

Edited by Sandra L. Judd. 638 pages. 2008. 978-0-7808-1007-5.

"An excellent book for patients, their families, or for those who are just curious about respiratory disease. Public libraries and physician offices would find this a valuable resource as well. 4 Stars! (out of 5)"
—Doody's Review Service, 2009

"A great addition for public and school libraries because it provides concise health information... readers can start with this reference source and get satisfactory answers before proceeding to other medical reference tools for

more in depth information... A good guide for health education on lung disorders."
—American Reference Books Annual, 2009

SEE ALSO Asthma Sourcebook, 2nd Edition, Lung Disorders Sourcebook

Sexually Transmitted Diseases Sourcebook, 4th Edition

Basic Consumer Health Information about Chlamydial Infections, Gonorrhea, Hepatitis, Herpes, HIV/AIDS, Human Papillomavirus, Pubic Lice, Scabies, Syphilis, Trichomoniasis, Vaginal Infections, and Other Sexually Transmitted Diseases, Including Facts about Risk Factors, Symptoms, Diagnosis, Treatment, and the Prevention of Sexually Transmitted Infections

Along with Updates on Current Research Initiatives, a Glossary of Related Terms, and Resources for Additional Help and Information

Edited by Laura Larsen. 623 pages. 2009. 978-0-7808-1073-0.

"Extremely beneficial... The question-and-answer format along with the index and table of contents make this well-organized resource extremely easy to reference, read, and comprehend... an invaluable medical reference source for lay readers, and a highly appropriate addition for public library collections, health clinics, and any library with a consumer health collection"
—ARBAOnline, Oct '09

SEE ALSO AIDS Sourcebook, 4th Edition, Contagious Diseases Sourcebook, 2nd Edition, Men's Health Concerns Sourcebook, 3rd Edition, Women's Health Concerns Sourcebook, 3rd Edition

Sleep Disorders Sourcebook, 3rd Edition

Basic Consumer Health Information about Sleep Disorders, Including Insomnia, Sleep Apnea and Snoring, Jet Lag and Other Circadian Rhythm Disorders, Narcolepsy, and Parasomnias, Such as Sleep Walking and Sleep Talking, and Featuring Facts about Other Health Problems that Affect Sleep, Why Sleep Is Necessary, How Much Sleep Is Needed, the Physical and Mental Effects of Sleep Deprivation, and Pediatric Sleep Issues

Along with Tips for Diagnosing and Treating Sleep Disorders, a Glossary of Related Terms, and a List of Resources for Additional Help and Information

Edited by Sandra J. Judd. 600 pages. 2010. 978-0-7808-1084-6.

Smoking Concerns Sourcebook

Basic Consumer Health Information about Nicotine Addiction and Smoking Cessation, Featuring Facts about the Health Effects of Tobacco Use, Including Lung and Other Cancers, Heart Disease, Stroke, and Respiratory Disorders, Such as Emphysema and Chronic Bronchitis

Along with Information about Smoking Prevention Programs, Suggestions for Achieving and Maintaining a Smoke-Free Lifestyle, Statistics about Tobacco Use, Reports on Current Research Initiatives, a Glossary of Related Terms, and Directories of Resources for Additional Help and Information

Edited by Karen Bellenir. 595 pages. 2004. 978-0-7808-0323-7.

"Provides everything needed for the student or general reader seeking practical details on the effects of tobacco use."
—The Bookwatch, Mar '05

"Public libraries and consumer health care libraries will find this work useful."
—American Reference Books Annual, 2005

SEE ALSO Respiratory Disorders Sourcebook, 2nd Edition

Sports Injuries Sourcebook, 3rd Edition

Basic Consumer Health Information about Sprains and Strains, Fractures, Growth Plate Injuries, Overtraining Injuries, and Injuries to the Head, Face, Shoulders, Elbows, Hands, Spinal Column, Knees, Ankles, and Feet, and with Facts about Heat-Related Illness, Steroids and Sport Supplements, Protective Equipment, Diagnostic Procedures, Treatment Options, and Rehabilitation

Along with a Glossary of Related Terms and a Directory of Resources for Additional Help and Information

Edited by Sandra J. Judd. 623 pages. 2007. 978-0-7808-0949-9.

SEE ALSO Fitness and Exercise Sourcebook, 3rd Edition, Podiatry Sourcebook, 2nd Edition

Stress-Related Disorders Sourcebook, 2nd Edition

Basic Consumer Health Information about Stress and Stress-Related Disorders, Including Types of Stress, Sources of Acute and Chronic Stress, the Impact of Stress on the Body's Systems, and Mental and Emotional Health Problems Associated with Stress, Such as Depression, Anxiety Disorders, Substance Abuse, Posttraumatic Stress Disorder, and Suicide

Along with Advice about Getting Help for Stress-Related Disorders, Information about Stress Management Techniques, a Glossary of Stress-Related Terms, and a Directory of Resources for Additional Help and Information

Edited by Amy L. Sutton. 608 pages. 2007. 978-0-7808-0996-3.

"Accessible to the lay reader. Highly recommended for medical and psychiatric collections."
—Library Journal, Mar '08

"Well-written for a general readership, the 2ⁿᵈ Edition of Stress-Related Disorders Sourcebook is a useful addition to the health reference literature."
—American Reference Books Annual, 2008

SEE ALSO Mental Health Disorders Sourcebook, 4th Edition

Stroke Sourcebook, 2nd Edition

Basic Consumer Health Information about Stroke, Including Ischemic, Hemorrhagic, and Mini Strokes, as Well as Risk Factors, Prevention Guidelines, Diagnostic Tests, Medications and Surgical Treatments, and Complications of Stroke

Along with Rehabilitation Techniques and Innovations, Tips on Staying Healthy and Maintaining Independence after Stroke, a Glossary of Related Terms, and a Directory of Resources for Stroke Survivors and Their Families

Edited by Amy L. Sutton. 626 pages. 2008. 978-0-7808-1035-8.

"An encyclopedic handbook on stroke that is written in a language the layperson can understand... This is one of the most helpful, readable books on stroke. This volume is highly recommended and should be in every medical, hospital and public library; in addition, every family practitioner should have a copy in his or her office."
—American Reference Books Annual, 2009

SEE ALSO Brain Disorders Sourcebook, 3rd Edition, Hypertension Sourcebook

Surgery Sourcebook, 2nd Edition

Basic Consumer Health Information about Common Inpatient and Outpatient Surgeries, Including Critical Care and Trauma, Gastrointestinal, Gynecologic and Obstetric, Cardiac and Vascular, Neurologic, Ophthalmologic, Orthopedic, Reconstructive and Cosmetic, and Other Major and Minor Surgeries

Along with Information about Anesthesia and Pain Relief Options, Risks and Complications, Postoperative Recovery Concerns, and Innovative Surgical Techniques and Tools, a Glossary of Related Terms, and a Directory of Additional Resources

Edited by Amy L. Sutton. 645 pages. 2008. 978-0-7808-1004-4.

"Large public libraries and medical libraries would benefit from this material in their reference collections."
—American Reference Books Annual, 2009

SEE ALSO Cosmetic and Reconstructive Surgery Sourcebook, 2nd Edition

Thyroid Disorders Sourcebook

Basic Consumer Health Information about Disorders of the Thyroid and Parathyroid Glands, Including Hypothyroidism, Hyperthyroidism, Graves Disease, Hashimoto Thyroiditis, Thyroid Cancer, and Parathyroid Disorders, Featuring Facts about Symptoms, Risk Factors, Tests, and Treatments

Along with Information about the Effects of Thyroid Imbalance on Other Body Systems, Environmental Factors That Affect the Thyroid Gland, a Glossary, and a Directory of Additional Resources

650

Edited by Joyce Brennfleck Shannon. 573 pages. 2005. 978-0-7808-0745-7.

"Recommended for consumer health collections."
—American Reference Books Annual, 2006

"Highly recommended pick for Basic Consumer health reference holdings at all levels."
—The Bookwatch, Aug '05

SEE ALSO Endocrine and Metabolic Disorders Sourcebook, 2nd Edition

■

Transplantation Sourcebook
Basic Consumer Health Information about Organ and Tissue Transplantation, Including Physical and Financial Preparations, Procedures and Issues Relating to Specific Solid Organ and Tissue Transplants, Rehabilitation, Pediatric Transplant Information, the Future of Transplantation, and Organ and Tissue Donation

Along with a Glossary and Listings of Additional Resources

Edited by Joyce Brennfleck Shannon. 610 pages. 2002. 978-0-7808-0322-0.

"Recommended for libraries with an interest in offering consumer health information."
—E-Streams, Jul '02

"This is a unique and valuable resource for patients facing transplantation and their families."
—Doody's Review Service, Jun '02

■

Traveler's Health Sourcebook
Basic Consumer Health Information for Travelers, Including Physical and Medical Preparations, Transportation Health and Safety, Essential Information about Food and Water, Sun Exposure, Insect and Snake Bites, Camping and Wilderness Medicine, and Travel with Physical or Medical Disabilities

Along with International Travel Tips, Vaccination Recommendations, Geographical Health Issues, Disease Risks, a Glossary, and a Listing of Additional Resources

Edited by Joyce Brennfleck Shannon. 619 pages. 2000. 978-0-7808-0384-8.

"Recommended reference source."
—Booklist, Feb '01

"This book is recommended for any public library, any travel collection, and especially any collection for the physically disabled."
—American Reference Books Annual, 2001

SEE ALSO Worldwide Health Sourcebook

■

Urinary Tract and Kidney Diseases and Disorders Sourcebook, 2nd Edition
Basic Consumer Health Information about the Urinary System, Including the Bladder, Urethra, Ureters, and Kidneys, with Facts about Urinary Tract Infections, Incontinence, Congenital Disorders, Kidney Stones, Cancers of the Urinary Tract and Kidneys, Kidney Failure, Dialysis, and Kidney Transplantation

Along with Statistical and Demographic Information, Reports on Current Research in Kidney and Urologic Health, a Summary of Commonly Used Diagnostic Tests, a Glossary of Related Terms, and a Directory of Resources for Additional Help and Information

Edited by Ivy L. Alexander. 621 pages. 2005. 978-0-7808-0750-1.

"A good choice for a consumer health information library or for a medical library needing information to refer to their patients."
—American Reference Books Annual, 2006

SEE ALSO Prostate and Urological Disorders Sourcebook

■

Vegetarian Sourcebook
Basic Consumer Health Information about Vegetarian Diets, Lifestyle, and Philosophy, Including Definitions of Vegetarianism and Veganism, Tips about Adopting Vegetarianism, Creating a Vegetarian Pantry, and Meeting Nutritional Needs of Vegetarians, with Facts Regarding Vegetarianism's Effect on Pregnant and Lactating Women, Children, Athletes, and Senior Citizens

Along with a Glossary of Commonly Used Vegetarian Terms and Resources for Additional Help and Information

Edited by Chad T. Kimball. 337 pages. 2002. 978-0-7808-0439-5.

"Organizes into one concise volume the answers to the most common questions concerning vegetarian diets and lifestyles. This title is

651

recommended for public and secondary school libraries."

—*E-Streams, Apr '03*

"Invaluable reference for public and school library collections alike."
—*Library Bookwatch, Apr '03*

"The articles in this volume are easy to read and come from authoritative sources. The book does not necessarily support the vegetarian diet but instead provides the pros and cons of this important decision... Recommended for public libraries and consumer health libraries."
—*American Reference Books Annual, 2003*

SEE ALSO *Diet and Nutrition Sourcebook, 3rd Edition*

Women's Health Concerns Sourcebook, 3rd Edition

Basic Consumer Health Information about Issues and Trends in Women's Health and Health Conditions of Special Concern to Women, Including Endometriosis, Uterine Fibroids, Menstrual Irregularities, Menopause, Sexual Dysfunction, Infertility, Cancer in Women, and Other Such Chronic Disorders as Lupus, Fibromyalgia, and Thyroid Disease

Along with Statistical Data, Tips for Maintaining Wellness, a Glossary, and a Directory of Resources for Further Help and Information

Edited by Sandra J. Judd. 679 pages. 2009. 978-0-7808-1036-5.

"This useful resource provides information about a wide range of topics that will help women understand their bodies, prevent or treat disease, and maintain health... A detailed index helps readers locate information. This is a useful addition to public and consumer health library collections"
—*ARBAOnline, Jun '09*

SEE ALSO *Breast Cancer Sourcebook, 3rd Edition, Cancer Sourcebook for Women, 4th Edition, Healthy Heart Sourcebook for Women*

Workplace Health and Safety Sourcebook

Basic Consumer Health Information about Workplace Health and Safety, Including the Effect of Workplace Hazards on the Lungs,

Skin, Heart, Ears, Eyes, Brain, Reproductive Organs, Musculoskeletal System, and Other Organs and Body Parts

Along with Information about Occupational Cancer, Personal Protective Equipment, Toxic and Hazardous Chemicals, Child Labor, Stress, and Workplace Violence

Edited by Chad T. Kimball. 610 pages. 2000. 978-0-7808-0231-5.

"As a reference for the general public, this would be useful in any library."
—*E-Streams, Jun '01*

"Provides helpful information for primary care physicians and other caregivers interested in occupational medicine... General readers; professionals."
—*CHOICE, May '01*

Worldwide Health Sourcebook

Basic Information about Global Health Issues, Including Malnutrition, Reproductive Health, Disease Dispersion and Prevention, Emerging Diseases, Risky Health Behaviors, and the Leading Causes of Death

Along with Global Health Concerns for Children, Women, and the Elderly, Mental Health Issues, Research and Technology Advancements, and Economic, Environmental, and Political Health Implications, a Glossary, and a Resource Listing for Additional Help and Information

Edited by Joyce Brennfleck Shannon. 597 pages. 2001. 978-0-7808-0330-5.

"Named an Outstanding Academic Title."
—*CHOICE, Jan '02*

"Yet another handy but also unique compilation in the extensive Health Reference Series, this is a useful work because many of the international publications reprinted or excerpted are not readily available. Highly recommended."
—*CHOICE, Nov '01*

SEE ALSO *Traveler's Health Sourcebook*

Teen Health Series
Complete Catalog
List price $69 per volume. School and library price $62 per volume.

Abuse and Violence Information for Teens
Health Tips about the Causes and Consequences of Abusive and Violent Behavior

Including Facts about the Types of Abuse and Violence, the Warning Signs of Abusive and Violent Behavior, Health Concerns of Victims, and Getting Help and Staying Safe

Edited by Sandra Augustyn Lawton. 411 pages. 2008. 978-0-7808-1008-2.

"A useful resource for schools and organizations providing services to teens and may also be a starting point in research projects."
—*Reference and Research Book News, Aug '08*

"Violence is a serious problem for teens... This resource gives teens the information they need to face potential threats and get help—either for themselves or for their friends."
—*American Reference Books Annual, 2009*

Accident and Safety Information for Teens
Health Tips about Medical Emergencies, Traumatic Injuries, and Disaster Preparedness

Including Facts about Motor Vehicle Accidents, Burns, Poisoning, Firearms, Natural Disasters, National Security Threats, and More

Edited by Karen Bellenir. 420 pages. 2008. 978-0-7808-1046-4.

"Aimed at teenage audiences, this guide provides practical information for handling a comprehensive list of emergencies, from sport injuries and auto accidents to alcohol poisoning and natural disasters."
—*Library Journal, Apr 1, '09*

"Useful in the young adult collections of public libraries as well as high school libraries."
—*American Reference Books Annual, 2009*

SEE ALSO *Sports Injuries Information for Teens, 2nd Edition*

Alcohol Information for Teens, 2nd Edition
Health Tips about Alcohol and Alcoholism

Including Facts about Alcohol's Effects on the Body, Brain, and Behavior, the Consequences of Underage Drinking, Alcohol Abuse Prevention and Treatment, and Coping with Alcoholic Parents

Edited by Lisa Bakewell. 410 pages. 2009. 978-0-7808-1043-3.

"This handbook, written for a teenage audience, provides information on the causes, effects, and preventive measures related to alcohol abuse among teens... The chapters are quick to make a connection to their teenage reading audience. The prose is straightforward and the book lends itself to spot reading. It should be useful both for practical information and for research, and it is suitable for public and school libraries."
—*ARBAOnline, Jun '09*

SEE ALSO *Drug Information for Teens, 2nd Edition*

Allergy Information for Teens
Health Tips about Allergic Reactions Such as Anaphylaxis, Respiratory Problems, and Rashes

Including Facts about Identifying and Managing Allergies to Food, Pollen, Mold, Animals, Chemicals, Drugs, and Other Substances

Edited by Karen Bellenir. 410 pages. 2006. 978-0-7808-0799-0.

"This is a comprehensive, readable text on the subject of allergic diseases in teenagers. 5 Stars (out of 5)!"
—*Doody's Review Service, Jun '06*

"This authoritative and useful self-help title is a solid addition to YA collections, whether for personal interest or reports."
—*School Library Journal, Jul '06*

Asthma Information for Teens, 2nd Ed.
Health Tips about Managing Asthma and Related Concerns

Including Facts about Asthma Causes, Triggers and Symptoms, Diagnosis, and Treatment

Edited by Kim Wohlenhaus. 400 pages. 2010. 978-0-7808-1086-0.

Body Information for Teens
Health Tips about Maintaining Well-Being for a Lifetime
Including Facts about the Development and Functioning of the Body's Systems, Organs, and Structures and the Health Impact of Lifestyle Choices

Edited by Sandra Augustyn Lawton. 458 pages. 2007. 978-0-7808-0443-2.

Cancer Information for Teens, 2nd Edition
Health Tips about Cancer Awareness, Symptoms, Prevention, Diagnosis, and Treatment
Including Facts about Common Cancers Affecting Teens, Causes, Detection, Coping Strategies, Clinical Trials, Nutrition and Exercise, Cancer in Friends or Family, and More

Edited by Karen Bellenir and Lisa Bakewell. 445 pages. 2010. 978-0-7808-1085-3.

Complementary and Alternative Medicine Information for Teens
Health Tips about Non-Traditional and Non-Western Medical Practices
Including Information about Acupuncture, Chiropractic Medicine, Dietary and Herbal Supplements, Hypnosis, Massage Therapy, Prayer and Spirituality, Reflexology, Yoga, and More

Edited by Sandra Augustyn Lawton. 407 pages. 2007. 978-0-7808-0966-6.

"This volume covers CAM specifically for teenagers but of general use also. It should be a welcome addition to both public and academic libraries."
—*American Reference Books Annual, 2008*

"This volume provides a solid foundation for further investigation of the subject, making it useful for both public and high school libraries."
—*VOYA: Voice of Youth Advocates, Jun '07*

Diabetes Information for Teens
Health Tips about Managing Diabetes and Preventing Related Complications
Including Information about Insulin, Glucose Control, Healthy Eating, Physical Activity, and Learning to Live with Diabetes

Edited by Sandra Augustyn Lawton. 410 pages. 2006. 978-0-7808-0811-9.

"A comprehensive instructional guide for teens... some of the material may also be directed towards parents or teachers. 5 stars (out of 5)!"
—*Doody's Review Service, 2006*

"Students dealing with their own diabetes or that of a friend or family member or those writing reports on the topic will find this a valuable resource."
—*School Library Journal, Aug '06*

"This text is directed to the teen population and would be an excellent library resource for a health class or for the teacher as a reference for class preparation. It can, however, serve a much wider audience. The clinical educator on diabetes may find it valuable to educate the newly diagnosed client regardless of age. It also would be an excellent reference and education tool for a preventive medicine seminar on diabetes."
—*Physical Therapy, Mar '07*

Diet Information for Teens, 2nd Edition
Health Tips about Diet and Nutrition
Including Facts about Dietary Guidelines, Food Groups, Nutrients, Healthy Meals, Snacks, Weight Control, Medical Concerns Related to Diet, and More

Edited by Karen Bellenir. 432 pages. 2006. 978-0-7808-0820-1.

"A very quick and pleasant read in spite of the fact that it is very detailed in the information it gives... A book for anyone concerned about diet and nutrition."
—*American Reference Books Annual, 2007*

SEE ALSO *Eating Disorders Information for Teens, 2nd Edition*

Drug Information for Teens, 2nd Edition
Health Tips about the Physical and Mental Effects of Substance Abuse
Including Information about Marijuana, Inhalants, Club Drugs, Stimulants, Hallucinogens, Opiates, Prescription and Over-the-Counter Drugs, Herbal Products, Tobacco, Alcohol, and More

Edited by Sandra Augustyn Lawton. 468 pages. 2006. 978-0-7808-0862-1.

"As with earlier installments in Omnigraphics' Teen Health Series, Drug Information for Teens is designed specifically to meet the needs and interests of middle and high school students... Strongly recommended for both academic and public libraries."
—*American Reference Books Annual, 2007*

"Solid thoughtful advice is given about how to handle peer pressure, drug-related health concerns, and treatment strategies."
—*School Library Journal, Dec '06*

SEE ALSO *Alcohol Information for Teens, 2nd Edition, Tobacco Information for Teens, 2nd Edition*

Eating Disorders Information for Teens, 2nd Edition
Health Tips about Anorexia, Bulimia, Binge Eating, And Other Eating Disorders
Including Information about Risk Factors, Diagnosis and Treatment, Prevention, Related Health Concerns, and Other Issues

Edited by Sandra Augustyn Lawton. 377 pages. 2009. 978-0-7808-1044-0.

"This handy reference offers basic information and addresses specific disorders, consequences, prevention, diagnosis and treatment, healthy eating, and more. It is written in a conversational style that is easy to understand... Will provide plenty of facts for reports as well as browsing potential for students with an interest in the topic.
—*School Library Journal, Jun '09*

"Written in a straightforward style that will appeal to its teenage audience. The author does not play down the danger of living with an eating disorder and urges those struggling with this problem to seek professional help.

This work, as well as others in this series, will be a welcome addition to high school and undergraduate libraries."
—*American Reference Books Annual, 2009*

SEE ALSO *Diet Information for Teens, 2nd Edition*

Fitness Information for Teens, 2nd Edition
Health Tips about Exercise, Physical Well-Being, and Health Maintenance
Including Facts about Conditioning, Stretching, Strength Training, Body Shape and Body Image, Sports Nutrition, and Specific Activities for Athletes and Non-Athletes

Edited by Lisa Bakewell. 432 pages. 2009. 978-0-7808-1045-7.

"This no-nonsense guide packs a great deal into its pages... This is a helpful reference for basic diet and exercise information for health reports or personal use."
—*School Library Journal, April 2009*

"An excellent source for general information on why teens should be active, making time to exercise, the equipment people might need, various types of activities to try, how to maintain health and wellness, and how to avoid barriers to becoming healthier... This would still be an excellent addition to a public library ready-reference collection or a high school health library collection."
—*American Reference Books Annual, 2009*

"This easy to read, well-written, up-to-date overview of fitness for teenagers provides excellent wellness and exercise tips, information, and directions... It is a useful tool for them to obtain a base knowledge in fitness topics and different sports."
—*Doody's Review Service, 2009*

SEE ALSO *Diet Information for Teens, 2nd Edition, Sports Injuries Information for Teens, 2nd Edition*

Learning Disabilities Information for Teens
Health Tips about Academic Skills Disorders and Other Disabilities That Affect Learning

Including Information about Common Signs of Learning Disabilities, School Issues, Learning to Live with a Learning Disability, and Other Related Issues

Edited by Sandra Augustyn Lawton. 400 pages. 2006. 978-0-7808-0796-9.

"This book provides a wealth of information for any reader interested in the signs, causes, and consequences of learning disabilities, as well as related legal rights and educational interventions... Public and academic libraries should want this title for both students and general readers."
—*American Reference Books Annual, 2006*

Mental Health Information for Teens, 3rd Edition
Health Tips about Mental Wellness and Mental Illness
Including Facts about Mental and Emotional Health, Depression and Other Mood Disorders, Anxiety Disorders, Behavior Disorders, Self-Injury, Psychosis, Schizophrenia, and More

Edited by Karen Bellenir. 400 pages. 2010. 978-0-7808-1087-7.

SEE ALSO *Stress Information for Teens, Suicide Information for Teens, 2nd Edition*

Pregnancy Information for Teens
Health Tips about Teen Pregnancy and Teen Parenting
Including Facts about Prenatal Care, Pregnancy Complications, Labor and Delivery, Postpartum Care, Pregnancy-Related Lifestyle Concerns, and More

Edited by Sandra Augustyn Lawton. 434 pages. 2007. 978-0-7808-0984-0.

Sexual Health Information for Teens, 2nd Edition
Health Tips about Sexual Development, Reproduction, Contraception, and Sexually Transmitted Infections
Including Facts about Puberty, Sexuality, Birth Control, Chlamydia, Gonorrhea, Herpes, Human Papillomavirus, Syphilis, and More

Edited by Sandra Augustyn Lawton. 430 pages. 2008. 978-0-7808-1010-5.

"This offering represents the most up-to-date information available on an array of topics including abstinence-only sexual education and pregnancy-prevention methods... The range of coverage—from puberty and anatomy to sexually transmitted diseases—is thorough and extensive. Each chapter includes a bibliographic citation, and the three back sections containing additional resources, further reading, and the index are all first-rate... This volume will be well used by students in need of the facts, whether for educational or personal reasons."
—*School Library Journal, Nov '08*

"Presents information related to the emotional, physical, and biological development of both males and females that occurs during puberty. It also strives to address some of the issues and questions that may arise... The text is easy to read and understand for young readers, with satisfactory definitions within the text to explain new terms."
—*American Reference Books Annual, 2009*

Skin Health Information for Teens, 2nd Edition
Health Tips about Dermatological Concerns and Skin Cancer Risks
Including Facts about Acne, Warts, Hives, and Other Conditions and Lifestyle Choices, Such as Tanning, Tattooing, and Piercing, That Affect the Skin, Nails, Scalp, and Hair

Edited by Edited by Kim Wohlenhaus. 418 pages. 2009. 978-0-7808-1042-6.

"The material in this work will be easily understood by teenagers and young adults. The publisher has liberally used bulleted lists and sidebars to keep the reader's attention... A useful addition to school and public library collections."
—*ARBAOnline, Oct '09*

Sleep Information for Teens
Health Tips about Adolescent Sleep Requirements, Sleep Disorders, and the Effects of Sleep Deprivation
Including Facts about Why People Need Sleep, Sleep Patterns, Circadian Rhythms, Dreaming, Insomnia, Sleep Apnea, Narcolepsy, and More

Edited by Karen Bellenir. 355 pages. 2008. 978-0-7808-1009-9.

"Clear, concise, and very readable and would be a good source of sleep information for anyone—not just teenagers. This work is highly recommended for medical libraries, public school libraries, and public libraries."
—*American Reference Books Annual, 2009*

SEE ALSO *Body Information for Teens*

Sports Injuries Information for Teens, 2nd Edition
Health Tips about Acute, Traumatic, and Chronic Injuries in Adolescent Athletes
Including Facts about Sprains, Fractures, and Overuse Injuries, Treatment, Rehabilitation, Sport-Specific Safety Guidelines, Fitness Suggestions, and More

Edited by Karen Bellenir. 429 pages. 2008. 978-0-7808-1011-2.

"An engaging selection of informative articles about the prevention and treatment of sports injuries... The value of this book is that the articles have been vetted and are often augmented with inserts of useful facts, definitions of technical terms, and quick tips. Sensitive topics like injuries to genitalia are discussed openly and responsibly. This revised edition contains updated articles and defines sport more broadly than the first edition."
—*School Library Journal, Nov '08*

"This work will be useful in the young adult collections of public libraries as well as high school libraries... A useful resource for student research."
—*American Reference Books Annual, 2009*

SEE ALSO *Accident and Safety Information for Teens*

Stress Information for Teens
Health Tips about the Mental and Physical Consequences of Stress
Including Information about the Different Kinds of Stress, Symptoms of Stress, Frequent Causes of Stress, Stress Management Techniques, and More

Edited by Sandra Augustyn Lawton. 392 pages. 2008. 978-0-7808-1012-9.

"Understanding what stress is, what causes it, how the body and the mind are impacted by it, and what teens can do are the general categories addressed here... The chapters are brief but informative, and the list of community-help organizations is exhaustive. Report writers will find information quickly and easily, as will those who have personal concerns. The print is clear and the format is readable, making this an accessible resource for struggling readers and researchers."
—*School Library Journal, Dec '08*

"The articles selected will specifically appeal to young adults and are designed to answer their most common questions."
— *American Reference Books Annual, 2009*

SEE ALSO *Mental Health Information for Teens, 3rd Edition*

Suicide Information for Teens, 2nd Edition
Health Tips about Suicide Causes and Prevention
Including Facts about Depression, Risk Factors, Getting Help, Survivor Support, and More

Edited by Kim Wohlenhaus. 400 pages. 2010. 978-0-7808-1088-4.

SEE ALSO *Mental Health Information for Teens, 3rd Edition*

Tobacco Information for Teens, 2nd Edition
Health Tips about the Hazards of Using Cigarettes, Smokeless Tobacco, and Other Nicotine Products
Including Facts about Nicotine Addiction, Nicotine Delivery Systems, Secondhand Smoke, Health Consequences of Tobacco Use, Related Cancers, Smoking Cessation, and Tobacco Use Statistics

Edited by Karen Bellenir. 400 pages. 2010. 978-0-7808-1153-9.

SEE ALSO *Drug Information for Teens, 2nd Edition*

Health Reference Series